What's hype and what's science?

HOW MUCH DO YOU REALLY KNOW ABOUT NATURAL REMEDIES?

✳ *Can you relieve symptoms of menopause without hormone replacement therapy?*

YES. Black cohosh, sold as Remifemin, actually performed better than hormones in scientific tests— with an A rating for safety.

✳ *Can hemorrhoids be helped without surgery?*

YES. Citrus bioflavonoids rate an A for effectiveness as shown in double-blind studies—and get the highest safety rating.

✳ *Can you get relief from insomnia without dangerous prescription drugs?*

YES. Take your pick from valerian (rated A for effectiveness), melatonin (B+), or 5-HTP (B+).

✳ *Can a natural prohormone, androstenedione, help young athletes increase strength?*

NO. It not only doesn't build muscle in those under thirty, it is HIGHLY dangerous—even though it's "natural"!

THE BOOK NO CONSUMER OF NATURAL PRODUCTS SHOULD BE WITHOUT!

THE
PILL BOOK GUIDE
TO
NATURAL MEDICINES

*Vitamins, Minerals, Nutritional
Supplements, Herbs, and Other
Natural Products*

Michael T. Murray, N.D.

BANTAM BOOKS
New York   Toronto   London   Sydney   Auckland

THE PILL BOOK GUIDE TO NATURAL MEDICINES:
VITAMINS, MINERALS, NUTRITIONAL SUPPLEMENTS, HERBS,
AND OTHER NATURAL PRODUCTS

A Bantam Book/April 2002

All rights reserved.

ISBN: 0-553-58194-5

Published simultaneously in the United States and Canada

PRINTED IN THE UNITED STATES OF AMERICA

OPM 10 9 8 7 6 5 4 3 2

Contents

Index of Health Conditions

Index of Natural Products

Introduction: Natural Medicine Today

According to the 1999 Gallup Study of Vitamin Use in the United States, nearly one out of two adults (48 percent) now report current use of nutritional supplements, with 42 percent of the adult population taking three or more supplements daily. These numbers have increased by a third since 1993. Today, vast amounts of information on natural products are available from a variety of sources. But how reliable is this information? And even with the best information, consumers are often confused about how to make the best choices. This book is designed to make the process easier by providing answers to the key questions consumers have about the proper use of natural products. This book will provide you with the facts about the role of natural products in promoting health for you and your family. You'll find answers to help guide you to the proper use of products in the prevention and treatment of over one hundred common health conditions, from acne to varicose veins.

The Science of Natural Medicine

You may have noticed the designation *N.D.* after my name. The *N.D.* signifies that I am a naturopathic doctor. I am a graduate of Bastyr University in Seattle, Washington, and licensed in the State of Washington as a primary care physician. Naturopathic medicine is a system of medicine that emphasizes the use of natural, nontoxic therapies to prevent and treat disease and to promote optimal health. The scope of practice of an N.D. includes all aspects of family and primary care, from pediatrics to geriatrics, as well as the full range of human health conditions, including cancer. The natural products described in this book are the medicines that many naturopathic physicians rely on.

It occurred to me very early on in my educational process that if natural medicines are truly effective, their value should be evident in well-designed clinical studies. With that in mind I began a data-gathering process that continues to this day. Over the past twenty-plus years I have collected over fifty thousand articles from medical journals and other scientific literature that provide strong evidence of the effectiveness of diet, vitamins, minerals, glandular extracts, herbs, and other natural measures in the maintenance of health and the treatment of disease. It is from this constantly expanding database that I base my recommendations on health and healing. This database is also the basis for the rating scales for effectiveness and safety that are a prominent feature of this book. (See "How to Use This Book" for a complete explanation of the criteria.)

It gives me a sense of great pride that I have played a significant role in bringing many safe and effective natural products to America, including:

Ginkgo biloba extract
Glucosamine sulfate
Silymarin (milk thistle extract)
Enteric-coated peppermint oil
Saw palmetto berry extract

These natural products are now household names because of their ability to make a difference in the health of the people who take them. They are prime examples of natural products whose efficacy is clearly demonstrated by solid, clinically based evidence. Unfortunately, not all natural products have the level of scientific and clinical support that these products have. And not all natural products are safe and effective.

When people refer to me as an expert in "alternative medicine," I usually correct them. I am a proponent of what I like to refer to as "rational medicine," which combines the best of both conventional medicine and alternative methods. We have all been helped by the wonders of modern, high-tech medicine. It can make a life-or-death difference when heroic measures are needed. As far as improving our general level of health, however, I believe it is woefully deficient. Modern medicine fails us most in the treatment of chronic degenerative diseases such as heart disease, high blood pressure, arthritis, and diabetes. In many diseases, the natural approach is simply a much more rational approach. Rather than relying on drugs and surgery to suppress symptoms, I believe it makes more sense to use natural, noninvasive techniques whenever possible to promote health and healing—especially when studies indicate that adverse reactions to conventional medicines may be the fourth leading cause of death in America.

Using Natural Products as "Drug Substitutes"

To illustrate the use of natural products as an alternative to drugs, let's take a look at the use of glucosamine sulfate versus the drug approach to osteoarthritis—the most common form of arthritis. Osteoarthritis is characterized by a breakdown of cartilage. Cartilage plays an important role in joint function. Its gel-like nature protects the ends of joints by acting as a shock absorber. When this cartilage degenerates, it causes inflammation, pain, deformity, and limitation of motion in the joint.

The primary drugs used to treat osteoarthritis are the nonsteroidal anti-inflammatory drugs, or NSAIDs, including aspirin, ibuprofen (Advil, Motrin), naproxen (Aleve, Naprosyn), piroxicam (Feldene), and diclofenac (Voltaren). These drugs are used extensively in the United States, but research indicates that while they may produce short-term benefits in the treatment of osteoarthritis, some of these drugs actually accelerate the progression of joint destruction and cause more problems down the road. NSAIDs are also associated with side effects such as gastrointestinal upset, headaches, and dizziness.

Simply stated, aspirin and other NSAIDs are designed to fight disease rather than promote health. Glucosamine sulfate, on the other hand, works by stimulating the manufacture of key cartilage components responsible for the shock-absorbing qualities of cartilage. The use of glucosamine sulfate in the treatment of osteoarthritis is consistent with the philosophy and practice of naturopathic medicine because of its action in facilitating the body's natural healing process. The clinical benefits of treating osteoarthritis with glucosamine sulfate are impressive. In head-to-head comparison studies, glucosamine sulfate has been shown to provide greater benefit than NSAIDs and to do so without any significant side effects.

The treatment of osteoarthritis with glucosamine sulfate is just one example in which a more natural approach produces better results and does so without side effects. Frankly, in my opinion it is a more rational approach than the drug approach.

Complementary Aspects of Naturopathic Medicine

In addition to being used as primary therapy, natural products are often useful as a complement to conventional medications. This situation is especially true with serious illnesses that require prescription drug and/or surgical treatments, such as cancer, angina, congestive heart failure, Parkinson's disease, and trauma. For example, a patient who has severe congestive heart failure that requires such drugs as digoxin and furosemide can benefit from the appropriate use of thiamin, carnitine, and coenzyme Q_{10} supplementation. Although there are double-blind studies demonstrating the value of these agents as complementary therapies in congestive heart failure, they are rarely prescribed by conventional medical doctors in the United States.

Natural Medicine Goes Mainstream

The astonishing increase in the popularity of natural products has several explanations. First, increased scientific investigation into the importance of nutrition and the value of antioxidant nutrients such as vitamins E and C led to more credible information on the value of nutritional supplementation. This information was well accepted by the early devotees of nutritional supplementation. Initially, demographic studies of supplement users indicated that they tended to be better educated and have a higher social status than nonusers. That is no longer the case, as more and more people from all walks of life have begun to use vitamin C to ward off a cold and vitamin E to possibly prevent heart disease.

The next major development was the tremendous influx into North America in the 1980s and early

1990s of high-quality products that actually produced noticeable results. Many of these products, such as *Ginkgo biloba* extract, St. John's wort extract, and glucosamine sulfate, carried with them significant scientific documentation of their safety and efficacy, leading to even greater credibility and acceptance.

Perhaps the biggest reason for the tremendous explosion in popularity for many products, however, occurred in 1994 when Congress passed the Dietary Supplement Health and Education Act (DSHEA). This landmark bill was the result of tremendous support from the American public. In passing DSHEA, Congress recognized that many people believe dietary supplements offer health benefits and that consumers want a greater opportunity to determine whether supplements may help them.

DSHEA essentially gave dietary supplement manufacturers freedom to market more products as dietary supplements and to provide information about their products' health-promoting benefits. Under DSHEA, the Food and Drug Administration (FDA) is still responsible for overseeing the supplement industry and the truthfulness of the claims that are being made. In addition, the Federal Trade Commission (FTC) regulates the advertising of dietary supplements.

How Natural Products Are Regulated

As with any food product, federal law requires manufacturers of dietary supplements to ensure that the products they put on the market are safe. It is the FDA's responsibility to police the safety of nutritional supplements. But under DSHEA, once a dietary supplement is marketed, the FDA has the responsibility for showing that a dietary supplement is unsafe before it can take action to restrict the product's use or take it off the market. In regard to supervising label claims, in response to DSHEA, the FDA instituted new requirements for the product labels of dietary supplements. All natural products that fall under DSHEA must meet these label requirements.

The FDA's Requirements for Dietary Supplement Labels

Information that is required on the labels of dietary supplements includes:

- Statement of identity (e.g., "ginseng").
- Net quantity of contents (e.g., "60 capsules").
- Structure-function claim (e.g., "promotes joint health") and the statement "This statement has not been evaluated by the Food and Drug Administration. This product is not intended to diagnose, treat, cure, or prevent any disease."
- Directions for use (e.g., "take one capsule daily").
- Supplement Facts panel (lists serving size, amount, and active ingredient[s]).
- Other ingredients in descending order of predominance and by common name or proprietary blend.
- Name and place of business of manufacturer, packer, or distributor. This information provides the address to write to for more product information.

The Limit of the Health Claims

What separates a dietary supplement from a drug is that a dietary supplement must not make a claim to treat, cure, or prevent disease even if it is obviously true that it does. For example, it is generally accepted in even the most conservative medical circles that vitamin E supplementation helps to prevent heart disease, that vitamin C can reduce the severity and duration of the common cold, and that *Ginkgo biloba* extract is quite helpful in treating cerebral vascular insufficiency (decreased blood supply to the brain). Even though these statements are true, a manufacturer may not put them on a label. To do so would constitute a drug claim. A product sold as a dietary supplement and touted in its labeling as a new treatment or cure for a specific disease or condition would be considered an unapproved—and thus illegal—drug. Labeling changes consistent with the provisions in DSHEA would be required to maintain the product's status as a dietary supplement. In the case of vitamin E, for example, under DSHEA a manufacturer could say only that vitamin E is necessary for proper heart and vascular function.

DSHEA allows supplement manufacturers to use claims referring to the supplement's effect on the body's structure or function, including its overall effect on a person's well-being. These are known as structure-function claims. Examples of structure-function claims are:

- Calcium builds strong bones.
- Antioxidants maintain cell integrity.
- Fiber maintains bowel regularity.

Manufacturers can use structure-function claims without FDA authorization, but like all label claims, structure-function claims must be true and not misleading. Otherwise the FDA or FTC will step in. Structure-function claims can be easy to spot because, on the label, they must be accompanied with the disclaimer "This statement has not been evaluated by the Food and Drug Administration. This product is not intended to diagnose, treat, cure, or prevent any disease."

Manufacturers who plan to use a structure-function claim on a particular product must inform the FDA of the use of the claim no later than thirty days after the product is first marketed. While the manufacturer must be able to substantiate its claim, it does not have to share the substantiation with the FDA or make it publicly available. If the submitted claims promote the products as drugs instead of supplements, the FDA can advise the manufacturer to change or delete the claim.

The Goal of This Book

Obviously the current situation regarding label claims and intended uses of natural products is less than ideal. There is a tremendous gap between the usefulness, safety, and effectiveness of many products and what the manufacturer is able to tell consumers. My goal in this book is to set the record straight on the value of virtually every natural product on the marketplace. As a person who has dedicated his life to understanding how these products work, both in my clinical practice and through my ongoing involvement in the natural products industry, I know firsthand the relative merits of a particular natural product compared to conventional drugs, and also how it compares to other natural products.

I am such a strong advocate of responsible self-care with natural products because I know they can make a huge difference in the quality of life of people who take them. I want to see the natural health movement flourish, and I believe the best way that I can contribute to this movement is for people to get real, positive results when they use natural products. I believe in the healing power of nature and natural products, but that power is available only if you use the right product for the right indication at the right dosage. All of the information in this book is meant to ensure that you have a good experience with natural medicine.

This book does not tell you which brand of a particular product to buy. Branded products are profiled individually only when they represent a special formulation or combination of substances. Other brand names are mentioned within the profiles when a brand has a substantial amount of original scientific research behind it or has established a dominant position through marketing and/or unique features. Compared to over-the-counter and prescription drugs, there are relatively few unique branded products within the natural products category. This constitutes one of the key differences between the pharmaceutical world and the natural products industry. Drug companies invest huge sums of money to create the required research support for their products. (It is estimated that achieving FDA approval for a new drug costs in excess of $300 million.) They spend even more money marketing their brand names. They can afford to make the investment because they have been granted patent protection for their product—exclusive rights to manufacture and sell it for a given number of years. Only after the patent has expired are generic versions made available, usually at much lower prices. However, a natural compound per se cannot be patented. Extraction or manufacturing techniques, and sometimes the use of a natural product for a specific application, may be patented, but not a naturally occurring plant, vitamin, or mineral.

Because of the lack of patent protection, when a particular manufacturer does invest in clinical research on a natural substance, it is often co-opted by other manufacturers to promote the sale of their knockoff product—which may or may not be identical to what was used in the study. In the supplement industry this is referred to as "borrowed science." For example, let's take one of the most popular natural products in North America, glucosamine sulfate. All of the clinical research on glucosamine sulfate was conducted using a compound developed by Rotta Pharmaceuticals of Milan, Italy. The Rotta product is available in the United States, but it is priced substantially higher than generic glucosamine sulfate.

Most physicians and pharmacists allow for generic substitutions for branded prescription drugs because a generic drug is legally required to contain the same level of the active ingredient as the branded drug. Theoretically, the same should be true for natural products, but quality control standards are still a problem within the natural products industry. For example, in December 1999 and January 2000 ConsumerLab.com purchased a total of twenty-five brands of glucosamine, chondroitin, and combined glucosamine/chondroitin products. These products were then tested to determine whether they contained the amounts of glucosamine and/or chondroitin stated on the label. Nearly one-third of the products tested did not pass.

Although I do not recommend particular brands, I can offer you a rule of thumb in making your purchases: Buy from respected manufacturers that employ good manufacturing practices (GMP). A manufacturer that follows FDA (or HPB in Canada) guidelines for GMP for a drug manufacturing facility is the most likely to have a higher-quality product. In general, if one product is substantially cheaper than a seemingly identical product, buy the more expensive one. With nutritional and herbal products (as with many other things), you get what you pay for. Companies that follow appropriate GMP and have their own quality control laboratory will have higher overhead than manufacturers who do not follow GMP; as a result, they will have to charge more for their product.

In an effort to establish quality control standards for the supplement industry, the National Nutritional Foods Association (see www.nnfa.org)—the largest trade association in the natural products industry— is in the process of developing its own set of standards for GMP. The NNFA program currently in place, the TruLabel program, has been extremely successful. Members of the NNFA who manufacture dietary supplements and herbs under their own label are required to be members of NNFA's TruLabel program. More than seventeen thousand product labels are currently registered as part of the TruLabel program, the industry's most expansive and successful self-regulatory program. Since 1990, NNFA's TruLabel program has garnered national and international respect by promoting quality assurance, safety, and guideline compliance to dietary supplement suppliers.

Responsible Self-Care

With the use of natural products for self-care comes personal responsibility. Here are some important points to consider:

- Although this book discusses the use of natural products for numerous health conditions, it is not intended as a substitute for appropriate medical care.
- If you wish to try a nutritional supplement or herbal product as a therapeutic measure, discuss it with your physician first, especially if you are taking any prescription medication. Doing so can help avoid potential side effects and adverse interactions.
- Do not self-diagnose. Proper medical care is critical to good health. If you have symptoms that suggest an illness described in this book, please consult a physician or health care provider immediately.
- If you are currently taking a prescription medication, you absolutely must work with your doctor before discontinuing any drug or altering any drug regimen.
- Make sure your physician and pharmacist are aware of all the nutritional supplements or herbal products you are currently taking.
- Many nutritional supplements and herbal products are effective on their own, but they work best when they are used as part of a comprehensive natural approach to health that incorporates diet and lifestyle factors.

Michael T. Murray, N.D.

How to Use This Book

The Pill Book Guide to Natural Medicines profiles more than 275 of the most commonly used natural products available today. The entries are listed alphabetically within each of the following categories: vitamins, minerals, accessory nutrients and other natural products, herbal products, and topical preparations. If you are interested in a particular supplement and do not know to which category it belongs, please consult the Index of Natural Products at the front of the book.

Here is a brief description of each category. Particular issues related to each category are discussed in more depth at the beginning of each part. You will find it useful to read these overviews as well as the profile of the individual supplement that interests you.

Part I: Vitamins. Vitamins are essential nutrients that function along with enzymes in chemical reactions necessary for human bodily function, including energy production. Together, vitamins and enzymes work to act as catalysts in speeding up the making or breaking of chemical bonds that join molecules together.

Part II: Minerals. Minerals function, along with vitamins, as components of the body's enzymes. Minerals are also needed for proper composition of bone and blood and for the maintenance of normal cell function.

Part III: Accessory Nutrients and Other Natural Products. Accessory nutrients are food components and substances naturally produced in the body that are required for normal physiology. Other natural products include supplementary hormones, glandular preparations, amino acids, and helpful bacterial preparations such as *Lactobacillus acidophilus.*

Part IV: Herbal Products. These include not only crude herb preparations but also compounds composed of or derived from herbs and other medicinal plants.

Part V: Natural Ingredients Used in Topical Preparations. While Parts I–IV cover products for oral use, this part provides information on natural substances used in skin care products and topical medications.

You can also use this book to discover alternative medicines that may be helpful in treating a specific health condition. This information is contained in *Part VI: Common Health Conditions.* This part provides an alphabetical guide to more than sixty-five common health conditions; each entry includes both the prescription drugs and the natural medicines most often used for each condition.

Organization of the Natural Product Entries

Parts I–IV include natural products taken orally. Each product entry is organized according to the following outline:

Generic or Brand Name

The common name of the natural product is used for most entries (e.g., "vitamin C" instead of "ascorbic acid"). A supplement is listed by brand name only when a brand has established itself as a unique proprietary product.

Used For

A listing of the popular uses for each entry is given. In an effort to provide information on the effectiveness and safety of the entries, a rating system was developed based upon currently available information. The rating is based upon the level of scientific support for a particular application. The fact

---

Rating Scales Used in This Book

Effectiveness

A = Excellent results in multiple double-blind studies

B+ = Very good results in a small number of double-blind studies

B = Some clinical evidence of effectiveness

B– = Some clinical evidence of effectiveness, but also some studies showing no effect

C = Strong historical use or scientific rationale but no clinical trials to show effectiveness in humans

D = No significant documentation of historical use or scientific rationale, or majority of clinical studies show no effect

F = Documentation that it is *not* effective

Safety

A = Excellent safety profile

B = Good safety profile

C = Generally regarded as safe at recommended levels

D = Generally regarded as safe at recommended levels but must be used with caution

F = Potentially dangerous, should not be used

that a substance has not been scientifically investigated does not mean that it is without benefit. Likewise, the fact that a substance has been used for hundreds of years does not necessarily mean that it is either effective or safe. The scientific investigation of natural products is an ongoing effort, and new information is constantly validating or refuting claims about the therapeutic value of these preparations.

Here is an expanded explanation of the rating scales:

Effectiveness

A = Excellent results in multiple double-blind studies

In order to receive an A rating, the substance must have undergone a clinical trial—a study in which human subjects receive treatment. The studies with the most scientific weight are double-blind, controlled trials. In a double-blind study, neither the researchers nor the subjects know what is being given; all information is coded, and the code is not broken until the end of the trial. Double-blinding is important because researchers can give unconscious signals to test subjects if they know what the subject is receiving, and this can affect the results. In a controlled trial, at least two groups are compared.

In a double-blind, placebo-controlled trial, an inactive pill—the placebo—is given to a control group. *Placebo* is Latin for "I will please [you]." Placebos got their name because any treatment, even simple attention, tends to make people feel better. Overall, an average of one out of three subjects will report significant improvement from being given a placebo (usually a sugar pill), although this figure can be much lower or much higher depending upon the condition. Sometimes instead of a placebo, a substance will be compared to another active compound. For example, there have been several comparative studies of glucosamine sulfate and ibuprofen in the treatment of osteoarthritis.

The double-blind study is thought of as the gold standard. However, a good double-blind study must also have a large enough sample size (the bigger the better) to produce statistically significant results. Often a probability value (p value) is given. A p value less than 0.1 means that the probability that the results occurred by chance is less than 1 out of 100 (1 percent). A p value of less than 0.5 is generally regarded as being statistically significant. The lower the p value, the more significant the results.

When a number of small trials have provided conflicting or inconclusive results, a metanalysis can be performed in order to achieve a more statistically significant assessment.

In order for a substance to receive an effectiveness rating of A, it must have shown consistent benefit in double-blind, controlled trials or in a metanalysis.

B+ = Very good results in a small number of double-blind studies

The difference between an A and a B+ is that although there are double-blind studies showing that the substance rated as B+ is effective, these preliminary studies need to be followed up with larger, better-designed studies. Also, a substance would be given a score of B+ rather than A if the studies were poorly designed or did not produce a high degree of statistical significance.

B = Some clinical evidence of effectiveness

There are other types of clinical studies that are often conducted as preliminary studies. Sometimes, because of the lack of financing or other reasons, promising results are never followed up in better-designed studies. Examples of preliminary studies can range from a series of individual case histories to open clinical trials. In an open clinical trial, both the doctor and the subject know exactly what the subject is taking. Open trials are not as well respected in the scientific community because of the expectations of the patient and/or the physician.

B– = Some clinical evidence of effectiveness, but also some studies showing no effect

It is not uncommon for even established drugs to have some studies showing no or little effect. If the majority of the studies have been positive, the substance was given a rating of A or B+ depending upon the weight of evidence. However, if a number of preliminary studies showed positive results and a double-blind study showed little or no effect, the substance was given an effectiveness rating of B–. In the future it may be proven to be effective, but at present there is simply not enough evidence that is convincing.

C = Strong historical use or scientific rationale but no clinical trials to show effectiveness in humans

This rating is probably the most common in this book. There are numerous natural products that should be better evaluated in clinical trials but have not been. A rating of C does not indicate that a substance is any less effective than one with a rating of A or B; it simply signifies that we really do not know how effective it is, but there is reasonable probability that it may offer benefit.

D = No significant documentation of historical use or scientific rationale, or majority of clinical studies show no effect

A rating of D is cause for concern. In general, unless instructed to do so because of some extenuating circumstance by a health care professional, substances receiving a rating of D should not be used.

F = Documentation that it is *not* effective

A rating of F is straightforward and reflects considerable evidence that the product is not effective for a particular application. Unless new, convincing evidence becomes available in the future, these products offer no value for the noted application.

Safety

A = Excellent safety profile

In order to receive an A for safety, a substance must be generally regarded as safe by most authorities (e.g., the FDA or the National Academy of Sciences) or have been extensively evaluated in toxicology studies in animals or humans.

B = Good safety profile

Clinical studies have been conducted on the product and no significant side effects have been reported, or there are preliminary toxicology studies on the product.

C = Generally regarded as safe at recommended levels

Most often, products receiving this classification have a long history of use without any serious side effects at recommended levels.

D = Generally regarded as safe at recommended levels, but must be used with caution

A rating of D for safety does not mean that the product is unsafe; it simply implies that there may be situations where it should not be used or that it should be used with caution or under the supervision of a health care professional.

F = Potentially dangerous, should not be used

Products with a rating of an F should not be used unless recommended and closely monitored by a health care professional because they pose a significant health risk.

General Information

This entry will usually contain the most useful information to assist you in determining the merits of the product for a particular indication. It provides a full description of the product's effects and uses, including results from clinical trials in humans where available.

Available Forms

Natural products are available in many different physical forms (e.g., capsules, tablets, liquids, powders, etc.). In addition, there may be different forms of a specific nutrient or herb. For example, there are five major forms of calcium on the market. Information is provided to help you make an informed choice. Brand names are given when there has been a significant amount of scientific research conducted on it or the product has established a dominant position through marketing and/or unique features.

Cautions and Warnings

Although generally safe, some natural products carry warnings and cautions. This heading will alert you to any concerns.

Possible Side Effects

A description of possible side effects is presented to alert you to any problems that may occur when using a particular natural product.

Drug Interactions

One area that is particularly important for consumers is the interaction of drugs with natural products. If you are on any prescription medication, it is recommended that you talk to your physician or pharmacist about your use of natural products to avoid any adverse interaction. Although drug-nutrient interactions and drug-herb interactions are not as common as drug-drug interactions, all can have an impact on therapeutic outcome.

Most interactions are the result of a change in the pharmacokinetics of one of the substances. *Pharmacokinetics* refers to the absorption, distribution, metabolism, and excretion of compounds, whether they are drugs, nutrients, or herbs. The most straightforward interactions are those whereby one compound inhibits the absorption of the other. For example, the drug sulfasalazine (Azulfidine) decreases the absorption of folic acid. Such effects are often referred to as "drug-induced nutrient depletion" or "drug-induced nutrient deficiency." Of course, certain nutrients and herbs can also inhibit the absorption of drugs.

There are several other causes of interactions. In regard to herbal products, a particularly troublesome situation can occur when herbal constituents interfere with or enhance the manner in which the liver breaks down certain drugs. For example, recent medical case reports and pharmacological studies suggest that St. John's wort extracts may increase the rate at which the liver breaks down certain drugs and as a result reduce the blood levels of these drugs. Some of the drugs that may be affected include cyclosporine, digoxin, oral contraceptives, theophylline, and anticoagulants such as warfarin. The opposite effect—increasing blood levels of a drug—may also occur.

Some prescription drugs work by interfering with the body's utilization of nutrients. The best-known drug with this sort of action is the anticoagulant drug warfarin (Coumadin). This drug works to thin the blood by interfering with the body's ability to utilize vitamin K. Hence, people taking Coumadin are advised to avoid consuming green leafy vegetables and vitamin formulas that contain high levels of vitamin K.

While negative interactions get more attention, positive interactions between drugs and natural products can produce significant benefits. For example, there are numerous cases where natural products can reduce the severity of side effects or prevent them from developing in the first place. Perhaps the best-known example of this sort of interaction is the use of lactobacillus ("friendly" bacteria) supplementation to prevent or treat diarrhea induced by taking an antibiotic. You can use the general index to this book to look up a prescription drug you may be taking and find potentially helpful interactions. For example, if you are taking the chemotherapy drug paclitaxel (Taxol), the index would refer you to the entry for the amino acid glutamine, which has been shown to prevent the mouth ulcers (stomatitis), muscle and joint pain, and suppression of the immune system almost always seen in people taking paclitaxel.

I hope these examples make it clear why it is so important to inform your physician or pharmacist about any natural products you are taking, in addition to using this book to check for potential interactions.

Food and Nutrient Interactions

The presence of food in your stomach may interfere with or enhance the absorption or action of some natural products. This entry tells you whether a supplement should be taken with meals or on an empty stomach. It also includes a description of any interactions with other nutrients. For example, calcium supplements may inhibit the absorption of other minerals, including copper and zinc, while vitamin B_6 and magnesium work cooperatively. Thus, nutrient interactions may be either antagonistic (negative) or agonistic (positive).

Usual Dosage

In order for natural products to produce the best results, it is important to take them in the proper dosage. Such information is provided along with different dosages for particular applications or available forms.

Overdosage

A description of the symptoms of an overdose, when applicable, and information on what to do in an emergency situation are provided. *The fact that a substance is natural does not mean that it is not potentially dangerous.* Although most natural products are safe at recommended levels, accidental overdosages have occurred. Usually when there is any question of safety (such as with supplements that contain iron) manufacturers of natural products will use child-resistant containers.

Special Populations

Pregnant or breast-feeding women, children, and seniors have special concerns with natural products as well as prescription and over-the-counter drugs. Pregnant and breast-feeding women need to know if a product can harm the fetus or infant. Children are more susceptible to overdosage and side effects. In general, no supplement should be given to a child less than two years of age without specific approval from your physician, and some supplements should never be given to children. Seniors are often taking one or more prescription drugs; they need to be especially aware of potential interactions. Because of age-related changes in the body, they may also metabolize both natural products and prescription drugs differently than a younger person.

Note: • *Within each profile, other products that are profiled separately are highlighted in boldface type.*

        • *The organization of entries in Parts V and VI is different and is explained in the introduction to those parts.*

PART I
Vitamins

Vitamins are essential nutrients required for normal chemical processes to occur in the body. The key function of vitamins (and minerals) in the human body is to serve as essential components in enzymes and coenzymes. Enzymes are molecules involved in speeding up chemical reactions necessary for human bodily function such as energy production or the assembling of tissue components. Coenzymes are molecules that help the enzymes in their chemical reactions.

Enzymes and coenzymes work to either join molecules together or split them apart by making or breaking the chemical bonds that join molecules together. Most enzymes are composed of a protein along with an essential mineral and possibly a vitamin. If an enzyme is lacking the essential mineral or vitamin, it cannot function properly.

There are thirteen vitamins divided into two primary classes. Those that dissolve in fat (fat-soluble) are vitamins A, D, E, and K. Those that dissolve in water (water-soluble) are vitamin C, the B vitamins, biotin, and folic acid.

Fat-soluble vitamins can be stored in fat cells. For that reason your body is able to keep a supply of these vitamins available for use on demand. The downside is that they can build up to toxic levels in the body, leading to potentially severe side effects. Water-soluble vitamins, on the other hand, are stored in only small amounts. Normally any quantity of these vitamins that your body does not use is excreted in the urine. While it is harder to build up toxic amounts of water-soluble vitamins, it is also easier to develop deficiencies of them.

The RDA and DRIs

Included in the description of each vitamin is the Recommended Dietary Allowance (RDA). The RDAs for vitamins and minerals have been prepared by the Food and Nutrition Board of the National Research Council since 1941. These guidelines were originally developed to help reduce the incidence of severe nutritional deficiency diseases such as scurvy (deficiency of vitamin C), pellagra (deficiency of niacin), and beriberi (deficiency of vitamin B_1). Another critical point is that the RDAs were designed to serve as the basis for evaluating the adequacy of diets of groups of people, not individuals. Individuals simply vary too widely in their nutritional requirements for one guideline to be adequate for everyone. As the Food and Nutrition Board states: "Individuals with special nutritional needs are not covered by the RDAs." Statistically speaking, RDAs would prevent deficiency diseases in 97 percent of a population, but there was no scientific basis for thinking that the RDAs would meet the needs of any given person.

In 1993, the Food and Nutrition Board put the RDA revision process into motion by holding a symposium and asking for scientific and public comment on how the RDAs should be revised. Utilizing feedback from this conference and other sources, the Food and Nutrition Board developed an ambitious framework for revamping the old RDAs: Rather than having a single group of scientists revise the existing set of RDAs, they had a number of expert panels review nutrient categories in much more detail than had ever been done before.

Not only did the definition of RDAs change, but three new values were also created: the Estimated Average Requirement (EAR), the Adequate Intake (AI), and the Tolerable Upper Intake Level (UL). All four values are collectively known as Dietary Reference Intakes or DRIs.

The Food and Nutrition Board partnered with Health Canada, the Canadian government agency responsible for nutrition policy, to jointly appoint the Standing Committee on the Scientific Evaluation of Dietary Reference Intakes of the Food and Nutrition Board.

The DRIs reflect a shift in emphasis from preventing deficiency to decreasing the risk of chronic disease through nutrition and proper nutritional supplementation. The RDAs were based on the amounts needed to protect against deficiency diseases. Where adequate scientific data exist, the DRIs strive to include levels that can help prevent certain cancers, cardiovascular disease, osteoporosis, and other diseases that are diet-related.

Definitions

"Dietary Reference Intakes" (DRIs) is the umbrella term that includes the following values:

Estimated Average Requirement (EAR): A nutrient intake value that is estimated to meet the requirement of half the healthy individuals in a group. It is used to assess nutritional adequacy of intakes of population groups. In addition, EARs are used to calculate RDAs.

Recommended Dietary Allowance (RDA): This value is a goal for individuals and is based upon the EAR. It is the daily dietary intake level that is sufficient to meet the nutrient requirement of 97–98 percent of all healthy individuals in a group. If an EAR cannot be set, no RDA value can be proposed.

Adequate Intake (AI): This is used when an RDA cannot be determined. It is a recommended daily intake level based on an observed or experimentally determined approximation of nutrient intake for a group (or groups) of healthy people.

Tolerable Upper Intake Level (UL): The highest level of daily nutrient intake that is likely to pose no risks of adverse health effects to almost all individuals in the general population. As intake increases above the UL, the risk of adverse effects increases.

The DRIs are intended to apply to the healthy general population. They do not apply to individuals who are deficient in a particular nutrient and want to restore proper levels, nor do they apply to individuals with diseases associated with increased nutritional requirements.

For all vitamins and minerals in this book, either the RDA or AI will be given. Information regarding UL is included in the Possible Side Effects and Overdosage sections for selected nutrients.

Beta-carotene

Used For

Antioxidant effects in the prevention of cancer and cardiovascular disease
Effectiveness: B–   Safety: A

Leukoplakia
Effectiveness: A   Safety: A

Low immunity and immune support
Effectiveness: B+   Safety: A

Photosensitivity disorders
Effectiveness: A   Safety: A

General Information

Beta-carotene is a member of the carotene family, the most widespread group of naturally occurring pigments in nature. Carotenes are a highly colored (red, orange, and yellow) group of fat-soluble antioxidants. Some carotenes, such as beta-carotene, can also be converted in the body to vitamin A (that is why it is categorized as a vitamin). Over six hundred carotenoids have been identified, but only between thirty and fifty are believed to have vitamin A activity. Beta-carotene has long been considered the most important carotene because it can easily be converted into vitamin A. However, although it has excellent antioxidant activity, several other carotenes (e.g., **lycopene** and **lutein**) have been shown to have greater antioxidant activity. Therefore, beta-carotene's claim to be the most important carotene may no longer be valid.

The conversion of beta-carotene to vitamin A is dependent on several factors, including protein status, thyroid hormones, zinc, and vitamin C. The rate of conversion diminishes as beta-carotene intake increases and when serum vitamin A levels are adequate. Therefore, beta-carotene does not lead to vitamin A toxicity.

In general, the carotenes are present in highest concentrations in highly colored vegetables and fruit. Beta-carotene is the predominant carotene in most green leaves; in general, the greater the intensity of the green color, the greater the concentration of beta-carotene. Orange-colored fruits and vegetables—carrots, apricots, mangoes, yams, squash, and so on—are also good food sources. The red and purple vegetables and fruits—such as tomatoes, red cabbage, berries, and plums—contain a large portion of other types of carotenes as well as another group of pigments known as flavonoids (see **bioflavonoids**).

Carotenes are used as antioxidants in the prevention of cancer and cardiovascular disease, as immune-enhancing agents, and in the treatment of leukoplakia and photosensitivity.

Prevention of cancer

Population-based (epidemiological) studies have clearly demonstrated that a diet high in beta-carotene is protective against a variety of cancers. The evidence is much stronger for beta-carotene than for Vitamin A, presumably because beta-carotene exerts greater antioxidant and immune-enhancing effects than vitamin A.

While there is little doubt that a diet high in carotenes is protective against cancer, the same cannot be said about beta-carotene. Based upon current evidence, it appears that on its own, synthetic beta-carotene supplementation does not prevent cancer. Large cancer prevention trials with synthetic beta-carotene in high-risk groups have produced negative results. In fact, the results of these studies indicate that synthetic beta-carotene supplementation may actually increase the risk for cancer and cardiovascular disease if people continue to smoke. The data strongly suggest that the protection offered by beta-carotene is apparent only when other important antioxidant nutrients (e.g., vitamins C and E and selenium) are provided. The results seem to indicate the need for a diet high in carotenes; if carotene supplementation is desired, people should not smoke, and they should protect against the formation of toxic beta-carotene derivatives by taking extra vitamin C and E and selenium.

Prevention of cardiovascular disease

A high dietary carotene intake is associated with a lower risk of cardiovascular disease. Beta-carotene may inhibit the oxidative damage to cholesterol and the lining of the arteries that initiates the process of hardening of the arteries (atherosclerosis). However, it appears that beta-carotene is less effective in protecting against cardiovascular disease than vitamin E, probably because vitamin E protects against oxidative damage to cholesterol better than beta-carotene.

Leukoplakia

Leukoplakias are white plaquelike lesions occurring anywhere in the mouth that are reactions to irritation, such as cigarette smoking or tobacco chewing. It is often a precancerous lesion that may develop into mouth or throat cancer. Beta-carotene has been found to be clinically effective in the treatment of leukoplakia. To date, there have been seven clinical trials showing that beta-carotene supplementation (30–180 mg per day) produces regression in anywhere from 15 to 71 percent of people with leukoplakia.

Low immunity and immune support

Beta-carotene has demonstrated a number of immune-enhancing effects. Originally it was thought that the immune-enhancing properties of beta-carotene were due to their being converted to vitamin A. Researchers now know that carotenes exert many immune-system-enhancing effects independent of any vitamin A activity. In addition to a great number of experimental studies showing immune-enhancing effects with beta-carotene supplementation, there are also several clinical studies in both healthy human volunteers and those with evidence of impaired immune function. For example, in one study with healthy subjects, beta-carotene given at a dosage of 180 mg daily (approximately 300,000 IU of vitamin A activity) significantly increased the frequency of helper/inducer T cells (white blood cells that play a critical role in fighting infection) by approximately 30 percent after only seven days.

However, rather than supplementing the diet with synthetic beta-carotene, it may be more advantageous to use carotene from natural sources or increase the intake of carotene-rich foods. For example, in a study in healthy college students, better results in improving immune function were shown in the group that consumed approximately 15 mg beta-carotene per day from carrots compared to those who took 15 mg of synthetic beta-carotene.

Photosensitivity disorders

Beta-carotene has become the treatment of choice for photosensitivity disorders (skin rashes induced by the sun) even in conventional medical circles. It is most effective in the treatment of a condition named erythropoietic protoporphyria (EPP), while its effectiveness in other photosensitivity disorders has also been demonstrated, but not to the same degree. For this application, it is recommended that you consult a physician.

Available Forms

There are two primary sources of beta-carotene on the market: synthetic beta-carotene and natural carotene extracts. Natural beta-carotene is available derived from carrot oil, the algae *Dunaliella salina* (e.g., Betatene), and from palm oil (e.g., Caroplex, Caromin). The natural forms appear to offer advantages over the synthetic form in that they contain a broader range of carotenes, exert more antioxidant protection, and are better absorbed. Beta-carotene, whether natural or synthetic, is available in capsules or tablets.

Cautions and Warnings

Supplementation may cause the skin to turn a yellow to orange hue (carotenodermia). This change is not harmful.

Possible Side Effects

Supplementing the diet with beta-carotene has not been shown to produce any significant side effects other than a possible yellowing of the skin. Dosages greater than 180 mg per day may produce loose stools, but this side effect usually clears quickly and does not necessitate stopping treatment.

Drug Interactions

The drugs cholestyramine (Questran), colestipol (Colestid), and orlistat (Xenical), all interfere with the absorption and/or metabolism of beta-carotene, as does mineral oil.

Food and Nutrient Interactions

Absorption of beta-carotene may be enhanced by taking it with food, particularly a meal with some fat or oil. High dosages of beta-carotene (e.g., greater than 15 mg/day) may increase the need for vitamin E. Olestra (a fat substitute) as well as sources of dietary fiber (psyllium, pectin, guar gum, etc.) may decrease the absorption of beta-carotene. Beta-carotene supplementation may decrease the absorption of other beneficial carotenes such as lutein and lycopene. A deficiency of zinc, vitamin C, protein, or thyroid hormone will impair the conversion of beta-carotene to vitamin A.

Usual Dosage

A daily dosage of 15 mg of beta-carotene (25,000 IU of vitamin A activity) appears to be reasonable for general health. For the treatment of precancerous lesions and immune enhancement, the dosage range is 25,000 to 300,000 IU. In the treatment of photosensitivity disorders (e.g., EPP), the dosage is based on maintaining blood carotene levels between 600 and 800 mcg/dl.

Overdosage

None known.

Special Populations

Pregnant/breast-feeding women
Considered safe during pregnancy and lactation.

Children
Suitable for children at one-half the adult dosage.

Seniors
No special precautions are known.

Biotin

Used For

Building strong nails and healthy hair
Effectiveness: B+   Safety: A

Diabetes
Effectiveness: C   Safety: A

Seborrheic dermatitis and diaper rash
Effectiveness: B+   Safety: A

General Information

Biotin is a member of the B vitamin family even though it can be produced by bacteria in the gut. It functions in the manufacture and utilization of fats and amino acids. A biotin deficiency in adults is characterized by dry, scaly skin; nausea; anorexia; and seborrhea. In infants under six months of age, the symptoms are seborrheic dermatitis (cradle cap), persistent diaper rash, and alopecia (hair loss).

Building strong nails and healthy hair

Biotin is a popular recommendation to increase the strength of nails and promote healthy hair. Early research on biotin in this application came from the veterinary literature, where it was shown to increase the strength and hardness of hooves in pigs and horses. Human studies have shown that biotin supplementation (2.5 mg per day) can produce a 25 percent increase in the thickness of the nail plate in patients diagnosed with brittle nails of unknown cause, and up to 91 percent of patients taking this dosage will experience definite improvement. The beneficial effects of biotin on the health of hair possibly reflect an ability to improve the metabolism of scalp oils, similar to its effects in seborrheic dermatitis.

Diabetes

Biotin supplementation has been shown to enhance insulin sensitivity and improve the utilization of blood sugar. This improvement is thought to be the result of an increase in the activity of the enzyme glucokinase, which is involved in the utilization of blood sugar by the liver. In one study, 8 mg of biotin twice daily resulted in significant lowering of fasting blood sugar levels and improvements in blood glucose control in type 1 diabetics. In a study of type 2 diabetics, similar effects were noted with 9 mg of biotin per day. High-dose biotin has also been reported to be very helpful in the treatment of severe diabetic nerve disease (diabetic neuropathy).

Seborrheic dermatitis

Seborrheic dermatitis is a common condition that may be associated with excessive oiliness (seborrhea) and dandruff. The scales of seborrhea may be yellowish and either dry or greasy. The scaly bumps may coalesce to form large plaques or patches. Seborrheic dermatitis usually occurs either in infancy (usually between two and twelve weeks of age) or in the middle-aged or elderly and has a prognosis of lifelong recurrence.

In infancy, seborrheic dermatitis is known as cradle cap. Several case histories have demonstrated successful treatment of cradle cap with biotin by either giving the mother the biotin if the baby is being breast-fed or giving it directly to the infant. Cases of persistent diaper rash have also responded as well.

In adults with seborrheic dermatitis, treatment with biotin alone is usually of no value; it probably requires all of the necessary B vitamins.

Available Forms

Biotin is available commercially either as isolated biotin or as biocytin, a biotin complex made from brewer's yeast and composed of 65.6 percent biotin.

Cautions and Warnings

Individuals with diabetes should use caution when using high dosages (e.g., greater than 4 mg), as it may produce reductions in blood sugar levels requiring changes in the dosage of insulin or other medications.

Possible Side Effects

Biotin is extremely safe, and no side effects have ever been reported with biotin supplementation.

Drug Interactions

Antibiotics, phenytoin, and phenobarbital may decrease biotin levels due to the drugs' destruction of biotin-producing bacteria in the intestines.

Food and Nutrient Interactions

Biotin works synergistically with other B vitamins as well as coenzyme Q_{10} and carnitine. Alcohol inhibits the absorption and utilization of biotin. High dosages of pantothenic acid may inhibit biotin absorption.

Usual Dosage

The estimated safe and adequate dietary intake for adults is 30–100 mcg. To promote stronger nails and healthy hair, a typical dosage range is 1,000 to 3,000 mcg (1 to 3 mg) per day. In the treatment of seborrheic dermatitis, the dosage to administer to nursing mothers is 3,000 mcg (3 mg) twice daily. For infants not being breast-fed, an effective dosage is estimated to be 100–300 mcg daily. In the treatment of diabetes and diabetic neuropathy, dosages of 4,000 to 8,000 mcg (4–8 mg) twice daily can be used.

Overdosage

No overdoses or serious adverse events have been reported with biotin use.

Special Populations

Pregnant/breast-feeding women
Considered safe during pregnancy and lactation.

Children
Suitable for children at one-half the adult dosage.

Seniors
No special precautions are known.

Enada (*see* NADH)

General Information
Enada is a patented form of NADH (niacinamide adenine dinucleotide), the activated form of vitamin B_3 (niacin). Preliminary research indicates that NADH may enhance brain chemistry in Parkinson's disease, Alzheimer's disease, and depression, and may help boost energy levels in chronic fatigue syndrome.

Ester-C (*see* Vitamin C)

General Information
Ester-C is a patented combination of vitamin C (as calcium ascorbate) along with various metabolites of vitamin C, such as threonate and aldonic acid. Ester-C is claimed to be better absorbed and utilized compared to other forms of vitamin C. However, absorption studies have not shown it to be better absorbed. Because it is a buffered vitamin C, it tends to be less irritating to the stomach.

Folic Acid

Used For

Cervical dysplasia
Effectiveness: B+   Safety: A

Depression
Effectiveness: B   Safety: A

Heart disease (atherosclerosis) prevention
Effectiveness: A   Safety: A

Prevention of birth defects
Effectiveness: A   Safety: A

General Information

Folic acid, also known as folate and folacin, functions together with vitamin B_{12} in many body processes. It is essential to cellular division because it is necessary in DNA synthesis; without folic acid cells do not divide properly. Folic acid is critical to the development of the nervous system of the fetus. Deficiency of folic acid during pregnancy has been linked to several birth defects, including neural tube defects such as spina bifida. Folic acid deficiency is also being linked to depression, atherosclerosis, and osteoporosis.

Folic acid, vitamin B_{12}, and a form of the amino acid methionine known as SAMe **(S-adenosylmethionine)** function as "methyl donors," that is, they carry and donate methyl molecules to facilitate biochemical reactions, including the manufacture of DNA and brain neurotransmitters.

Folic acid and other methyl donors reduce body

concentrations of homocysteine, which has been implicated in a variety of conditions including atherosclerosis and osteoporosis. Homocysteine is thought to promote atherosclerosis by directly damaging the artery as well as reducing the integrity of the vessel wall. In osteoporosis, elevated homocysteine levels lead to a defective bone matrix by interfering with the proper formation of collagen (the main protein in bone).

Cervical dysplasia

Cervical dysplasia is an abnormal condition of the cells of the cervix. It is generally regarded as a precancerous lesion, and has risk factors similar to those of cervical cancer. It is quite probable that many abnormal Pap smears reflect folate deficiency rather than true dysplasia, especially in women who are pregnant or taking oral contraceptives, because estrogens antagonize folic acid. Folic acid supplementation (10 mg per day) has resulted in improvement or normalization of Pap smears in patients with cervical dysplasia in clinical studies.

Depression

Folic acid exerts a mild antidepressant effect, presumably via its function as a methyl donor, which helps increase levels of serotonin in the brain. Folic acid supplementation in depressed patients taking antidepressant drugs such as fluoxetine (Prozac) was found to enhance the antidepressant action of the drugs.

Heart disease (atherosclerosis) prevention

Elevated homocysteine levels are an independent risk factor for heart attack, stroke, or peripheral vascular disease. Elevations in homocysteine are found in approximately 20 to 40 percent of patients with heart disease. It is estimated that folic acid supplementation (400 mcg daily) alone would reduce the number of heart attacks suffered by Americans each year by 10 percent.

Prevention of birth defects

Numerous studies have now demonstrated the benefit of folic acid supplementation in pregnancy—beginning either before conception or very early on in the pregnancy, and continuing throughout—in preventing a type of birth defect known as a neural tube defect (e.g., spina bifida). The evidence became so overwhelming that the FDA finally had to reverse its previous position, acknowledging the association and allowing folic acid supplements and foods fortified with folic acid to claim that "daily consumption of folic acid by women of childbearing age may reduce the risk of neural tube defects."

Available Forms

Folic acid is available as folic acid (folate) and folinic acid (5-methyltetrahydrofolate). In order to utilize folic acid, the body must convert it to folinic acid. Therefore, supplying the body with folinic acid allows it to bypass this process. Folinic acid is the most active form and has been shown to be more efficient at raising body stores than folic acid.

Cautions and Warnings

Folic acid supplementation should always include vitamin B_{12} supplementation (400 to 1,000 mcg daily), because folic acid supplementation can mask an underlying vitamin B_{12} deficiency. This is why the FDA restricts the amount of folic acid available in dietary supplements to 800 mcg. The danger is that while the folic acid will reverse the pernicious anemia caused by the B_{12} deficiency, it will not prevent or reverse the related neurological symptoms.

Dosages greater than 4,000 mcg must be used with extreme caution by epileptics, as occasionally seizure activity may be increased.

Possible Side Effects

In high dosages (e.g., 5,000 to 10,000 mcg daily) folic acid may cause increased flatulence, nausea, and loss of appetite. No side effects have been reported at lower dosages.

Drug Interactions

Estrogens, alcohol, various chemotherapy drugs (especially methotrexate), sulfasalazine (a drug used in the treatment of Crohn's disease and ulcerative colitis), barbiturates, cholestyramine, and anticonvulsant drugs all interfere with folic acid absorption or function. Folic acid supplementation is usually recommended when taking any of these drugs. Folic acid enhances the effectiveness of antidepressant drugs.

Oral pancreatic extracts may reduce folic acid absorption, so they should be administered several hours before or after folate supplementation.

Food and Nutrient Interactions

Folic acid supplements are generally better absorbed than the folic acid naturally present in foods.

Usual Dosage

For general health and the prevention of atherosclerosis and neural tube defects: 400 mcg to 1,000 mcg daily. For the treatment of cervical dysplasia and depression: 10 mg (10,000 mcg) daily. *(Note:* Since the FDA restricts the amount of folic acid available in nutritional supplements to 800 mcg, higher dosages are best achieved with a prescription from a health care provider.)

Overdosage

None known.

Special Populations

Pregnant/breast-feeding women
The importance of folic acid supplementation (400 to 1,000 mcg) during pregnancy cannot be overstated.

Children
Suitable for children at the adult dosage.

Seniors
No special precautions are known.

Inositol Hexaniacinate (*see* Niacin)

General Information

Inositol hexaniacinate (also referred to as hexanicotinate) is a special form of niacin composed of six nicotinic acid molecules bound to and surrounding one molecule of inositol, an unofficial member of the B vitamin group. Inositol hexaniacinate has been shown to exert the benefits of niacin without flushing or other side effects. It has been used in Europe for over thirty years not only to lower cholesterol but also to improve blood flow in the treatment of intermittent claudication (a painful cramp in the calf produced when walking, caused by a decreased oxygen supply to the calf muscle) and Raynaud's phenomenon (a painful response of the hands or feet to cold exposure due to constriction of blood vessels). The dosage and safety aspects of inositol hexaniacinate mirror those of niacin.

NADH (niacinamide adenine dinucleotide)

Used For

Alzheimer's disease and aging-related memory impairment
Effectiveness: B   Safety: A

Chronic fatigue syndrome
Effectiveness: B   Safety: A

Parkinson's disease
Effectiveness: B   Safety: A

General Information

NADH (niacinamide adenine dinucleotide) is the activated form of vitamin B_3 (niacin). NADH is required by the brain to make various neurotransmitters as well as chemical energy. Typically as one ages, the level of NADH declines. This reduced level of NADH leads to reduced energy production and decreased levels of important brain chemicals. Correcting this state of low NADH may lead to significant improvements in mental function and energy levels. Preliminary research showed modest effects in Alzheimer's disease, chronic fatigue syndrome, and Parkinson's disease, but more definitive research is needed.

Available Forms

NADH is available as the brand-name product Enada, found in tablets marketed by several different manufacturers.

Cautions and Warnings

None known.

Possible Side Effects

None known.

Drug Interactions

None known.

Food and Nutrient Interactions

None known.

Usual Dosage

The typical dosage for NADH is 5 to 20 mg daily, depending upon the severity of the symptoms.

Overdosage
None known.

Special Populations

Pregnant/breast-feeding women
Considered safe during pregnancy and lactation.

Children
Suitable for children at one-half the adult dosage.

Seniors
No special precautions are known.

Niacin (Vitamin B₃)

Used For

Lowering cholesterol and triglyceride levels
Effectiveness: A   Safety: D

Raynaud's phenomenon and intermittent claudication
Effectiveness: B+   Safety: D

General Information
The niacin or nicotinic acid form of vitamin B_3 has been known to be an effective method for lowering blood cholesterol levels since the 1950s. In the 1970s, the famed Coronary Drug Project demonstrated that niacin was the only cholesterol-lowering

agent to actually reduce overall mortality. Niacin typically lowers LDL cholesterol levels by 16 to 23 percent while raising HDL cholesterol levels by 20 to 33 percent. These effects, especially the effect on HDL, compare quite favorably to conventional cholesterol-lowering drugs.

Raynaud's phenomenon and intermittent claudication

Inositol hexaniacinate, a form of niacin that has been used in Europe for over thirty years, has been shown not only to lower cholesterol but also to improve blood flow in the treatment of Raynaud's phenomenon (a painful response of the hands or feet to cold exposure, due to constriction of blood vessels supplying the hands) and intermittent claudication (a painful cramp in the calf produced when walking, a result of decreased oxygen supply to the calf muscle). Double-blind studies have verified the beneficial effects of this form of niacin in these peripheral vascular disorders.

Available Forms

Vitamin B_3 is available as niacin (nicotinic acid or nicotinate); **inositol hexaniacinate**; and **niacinamide**. Niacin and inositol hexaniacinate are useful in lowering blood cholesterol levels, while niacinamide is useful in arthritis and early-onset type 1 diabetes.

Niacin is available as pure crystalline niacin and in sustained- or timed-release preparations. Because of the significant risk of liver toxicity, sustained-release niacin should not be used unless prescribed by a physician. Inositol hexaniacinate yields slightly better results than standard niacin but is much better tolerated in terms both of flushing and, more important, long-term side effects.

Cautions and Warnings

Because niacin can damage the liver, periodic checking (minimum every three months) for liver enzyme levels in the blood is indicated. Please tell your physician that you are taking niacin and wish to be monitored.

Because niacin can impair glucose tolerance, it should probably not be used in diabetics unless they are under close observation.

Niacin should not be used in patients with preexisting liver disease or elevation in liver enzymes, gout, or peptic ulcers.

Possible Side Effects

Doses in excess of 50 mg of niacin typically produce a transient flushing of the skin. Other occasional side effects of niacin include gastric irritation, nausea, and liver damage. To get around the problem of skin flushing, drug and supplement manufacturers have developed timed-release products. However, while these preparations may effectively eliminate the problem of skin flushing, they are associated with greater liver destruction and serious side effects (discussed above). A better recommendation to eliminate the problem of skin flushing is to use inositol hexaniacinate. Both short- and long-term studies have shown it to be virtually free of side effects other than an occasional person experiencing mild gastric upset or mild flushing of the skin.

Drug Interactions

Niacin has been shown to potentiate the cholesterol-lowering effects of other lipid-lowering drugs, especially the statin drugs, such as atorvastatin (Lipitor), gemfibrozil (Lopid), lovastatin (Mevacor), pravastatin (Pravachol), and simvastatin (Zocor).

Because niacin can impair glucose tolerance, it may interfere with drugs used in the treatment of diabetes. If you are diabetic, consult a physician to discuss proper monitoring of blood sugar levels before taking niacin at therapeutic levels.

Aspirin and other nonsteroidal anti-inflammatory drugs can blunt the flushing effect of high-dosage niacin.

Food and Nutrient Interactions

Taking high doses of niacin with alcohol or hot beverages may exacerbate the skin flushing effect. Niacin can potentiate the cholesterol-lowering effect of red yeast rice.

Usual Dosage

Niacin is generally recommended at a dosage of 20 to 50 mg for general health purposes and to prevent deficiency. When being used to lower cholesterol levels, the dosage recommendation for crystalline niacin is to start with a dose of 100 mg three times a day and carefully increase the dosage over a period of four to six weeks to the full therapeutic dose of 1.5 to 3 g daily in divided dosages or as a single dosage at night. If inositol hexaniacinate is being used to lower cholesterol or improve blood flow in Raynaud's phenomenon or intermittent claudica-

ion, begin with 500 mg three times daily for two
weeks and then increase to 1,000 mg three times
daily. Either crystalline niacin or inositol hexaniacinate is best if taken with meals. Sustained-release
niacin should not be used unless prescribed by a
physician.

Overdosage

The toxic effects of a single ingestion of large quantities of niacin are not known. Do the following in
case of accidental overdose: If the victim is unconscious or having convulsions, call for an ambulance
immediately. If you take the victim to an emergency
room, be sure to bring the bottle or container with
you. If the victim is conscious, call your local poison
control center or a health care professional. The poison control center may suggest inducing vomiting
with ipecac syrup (available without a prescription
at any pharmacy). *Do not* induce vomiting unless
specifically instructed to do so.

Special Populations

Pregnant/breast-feeding women
Considered safe during pregnancy and lactation at
dosages below 100 mg. Dosages above 100 mg are
not indicated unless directed by a physician.

Children
Suitable for children at or near the level of the
Recommended Dietary Allowance (RDA).

Recommended Dietary Allowance for Niacin

Infants
Birth–6 months   5 mg
6 months–1 year   6 mg

Children
1–3 years   9 mg
4–8 years   8 mg
9–13 years   12 mg
14–18 years   14 mg

Young Adults and Adults
Males 11–14 years   17 mg
Males 15–18 years   20 mg
Males 19–50 years   19 mg
Males 51+ years   15 mg
Females 11–50 years   15 mg
Females 51+ years   13 mg
Pregnant women   17 mg
Lactating women   20 mg

Seniors
No special precautions are known.

Niacinamide

Used For

Diabetes
Effectiveness: B+   Safety: B

Osteoarthritis
Effectiveness: B+   Safety: B

Rheumatoid arthritis
Effectiveness: B   Safety: B

General Information

Niacinamide (nicotinamide) is a form of vitamin B_3 that has different effects compared to other forms such as niacin (nicotinic acid or nicotinate) or inositol hexaniacinate. The primary applications of niacinamide are in recent-onset type 1 diabetes, osteoarthritis, and rheumatoid arthritis.

Diabetes
Type 1 diabetes, or insulin-dependent diabetes mellitus (IDDM), is believed to be the result of immune-mediated destruction of the pancreatic beta cells that produce insulin. Niacinamide may block this attack. Niacinamide was first shown in the early 1950s to prevent the development of diabetes in experimental animals. Additional animal studies in the 1980s confirmed these earlier studies and ultimately led to several small clinical studies, including six double-blind studies. The results of the existing research suggests that niacinamide can prevent type 1 diabetes from progressing in some patients if given soon enough after the onset of the

disease by helping restore beta cells. Some newly diagnosed type 1 diabetics have experienced complete resolution of their diabetes with niacinamide supplementation. Larger clinical trials are in progress or have been proposed to better define responders to niacinamide therapy and better determine the success rate.

Osteoarthritis and rheumatoid arthritis

In the 1940s and 1950s, Dr. William Kaufman and later Dr. Abram Hoffer reported very good clinical results in the treatment of hundreds of patients with rheumatoid arthritis and osteoarthritis using high-dose niacinamide (900 to 4,000 mg per day in divided doses). Dr. Kaufman documented improvements in joint function and range of motion, increased muscle strength and endurance, and reduction in the sedimentation rate. Most patients achieved noticeable benefits within one to three months of use, with peak benefits noted between one and three years of continuous use.

These clinical results were upheld in a more recent double-blind study in patients with osteoarthritis. Researchers found that niacinamide produced a 29 percent improvement in all symptoms and signs compared to a 10 percent worsening in the placebo group. Pain levels did not change, but those on niacinamide reduced their use of pain-relieving drugs.

Available Forms

Niacinamide is available in capsules and tablets.

Cautions and Warnings

Niacinamide at pharmacological dosages (i.e., above 250 mg daily) should not be used in patients with preexisting liver disease or elevation in liver enzymes.

Individuals with diabetes need to be aware that taking niacinamide may alter insulin or drug requirements. Consult a physician to discuss proper monitoring of blood sugar levels before taking niacinamide.

Possible Side Effects

Niacinamide is generally well tolerated and without side effects. Unlike niacin, niacinamide does not produce flushing of the skin. At daily dosages greater than 1,000 mg, periodic (e.g., every three months) blood tests to determine any possible liver damage are advised.

Drug Interactions

Taking niacinamide at pharmacological dosages (i.e., above 250 mg daily) may result in the effectiveness of drugs that lower blood sugar levels, such as insulin, glyburide (Diabeta, Micronase), and metformin (Glucophage). Niacinamide may inhibit the breakdown of the drug carbamazepine (Tegretol).

Food and Nutrient Interactions

None known.

Usual Dosage

In recently diagnosed type 1 diabetics the daily dose
of nicotinamide is based on body weight, 25 mg per
kg (2.2 pounds). For osteoarthritis and rheumatoid
arthritis the typical dosage recommendation is 500
to 1,000 mg three times daily.

Overdosage

Overdosage is unlikely. But do the following in case
of accidental overdose: If the victim is unconscious
or having convulsions, call for an ambulance immediately. If you take the victim to an emergency room,
be sure to bring the bottle or container with you. If
the victim is conscious, call your local poison control center or a health care professional. The poison
control center may suggest inducing vomiting with
ipecac syrup (available without a prescription at any
pharmacy). *Do not* induce vomiting unless specifically instructed to do so.

Special Populations

Pregnant/breast-feeding women
   Niacinamide at dosages greater than 30 mg is not
advised during pregnancy and lactation.

Children
   The dosage for children with type 1 diabetes is 25
mg per kg (2.2 pounds) body weight.

Seniors
   No special precautions are known.

Pantethine

Used For

Lowering blood cholesterol and triglyceride levels
Effectiveness: B+   Safety: A

General Information

Pantethine is the most active stable form of pantothenic acid (vitamin B_5). Pantethine exerts significant cholesterol- and triglyceride-lowering effects, but for some reason pantothenic acid does not.

Patients most likely to respond to pantethine are those with elevated cholesterol and triglyceride levels who have diabetes or are on hemodialysis. Pantethine administration to patients in these categories has been shown to significantly reduce serum triglycerides (by 32 percent), total cholesterol (by 19 percent), and LDL cholesterol (by 21 percent) while increasing HDL cholesterol (by 23 percent) in patients.

In diabetics, pantethine has also been shown to act as an antioxidant and improve platelet function through correction of the derangement in cell membrane fatty acids characteristic of diabetes.

Available Forms

Pantethine is available in soft gelatin capsules and tablets.

Cautions and Warnings

None known.

Possible Side Effects

None known.

Usual Dosage

The typical recommendation is 300 mg three times daily.

Drug Interactions

None known.

Food and Nutrient Interactions

None known.

Special Populations

Pregnant/breast-feeding women
As the effects of pantethine during pregnancy and lactation have not been sufficiently evaluated, it should not be used during these times unless directed to do so by a physician.

Children
Suitable for children at one-half the adult dosage.

Seniors
No special precautions are known.

Pantothenic Acid

Adrenal support
Effectiveness: C   Safety: A

Rheumatoid arthritis
Effectiveness: B   Safety: A

General Information

Pantothenic acid, or vitamin B_5, is utilized in the manufacture of coenzyme A (CoA) and acyl carrier protein (ACP), two compounds that play critical roles in the utilization of fats and carbohydrates in energy production as well as the manufacture of adrenal hormones and red blood cells.

Adrenal support

Pantothenic acid supplementation is often recommended by nutritionally oriented physicians to support adrenal function. Although there are anecdotal reports of this benefit, no clinical trials exist to disprove or prove this application.

Rheumatoid arthritis

Lower blood levels of pantothenic acid levels have been reported in patients with rheumatoid arthritis compared to normal controls; the lower the level of pantothenic acid, the more severe the symptoms. Correction of low pantothenic acid levels to normal brought about some alleviation of symptoms. In one double-blind study, patients taking pantothenic acid (2 g daily) noted improvements in duration of morning stiffness, degree of disability, and severity of pain compared to a placebo group.

Available Forms

Pantothenic acid is available most often in capsules and tablets as calcium pantothenate. Another form, **pantethine,** is used to lower blood cholesterol and triglyceride levels.

Cautions and Warnings

None known.

Possible Side Effects

No significant side effects or adverse reactions have been reported with pantothenic acid.

Drug Interactions

None known.

Food and Nutrient Interactions

High dosages of pantothenic acid may inhibit the absorption of biotin.

Usual Dosage

For general adrenal support and possible benefit in allergies: 250 mg of pantothenic acid twice daily. For rheumatoid arthritis: 2 g of pantothenic acid daily.

Overdosage

None known.

Special Populations

Pregnant/breast-feeding women

Pantothenic acid is generally regarded as safe during pregnancy and lactation; however, because its effects during these times have not been sufficiently evaluated, it should not be used by pregnant or lactating women at dosages greater than 100 mg unless specifically directed to do so by a physician.

Children

Suitable for children at one-half the adult dosage.

Seniors

No special precautions are known.

Riboflavin (Vitamin B₂)

Used For

Cataracts
Effectiveness: C   Safety: A

Migraine headaches
Effectiveness: B   Safety: A

Sickle cell anemia
Effectiveness: B   Safety: A

General Information

Riboflavin (vitamin B₂) functions in two very important enzymes (FMN and FAD) involved in the pro-

duction of energy. Riboflavin deficiency is characterized by cracking of the lips and corners of the
mouth; an inflamed tongue; visual disturbances
such as sensitivity to light and loss of visual acuity;
cataract formation; burning and itching of the eyes,
lips, mouth, and tongue; and other signs of disorders of the mucous membranes.

As an important B vitamin, riboflavin is found in
many nutritional supplements, especially B complex
and multivitamin formulas. Low dietary levels of riboflavin have been linked to certain cancers.
Riboflavin supplementation is used specifically in
cataracts, prevention of migraine headaches, and
sickle cell anemia.

Cataracts

Early studies demonstrated an association between riboflavin deficiency and cataract formation.
However, later studies failed to demonstrate any association. In fact, more than 10 mg per day of riboflavin should not be used in individuals with
cataracts unless they take care to prevent sunlight
from hitting the eyes by wearing sunglasses that
block ultraviolet rays, as riboflavin interacts with
light and oxygen in a manner that can produce
highly reactive free radicals. In fact, riboflavin and
ultraviolet light have been used to induce cataracts
in experimental studies.

Migraine headaches

One hypothesis on why migraine headaches develop is that they are caused by a reduction of energy production within the cells of blood vessels in
the head. Because riboflavin has the potential to increase energy production, it was thought that it
might have preventive effects against migraine. A
few preliminary studies have shown excellent re-

sults. In one double-blind study, riboflavin (400 mg) or a placebo was given for three months to fifty-five patients with a history of migraine headaches. Riboflavin was shown to be superior to placebo in reducing attack frequency and duration. The proportion of patients who improved by at least 50 percent was 59 percent for the riboflavin group and only 15 percent for the placebo group.

Sickle cell anemia

Riboflavin supplementation (5 mg twice daily) was shown to be of benefit in patients with sickle cell disease in one small study (eighteen patients).

Available Forms

Riboflavin is available in pill form (capsules and tablets) as simple riboflavin and activated riboflavin (riboflavin-5-phosphate).

Cautions and Warnings

Because riboflavin has the potential to generate free radicals when exposed to sunlight, at dosages greater than 10 mg per day, a person should take care to prevent sunlight from hitting the eyes by wearing sunglasses that block ultraviolet rays.

Possible Side Effects

No immediate side effects are known even at higher dosages, although in the studies in patients with migraine headaches, high-dose (400 mg/day) riboflavin therapy may have produced the side effects of diarrhea and increased urinary frequency in two patients.

Drug Interactions

The chemotherapy drug adriamycin and drugs used in the treatment of malaria (e.g., quinacrine, chlorpromazine, and daunomycin) can interfere with riboflavin metabolism, while cholestyramine, colestipol, and metoclopramide may decrease the absorption of riboflavin. People taking these drugs may need to take additional riboflavin to prevent riboflavin deficiency.

Food and Nutrient Interactions

Taking riboflavin with food increases its absorption. Riboflavin is necessary to convert vitamin B_6 to its active form.

Usual Dosage

For general health, a daily dosage of 2 to 10 mg appears reasonable. For the prevention of migraine headaches, the dosage used has been 400 mg daily. However, it must be pointed out that absorption studies indicate that the capacity of the human gastrointestinal tract to absorb riboflavin may be less than 20 mg in a single oral dose, so it is not known whether this high dosage level is necessary.

Overdosage

No overdoses of riboflavin have been reported.

Recommended Dietary Allowance for Riboflavin

Infants	
Birth–6 months	0.4 mg
6 months–1 year	0.5 mg
Children	
1–3 years	0.5 mg
4–8 years	0.6 mg
Young Adults and Adults	
Males 9–13 years	0.9 mg
Males 14–18 years	1.0 mg
Males 19+ years	1.3 mg
Females 9–13 years	0.9 mg
Females 14–18 years	1.0 mg
Females +19 years	1.3 mg
Pregnant women	1.4 mg
Lactating women	1.6 mg

Special Populations

Pregnant/breast-feeding women
   Considered safe during pregnancy and lactation.

Children
   Suitable for children even at adult dosages.

Seniors
   No special precautions are known.

Thiamin (Vitamin B₁)

Used For

Alzheimer's disease and aging-related mental impairment
Effectiveness: B+   Safety: A

Congestive heart failure
Effectiveness: B+   Safety: A

Epilepsy (improving mental function in people on antiseizure drugs)
Effectiveness: B   Safety: A

General Information

Thiamin was the first B vitamin discovered, hence its designation as vitamin B_1. Thiamin is essential for proper energy production in every cell of the body, but especially in the heart and brain. Severe thiamin deficiency was discovered as the cause of a syndrome known as beriberi. Symptoms include mental confusion, muscle wasting (dry beriberi), fluid retention (wet beriberi), high blood pressure, difficulty walking, and heart disturbances.

Alzheimer's disease and aging-related mental impairment

Thiamin at high dosages mimics an important neurotransmitter involved in memory, acetylcholine. Alzheimer's disease is characterized by a severe loss of acetylcholine action within certain key areas of the brain. Positive clinical results have been noted for thiamin (3–8 g/day) in improving mental function in Alzheimer's disease and age-related impaired mental function (senility).

Congestive heart failure

Thiamin deficiency can result in the cardiovascular manifestations of wet beriberi, sodium retention, peripheral dilation of blood vessels, and heart failure. There is evidence that many individuals with congestive heart failure (CHF) suffer from reduced levels of thiamin in the heart muscle, especially if they are using furosemide (Lasix), the most widely prescribed diuretic, or taking digoxin (Lanoxin). These drugs are known to induce thiamin deficiency. The first study to look at thiamin as a potential therapy in the treatment of CHF showed only modest benefits. However, several subsequent studies have shown that daily doses of 80 to 240 mg of thiamin per day improved the clinical picture, as indicated by an increase of 13 to 22 percent in the amount of blood pumped by the heart. Such a significant increase is associated with a greater survival rate in patients with CHF.

Epilepsy (improving mental function in people on antiseizure drugs)

Thiamin supplementation has also been shown to improve mental function in patients with epilepsy who take the drug phenytoin (Dilantin). In one double-blind study, epileptic patients receiving phenytoin alone or in combination with phenobarbital for more than four years demonstrated significantly improved mental functions in both verbal and nonverbal IQ testing when given thiamin supplementation (50 mg daily).

Available Forms

Thiamin is available in most nutritional supplements as thiamin hydrochloride.

Cautions and Warnings

None known.

Possible Side Effects

None known.

Drug Interactions

Diuretics such as furosemide (Lasix) are known to induce thiamin deficiency. Digoxin (Lanoxin) interferes with thiamin in the heart muscle. Individuals on these drugs require thiamin supplementation (200 to 240 mg daily). Thiamin supplementation has also been shown to improve mental function in patients with epilepsy who take the drug phenytoin (Dilantin).

Food and Nutrient Interactions

Sulfites (used as food preservatives) and black tea may inactivate thiamin. Thiamin works along with other B vitamins, especially riboflavin and niacin, in energy production. Magnesium is required in the conversion of thiamin to its active form.

Usual Dosage

For general supplementation and in epileptics taking phenytoin, a daily dosage of 50 to 100 mg appears safe and appropriate. In elderly individuals suffering from either Alzheimer's disease or age-related mental impairment, the recommended dosage for therapeutic effects is 3 to 8 g daily. For individuals with CHF or taking either furosemide (Lasix) or digoxin (Lanoxin), the recommended dosage is 200 to 240 mg daily.

Recommended Dietary Allowance for Thiamin

Infants	
Birth–6 months	0.3 mg
6 months–1 year	0.4 mg
Children	
1–3 years	0.7 mg
4–6 years	0.9 mg
7–10 years	1.0 mg
Young Adults and Adults	
Males 11–14 years	1.3 mg
Males 15–50 years	1.5 mg
Males 51+ years	1.2 mg
Females 11–50 years	1.1 mg
Females 51+ years	1.0 mg
Pregnant women	1.5 mg
Lactating women	1.6 mg

Overdosage

Thiamin is not associated with any toxicity.

Special Populations

Pregnant/breast-feeding women
Thiamin appears to be safe during pregnancy and lactation at dosage levels less than 100 mg daily.

Children
Suitable for use in children in dosages of up to 50 mg daily.

Seniors
Seniors are more likely to suffer from thiamin deficiency for a multitude of reasons, including reduced intake and absorption of thiamin and the increased use of various drugs that antagonize or deplete thiamin stores.

Vitamin A

Used For

Low immunity and immune support
Effectiveness: B+   Safety: A

Skin disorders
Effectiveness: B   Safety: D

General Information

Vitamin A was the first fat-soluble vitamin to be discovered. Vitamin A is necessary for proper visual function, immune system activity, growth and development, reproduction, and integrity of the skin and mucous membranes.

Vitamin A deficiency may be due to inadequate dietary intake (primary deficiency) or some secondary factor that interferes with the absorption, storage, or transportation of vitamin A. Some factors known to induce a vitamin A deficiency include malabsorption due to bile acid or pancreatic insufficiency, liver disease, and zinc deficiency.

Low immunity and immune support

Vitamin A is necessary to mount an effective immune system response. Individuals deficient in vitamin A are more susceptible to infectious diseases in general, but especially viral infections. Vitamin A supplementation appears appropriate for childhood viral illnesses. For example, vitamin A supplementation has been shown to produce significant benefits in improving immune function in children suffering from measles. Studies have also shown vitamin A to produce positive effects in fighting respiratory syncytial virus (RSV), a common cause of severe respiratory disease in young children. Vitamin A supplementation also appears useful in individuals with human immunodeficiency virus (HIV) infections, as a vitamin A deficiency is quite common during HIV infection and is associated with a higher rate of mortality due to AIDS.

Skin disorders

The use of high-dose vitamin A therapy for a wide variety of skin disorders was introduced in dermatology in the late 1930s. However, since the development of the synthetic vitamin A derivatives (retinoids such as isotretinoin), it is rarely used. Vitamin A therapy has been shown to be quite effective in treating skin conditions associated with excessive formation of keratin (hyperkeratosis), a skin protein that can clog the pores of the skin to produce a goose-bump effect. Examples of some skin conditions associated with hyperkeratosis include acne, psoriasis, ichthyosis, lichen planus, Darier's disease, palmoplantar keratoderma, and pityriasis rubra pilaris. The dosages of vitamin A used to treat these conditions have typically been quite high (300,000–500,000 IU per day for five to six months in the treatment of acne, and 1 million–3.5 million IU per day for one to two weeks for the other conditions). The use of these high dosages usually results in the development of significant toxicity (see "Possible Side Effects," below) and cannot be recommended without strict medical supervision.

Available Forms

Vitamin A is available as either retinol or retinyl palmitate in tablet, capsule, and liquid forms. Absorption may be improved slightly by using vitamin A that is micellized or emulsified. Micellization is the process of making the fat-soluble vitamin A into very small droplets (micelles) so that the material can disperse in water. Emulsification is the process of emulsifying the vitamin A with another chemical (such as lecithin) so that it can mix with water.

Cautions and Warnings

Do not supplement with more than 5,000 IU of vitamin A per day if you are pregnant or at risk of becoming pregnant.

Do not supplement with vitamin A without consulting a physician if you suffer from cirrhosis of the liver, hepatitis, or any other serious liver disorder.

Possible Side Effects

At recommended levels in people with normal liver function, vitamin A is not associated with any side effects. Vitamin A toxicity may occur in adults when taking an excess of 50,000 IU per day for several years or extremely high dosages for shorter periods of time. Signs of vitamin A toxicity generally include dry, fissured skin; brittle nails; hair loss; gingivitis; cracking of the lips; loss of appetite; irritability; fatigue; and nausea.

Drug Interactions

The drugs cholestyramine (Questran), colestipol (Colestid), neomycin (Neo-Fradin), and orlistat (Xenical), all interfere with the absorption of vitamin A, as does mineral oil.

Using vitamin A at higher dosages in conjunction with synthetic vitamin A derivatives such as isotretinoin (Accutane) and etretinate (Tegison) can result in increased risk of toxicity.

Food and Nutrient Interactions

Vitamin E and zinc are particularly important to the proper function of vitamin A. Olestra (a fat substitute) and sources of dietary fiber (psyllium, pectin, guar gum, etc.) may decrease the absorption of vitamin A.

Usual Dosage

Dosage ranges for vitamin A reflect intent of use. For general health purposes, a dosage of 5,000 IU for men and 2,500 for women appears reasonable. During an acute viral infection, a single oral dosage of 50,000 IU daily for one or two days appears to be safe. For the treatment of acne and hyperkeratosis, high-dose therapy may be useful but should be monitored closely by a physician.

Overdosage

Acute toxicity with vitamin A is most often seen in children as a result of the accidental ingestion of a single large dose of vitamin A (more than 300,000 IU) and manifests as raised intracranial pressure with vomiting, headache, joint pain, and stupor. Symptoms rapidly subside upon withdrawal of the vitamin, and complete recovery always results. Do the following in case of accidental overdose: If the victim is unconscious or having convulsions, call for an ambulance immediately. If you take the victim to an emergency room, be sure to bring the bottle or container with you. If the victim is conscious, call your local poison control center or a health care professional. The poison control center may suggest inducing vomiting with ipecac syrup (available without a prescription at any pharmacy). *Do not* induce vomiting unless specifically instructed to do so.

Special Populations

Pregnant/breast-feeding women
Because high doses of vitamin A during pregnancy can cause birth defects, women of childbearing age should not supplement with more than 5,000 IU of vitamin A per day (beta-carotene is a suitable nontoxic alternative). The same warning applies during lactation.

Children
Suitable for supplementation in children at the level of the Recommended Dietary Allowance (RDA):

Age	Retinol Equivalents (RE)	International Units (IU)
Infants		
Birth–1 year	375	1,875
Children		
1–3 years	400	2,000
4–6 years	500	2,500
7–10 years	700	3,500

Seniors
Seniors may be more sensitive to vitamin A toxicity.

Vitamin B$_6$ (Pyridoxine)

Used For

Asthma
Effectiveness: B   Safety: A

Carpal tunnel syndrome
Effectiveness: B   Safety: A

Depression
Effectiveness: B   Safety: A

Diabetes (prevention of diabetic complications)
Effectiveness: B   Safety: A

Heart disease (atherosclerosis) prevention
Effectiveness: B   Safety: A

Kidney stones
Effectiveness: B+   Safety: A

Nausea and vomiting during pregnancy
Effectiveness: B+   Safety: A

Premenstrual syndrome
Effectiveness: B+   Safety: A

General Information

Vitamin B$_6$ (pyridoxine) is an extremely important B vitamin involved in the formation of body proteins and structural compounds, chemical transmitters in the nervous system, red blood cells, and prostaglandins. Vitamin B$_6$ is also critical in maintaining hormonal balance and proper immune function.

Deficiency of vitamin B$_6$ is characterized by depression, convulsions (especially in children), glucose intolerance, anemia, impaired nerve function, cracking of the lips and tongue, and seborrhea or eczema.

Asthma
Double-blind clinical studies have shown that some patients with asthma benefit from vitamin B$_6$ supplementation. In one study, oral supplementa-

tion with 50 mg of vitamin B$_6$ twice daily resulted in a dramatic decrease in frequency and severity of wheezing and asthmatic attacks.

Carpal tunnel syndrome

Vitamin B$_6$ supplementation has been shown to be helpful in many cases of carpal tunnel syndrome, but it may take as long as three months to produce a benefit. Given the safety and positive clinical studies with vitamin B$_6$ in reasonable dosages (e.g., 25–50 mg three times daily), a trial of vitamin B$_6$ should still be utilized, especially before opting for surgery.

Depression

B$_6$ levels are typically quite low in depressed patients, especially women taking birth control pills or estrogens (e.g., Premarin). Depressed individuals with low B$_6$ status usually respond very well to supplementation, according to results from clinical trials.

Diabetes (prevention of diabetic complications)

Individuals with diabetic neuropathy have been shown to be deficient in vitamin B$_6$ and to benefit from supplementation.

Heart disease (atherosclerosis) prevention

Individuals with low levels of pyridoxal-5-phosphate (one form of vitamin B$_6$) in their blood have a five times greater risk of having a heart attack than individuals with higher levels. A deficiency of pyridoxine leads to the accumulation of homocysteine, a metabolite of the amino acid methionine. Homocysteine is very damaging to the cells that line the arteries. Vitamin B$_6$ may also be important in other aspects of atherosclerosis (hardening of the arteries). Vitamin B$_6$ supplementation has been shown to produce modest effects in reducing excessive platelet aggregation, oxidative damage to LDL cholesterol, and blood pressure.

Kidney stones

Calcium oxalate kidney stones can be effectively prevented in most recurrent stone formers with vitamin B$_6$ supplementation along with supplemental magnesium. Vitamin B$_6$ reduces the production and urinary excretion of oxalates.

Nausea and vomiting during pregnancy

Vitamin B$_6$ is often recommended in the treatment of nausea and vomiting during pregnancy. Double-blind studies have substantiated this recommendation. In the largest study, 342 pregnant women (less than seventeen weeks gestation) were given either 30 mg of vitamin B$_6$ or placebo. Patients graded the severity of their nausea and recorded the number of vomiting episodes over the previous twenty-four hours before treatment and again during five consecutive days on treatment. Compared to the placebo group, there was a statistically significant reduction in nausea scores and vomiting episodes; however, more than a third of the patients still experienced vomiting and significant nausea.

Premenstrual syndrome

Since 1975 there have been more than a dozen double-blind studies of vitamin B$_6$ in the treatment of premenstrual syndrome (PMS). Most but not all of these studies have demonstrated a positive effect. For example, in one study 84 percent of the subjects had a lower level of symptoms during the B$_6$ treatment period. In another study premenstrual acne flare-ups were reduced in 72 percent of 106 affected young women taking 50 mg of vitamin B$_6$ daily for one week prior to and during the menstrual period.

Available Forms

Vitamin B$_6$ is available as pyridoxine hydrochloride and pyridoxal-5-phosphate. The latter form is the more active. However, it must be pointed out that most of the pyridoxal-5-phosphate ingested will have the phosphate molecule removed by intestinal cells before it is absorbed. Therefore, for most people the pyridoxine form is satisfactory as long as the necessary cofactors for conversion (riboflavin and magnesium) are available. The exception is people with liver disease. Since the activation of pyridoxine to pyridoxal-5-phosphate occurs in the liver, people with liver disease, particularly liver cirrhosis, may have difficulty converting pyridoxine to pyridoxal-5-phosphate. In patients with cirrhosis and possibly other liver disease, supplementation with injectable pyridoxal-5-phosphate may be more advantageous than oral pyridoxine.

Cautions and Warnings

Excessive dosages of vitamin B$_6$ can lead to significant toxicity. Follow dosage recommendations below unless directed to do otherwise by a physician.

Do not use vitamin B$_6$ with levodopa (Larodopa) unless it is also combined with carbidopa, as in Sinemet.

Possible Side Effects

Vitamin B$_6$ is associated with symptoms of nerve toxicity (tingling sensations in the feet, loss of muscle coordination, and degeneration of nerve tissue) when taken in large doses or in moderate dosages for long periods of time. There are a few rare reports of toxicity occurring at chronic long-term dosages as low as 150 mg a day, but most reports of significant side effects resulted from chronic intake of dosages greater than 500 mg daily. The toxicity is thought to be a result of supplemental pyridoxine overwhelming the liver's ability to add a phosphate group to form the active form of vitamin B$_6$ (pyridoxal-5-phosphate). It is speculated that either pyridoxine is toxic to the nerve cells or it actually acts as an antimetabolite by binding to pyridoxal-5-phosphate receptors, thereby creating a relative deficiency of vitamin B$_6$. Again, it appears to make sense to limit dosages to 50 mg. If more than 50 mg is desired, then the dosages should be spread out throughout the day.

Drug Interactions

The asthma drug theophylline significantly depresses blood levels of active vitamin B$_6$ (pyridoxal-5-phosphate). Vitamin B$_6$ supplementation has been shown to significantly reduce the typical side effects of theophylline (headaches, nausea, irritability, sleep disorders, etc.).

Do not use vitamin B$_6$ with levodopa (Larodopa) unless it is also combined with carbidopa, as in Sinemet.

Vitamin B$_6$ may increase the risk for sun reactions (photosensitivity) in patients taking amiodarone (Cordarone).

Vitamin B$_6$ may lower blood levels of anticonvulsant drugs such as phenytoin (Dilantin) and phenobarbital.

Drugs that antagonize (interfere with) vitamin B$_6$

include isoniazid (Laniazid, Nydrazid), hydralazine (Apresoline), and penicillamine (Cuprimine, Depen). Individuals taking these drugs need to supplement with vitamin B$_6$ at recommended levels.

Food and Nutrient Interactions

Tartrazine (yellow dye #5), alcohol, and excessive protein intake antagonize the effects of vitamin B$_6$. Vitamin B$_6$ interacts significantly with magnesium and zinc; supplementation with B$_6$ may increase the intracellular concentrations of these essential minerals. Riboflavin and magnesium are necessary to convert pyridoxine to pyridoxal-5-phosphate.

Usual Dosage

For general health purposes the recommended dosage is 2.5 to 5 mg daily. For other indications the recommended dosage of vitamin B$_6$ is 25 to 100 mg daily. When using dosages greater than 50 mg, it is important to divide it into 50 mg dosages throughout the day. A single dosage of 100 mg of pyridoxine did not lead to a significant increase in pyridoxal-5-phosphate levels in the blood compared to a 50 mg dosage, indicating that a 50 mg oral dosage of pyridoxine is the maximum amount the body can utilize as a single dosage. The Tolerable Upper Intake Level (UL) for adults is 100 mg per day.

Overdosage

Doses greater than 2,000 mg per day can produce symptoms of nerve toxicity (tingling sensations in the feet, loss of muscle coordination, and degeneration of nerve tissue) in some individuals.

Special Populations

Pregnant/breast-feeding women

Vitamin B_6 supplementation at recommended levels is generally regarded as safe during pregnancy and lactation. The RDA for vitamin B_6 during pregnancy is 1.9 mg, it is 2.2 mg during lactation.

Children

Suitable for children at the level of the Recommended Dietary Allowance (RDA) as a general supplement and at the Tolerable Upper Intake Level (UL) for other applications.

Age	RDA	UL
Infants		
Birth–6 months	0.3 mg	Not determined
6 months–1 year	0.5 mg	Not determined
Children		
1–3 years	0.5 mg	30 mg
4–8 years	0.6 mg	40 mg
9–13 years	1.0 mg	60 mg
14–18 years	1.3 mg	80 mg

Seniors

No special precautions are known.

Vitamin B$_{12}$

Used For

B$_{12}$ deficiency
Effectiveness: A   Safety: A

Depression
Effectiveness: B+   Safety: A

Diabetic neuropathy
Effectiveness: B+   Safety: A

HIV infection and AIDS
Effectiveness: B   Safety: A

Impaired mental function in the elderly
Effectiveness: B+   Safety: A

Low sperm count
Effectiveness: B+   Safety: A

Multiple sclerosis
Effectiveness: B   Safety: A

Tinnitus (ringing in the ears)
Effectiveness: B   Safety: A

General Information

Vitamin B$_{12}$, or cobalamin, was isolated from a liver extract in 1948 and identified as the nutritional factor in the liver that prevented pernicious anemia—a deadly type of anemia characterized by large, immature red blood cells. Vitamin B$_{12}$ works with folic acid in many body processes, including the synthesis of DNA, red blood cells, and the insulation (myelin sheath) that surrounds nerve cells and speeds the conduction of the signals along nerve cells.

Vitamin B$_{12}$ is found in significant quantities only in animal foods. The richest sources are liver and kidney, followed by eggs, fish, cheese, and meat. Therefore, it is very important that vegetarians supplement their diets with vitamin B$_{12}$.

B$_{12}$ deficiency

Unlike other water-soluble nutrients, vitamin B$_{12}$ is stored in the liver, kidney, and other body tissues. As a result, signs and symptoms of vitamin B$_{12}$ deficiency may not show themselves until after five to six years of poor dietary intake or inadequate secretion of intrinsic factor, a substance that binds vitamin B$_{12}$ and facilitates its absorption. The classic symptom of vitamin B$_{12}$ deficiency is pernicious anemia. However, it appears that a deficiency of vitamin B$_{12}$ affects the brain and nervous system as well. Vitamin B$_{12}$ deficiency can produce symptoms such as numbness, a pins-and-needles sensation, or a burning feeling in the feet as well as impaired mental function that in the elderly can mimic Alzheimer's disease. In addition to anemia and nervous system symptoms, a vitamin B$_{12}$ deficiency will also result in a smooth, beefy-looking red tongue. Diarrhea is another symptom; it is due to the fact that rapidly reproducing cells such as those lining the mouth and entire gastrointestinal tract will not be able to replicate without vitamin B$_{12}$ (folic acid supplementation will mask this deficiency symptom).

Although it is popular to inject vitamin B$_{12}$ in the treatment of anemia and B$_{12}$ deficiency, injection is not required, as the oral administration of an appropriate dosage has been shown to produce results as good as those of injectable preparations.

Depression

Vitamin B$_{12}$ deficiency can cause depression, especially in the elderly. Correcting an underlying vitamin B$_{12}$ deficiency usually results in a dramatic improvement in mood.

Diabetic neuropathy

Vitamin B$_{12}$ supplementation has been used with some success in treating diabetic neuropathy. It is not clear if this is because it corrects a deficiency state or because it normalizes the deranged vitamin B$_{12}$ metabolism seen in diabetics. Clinically, diabetic neuropathy is very similar to the neuropathy associated with vitamin B$_{12}$ deficiency.

HIV infection and AIDS

Vitamin B$_{12}$ deficiency is seen in 10 to 35 percent of all patients with human immunodeficiency virus (HIV), presumably as a result of either decreased intake, reduced absorption, or antagonism by the drug azidothymidine (AZT). As blood levels decrease, progression to AIDS increases and neurological symptoms worsen. In addition, vitamin B$_{12}$ (in the forms of cyanocobalamin, methylcobalamin, and adenosylcobalamin) has been shown to inhibit HIV replication in vitro. Given the ability to achieve high blood and tissue levels of vitamin B$_{12}$ without toxicity, vitamin B$_{12}$ therapy for HIV infection holds great promise.

Impaired mental function in the elderly

Supplementation with vitamin B$_{12}$ has shown benefit in reversing impaired mental function in the elderly with low levels of vitamin B$_{12}$. In one large double-blind study, a complete recovery was observed in 61 percent of cases of mental impairment due to low levels of vitamin B$_{12}$. It was thought the remaining 39 percent did not respond due to irreversible damage to the brain as a result of long-term low levels of vitamin B$_{12}$. Several studies have shown the best clinical responders are those who have been showing signs of impaired mental function for less than six months.

Low sperm count

Since vitamin B$_{12}$ is critically involved in cellular replication, a deficiency leads to reduced sperm count and decreased sperm motility. Even in the absence of a vitamin B$_{12}$ deficiency, supplementation appears to be worthwhile in men with a sperm count of less than 20 million per ml or a motility rate of less than 50 percent. In one study, 27 percent of men with a sperm count of less than 20 million given 1,000 mcg per day of vitamin B$_{12}$ were able to achieve a total count in excess of 100 million.

Multiple sclerosis

A vitamin B$_{12}$ deficiency in multiple sclerosis (MS) may aggravate the disease and accelerate the progressive deterioration of the myelin sheath. There is evidence that individuals with MS have a defect in the utilization of vitamin B$_{12}$. In preliminary studies, the oral administration of 60 mg per day of vitamin B$_{12}$ (as methylcobalamin) improved sensory nerve function in MS patients by nearly 30 percent. However, motor (muscular) function did not improve. Methylcobalamin appears to be the superior form of vitamin B$_{12}$ to use in MS, as hydroxocobalamin produces no apparent benefit in MS.

Tinnitus

Individuals with tinnitus (ringing in the ears) are often deficient in vitamin B$_{12}$. Vitamin B$_{12}$ supplementation in these individuals results in some improvement in tinnitus, but it is not likely to produce any significant benefit in people who have tinnitus but do not have vitamin B$_{12}$ deficiency.

Available Forms

The most common forms are cyanocobalamin and hydroxocobalamin; however, vitamin B$_{12}$ is active in only two forms, methylcobalamin and adenosylcobalamin. These last two forms are preferred, as they are active immediately upon absorption, while cyanocobalamin and hydroxocobalamin must be converted to either methylcobalamin or adenosylcobalamin by the body. Methylcobalamin and adenosylcobalamin are supplied in sublingual tablets or as a nasal spray.

Cautions and Warnings

None known.

Possible Side Effects

None known.

Drug Interactions

The following drugs can interfere with the absorption or utilization of vitamin B$_{12}$: antibiotics, methyldopa (Aldomet), clofibrate (Atromid-S), azidothymidine (AZT), sulfasalazine (Azulfidine), birth control pills, cimetidine (Tagamet), metformin (Glucophage), isoniazid (Laniazid, Nydrazid), famotidine (Pepcid), lansoprazole (Prevacid), omeprazole (Prilosec), and rantidine (Zantac).

Food and Nutrient Interactions

Vitamin B$_{12}$ works to reactivate folic acid. Therefore, a high intake of folic acid may mask a vitamin B$_{12}$ deficiency. This situation is potentially quite serious because the folic acid will prevent any deficiency-related changes in red blood cells but will not counteract the deficiency of vitamin B$_{12}$ in the brain.

Usual Dosage

Vitamin B$_{12}$ is necessary in only very small quantities. The RDA is 2 mcg. In the treatment of vitamin B$_{12}$ deficiency with oral preparations, the recommended dosage is 2,000 mcg daily for at least one month followed by a daily intake of 1,000 mcg. This dosage schedule is suitable for other applications of vitamin B$_{12}$ except high-dose therapy for MS. For vegetarians, a dosage of at least 100 mcg per day is recommended to ensure adequate levels are absorbed.

Overdosage

None known.

Special Populations

Pregnant/breast-feeding women
Vitamin B$_{12}$ supplementation is generally regarded as safe during pregnancy and lactation.

Children
Suitable for children even at the adult dosage.

Seniors
No special precautions are known.

Vitamin C

Used For

Antioxidant effects
Effectiveness: A   Safety: A

Asthma and other allergies
Effectiveness: B+   Safety: A

Cancer prevention
Effectiveness: B   Safety: A

Cataracts
Effectiveness: B+   Safety: A

Common cold and other infections
Effectiveness: A   Safety: A

Diabetes
Effectiveness: B+   Safety: A

Gingivitis and periodontal disease
Effectiveness: B   Safety: A

Heart disease (atherosclerosis) prevention
Effectiveness: B   Safety: A

High blood pressure
Effectiveness: B+   Safety: A

Low immunity and immune support
Effectiveness: A   Safety: A

Low sperm count
Effectiveness: B+   Safety: A

Pregnancy complications
Effectiveness: B+   Safety: A

Wound healing
Effectiveness: B   Safety: A

General Information

The primary function of vitamin C is the manufacture of collagen, the main protein substance in the human body. Since collagen is such an important protein for the structures that hold our body together (connective tissue, cartilage, tendons, etc.), vitamin C is vital for wound repair, healthy gums, and the prevention of easy bruising.

In addition to its role in collagen metabolism, vitamin C is also critical to immune function, the manufacture of certain nerve-impulse-transmitting substances and hormones, carnitine synthesis, and the absorption and utilization of other nutritional factors.

Antioxidant effects

Vitamin C is one of the body's most important antioxidants. It works in aqueous (watery) environments in the body, both outside and inside human cells. It is the first line of antioxidant protection in the body. As an antioxidant, vitamin C is showing promise in the prevention of diseases associated with oxidative damage, such as heart disease, cancer, Alzheimer's disease, Parkinson's disease, cataracts, and macular degeneration.

Asthma and other allergies

Low vitamin C levels in the diet and the blood are an independent risk factor for asthma. Since 1973 there have been eleven clinical studies of vitamin C supplementation in asthma. Seven of these studies showed significant improvements in respiratory measures and asthma symptoms as a result of supplementing the diet with 1 to 2 g of vitamin C daily. This dosage recommendation appears extremely wise based on the increasing exposure to inhaled oxidants along with the growing appreciation of the antioxidant function of vitamin C in the respiratory system.

High-dose vitamin C therapy may also help asthma and other allergies by lowering histamine levels. Vitamin C prevents the secretion of histamine by white blood cells and increases the breakdown of histamine.

Cancer prevention

Vitamin C exerts many functions that may offer protection against cancer, including acting as an antioxidant. Vitamin C also helps the body deal with environmental pollution and toxic chemicals, enhances immune function, and inhibits the formation of cancer-causing compounds in the body. The population-based (epidemiological evidence) of a protective effect of vitamin C against cancer is undeniable. A high dietary intake of vitamin C reduces the risk for virtually all forms of cancer, including cancers of the lung, colon, breast, cervix, esophagus, oral cavity, and pancreas. While most of this evidence is based upon a high vitamin C intake from foods also rich in carotenes and other nutrients protective against cancer, a few of the studies looked at supplementation as well.

Cataracts

Individuals with higher dietary intakes of vitamin C have a much lower risk for developing cataracts and macular degeneration. In addition to offering protective effects, several clinical studies have demonstrated that vitamin C supplementation can halt cataract progression and, in some cases, significantly improve vision.

Common cold

Many claims have been made about the role of vitamin C (ascorbic acid) in regard to the prevention and treatment of the common cold. Since 1970, there have been over twenty double-blind studies designed to assess what role vitamin C can play in the common cold. In the majority of the studies vitamin C supplementation produced a decrease in either duration or symptom severity. Analysis of all studies indicates that vitamin C at a dosage of 1–6 g daily decreased the duration of the cold episodes by 0.93 days, or roughly 21 percent.

Diabetes

Since the transport of vitamin C into cells is facilitated by insulin, most diabetics suffer from a deficiency of intracellular vitamin C. A relative vitamin C deficiency exists in many diabetics despite an adequate dietary intake of the vitamin, as the diabetic simply needs more vitamin C. Failure to correct a chronic, latent intracellular vitamin C deficiency will lead to a number of problems for the diabetic, including increased capillary permeability, poor wound healing, elevation in cholesterol levels, and a depressed immune system.

Gingivitis and periodontal disease

Vitamin C plays a major role in preventing gingivitis and periodontal disease. Vitamin C helps maintain the integrity and immune function of the gums. Deficiency of vitamin C is associated with inflamed and bleeding gums.

Heart disease (atherosclerosis) prevention

A high dietary intake of vitamin C has been shown to significantly reduce the risk of death from heart attacks and strokes. There is some evidence that higher intakes of vitamin C are associated with decreased LDL cholesterol and higher levels of the protective HDL cholesterol. However, results from double-blind studies examining the benefit of high dosage vitamin C supplementation (usually 1,000 mg) on lowering total cholesterol while raising HDL cholesterol levels have been inconsistent. More recent studies have determined that only in subjects with low or marginal vitamin C status does high-dosage supplementation produce an effect.

High blood pressure

Population studies have shown that the higher the dietary intake of vitamin C, the lower the blood pressure. Several preliminary studies have shown a modest blood-pressure-lowering effect (e.g., a drop of 5 mm Hg systolic and diastolic) of vitamin C supplementation in people with mild elevations of blood pressure.

Low immunity and immune support

Vitamin C has been shown to enhance many different immune functions, including improving white blood cell function and activity and increasing interferon levels, antibody responses, antibody levels, secretion of thymic hormones, and integrity of collagen structures that serve as barriers to infection. Vitamin C also possesses many biochemical effects very similar to those of interferon, the body's natural antiviral and anticancer compound. During times of infection and stress, vitamin C requirements increase. Double-blind studies have shown vitamin C to improve many aspects of immune function and reduce the duration of infections, particularly in patients in hospitals.

Low sperm count

Vitamin C appears to play an important role in normal sperm formation. There is much more vitamin C in seminal fluid compared to other body fluids, including the blood. When dietary vitamin C was reduced from 250 mg to 5 mg per day in healthy human subjects, the number of sperm that had damage to their genetic material (DNA) increased by 91 percent. Several double-blind studies have shown that vitamin C supplementation can increase sperm count. In one study, thirty infertile but otherwise healthy men received either 200 mg or 1,000 mg vitamin C or placebo daily. After one week the 1,000 mg group demonstrated a 140 percent increase in sperm count, the 200 mg group had a 112 percent increase, and the placebo group saw no change.

Pregnancy complications

Vitamin C supplementation appears indicated to prevent at least two complications of pregnancy: preeclampsia and premature rupture of the fetal membranes. Preeclampsia is a serious condition of pregnancy associated with elevations in blood pressure, fluid retention, and loss of protein in the urine. Free-radical damage to the lining of blood vessels (vascular endothelium) is known to play a key role in the development of preeclampsia. Antioxidants are critically involved in the protection of the vascular endothelium. Low antioxidant levels, including vitamin C, have been shown to be a predisposing factor in preeclampsia.

Premature rupture of the fetal membranes (PROM) is one of the major contributors of infant

morbidity and mortality. The cause of PROM is un-
clear but may in some cases be due to low levels of
vitamin C. In one study, PROM subjects had significantly lower levels of vitamin C in the amniotic fluid.

Wound healing

Vitamin C is critical to proper wound healing and
may be helpful in preventing and treating pressure
sores (bedsores) in the elderly. Up to 60 percent of
all elderly hospital patients suffer from pressure
sores. Analysis of vitamin C levels in patients admit-
ted to a hospital for hip fracture indicated that patients who developed bedsores had vitamin C levels
that were 50 percent lower than the patients who did
not develop bedsores.

Available Forms

Vitamin C is available in a number of different
forms—crystals, powders, capsules, tablets, timed-
release tablets, and others. It is also available combined with other nutrients, such as in the brand
name product E-mergen-C. The actual type of vitamin C in these different forms can also vary. Ascorbic
acid is the most widely used (and least expensive)
form. Buffered vitamin C, such as Ester-C, is sodium
ascorbate, magnesium ascorbate, calcium ascorbate, or potassium ascorbate. Buffered vitamin C is
popular because the acid content of nonbuffered
ascorbic acid may bother some people's stomachs.
However, absorption studies have not shown any
type of buffered vitamin C to be better absorbed than
ascorbic acid. Taking vitamin C with bioflavonoids
may offer benefits in absorption, but only if the product contains bioflavonoids in amounts equal to or
greater than the amount of vitamin C.

Cautions and Warnings

Vitamin C supplementation at daily dosages greater than 500 mg is not advised for people on hemodialysis or those who suffer from recurrent kidney stones, severe kidney disease, or gout, as higher dosages may possibly increase kidney stone formation in these patients.

Possible Side Effects

Vitamin C is extremely safe in most people. Diarrhea and intestinal distension or gas are the most common complaints at higher dosage levels.

Drug Interactions

Vitamin C may increase the absorption of aluminum from aluminum-containing antacids such as Alterna-Gel, Amphojel, Basaljel, Nephrox, Maalox, and Mylanta. Take vitamin C at least two hours before or after taking one of these products.

Food and Nutrient Interactions

Vitamin C increases the absorption of iron and copper. It may also interfere with the blood test for vitamin B_{12}. Vitamin C is intricately involved with other nutritional antioxidants, especially vitamin E, selenium, and beta-carotene.

Usual Dosage

In healthy individuals, a daily dosage of 100 to 500 mg is believed to be sufficient. However, higher dosages may be necessary in certain health conditions such as asthma, diabetes, and cataracts, and in infectious conditions including the common cold. In these health conditions the dosage range is typically 500 to 2,000 mg daily. The Tolerable Upper Level Intake (UL) has been set at 2 g daily for men and women over nineteen years of age.

Overdosage

Vitamin C has no acute toxicity. High dosages may produce excessive flatulence and/or diarrhea.

Special Populations

Pregnant/breast-feeding women
The dosage range during pregnancy and lactation is 100 to 500 mg daily.

Children
Suitable for children at one-half the adult dosage.

Seniors
No special precautions are known.

Vitamin D

Used For

Osteoporosis
Effectiveness: B+   Safety: A

Prevention of vitamin D deficiency
Effectiveness: A   Safety: A

General Information

It is well known that vitamin D stimulates the absorption of calcium. Since vitamin D can be produced in our bodies by the action of sunlight on the skin, many experts consider it more of a hormone than a vitamin. The sunlight changes a compound (7-dehydrocholesterol) in the skin into vitamin D_3 (cholecalciferol), which is then converted to more active forms by the liver and kidneys. Disorders of the liver or kidneys result in impaired conversion of cholecalciferol to these more potent vitamin D compounds.

Prevention of vitamin D deficiency

Vitamin D deficiency results in rickets in children and osteomalacia in adults. Rickets is characterized by an inability to calcify the bone matrix; this results in softening of the skull bones, bowing of the legs, spinal curvature, and increased joint size. Once common, these diseases are now extremely rare.

Vitamin D deficiency is now most often seen in elderly people who do not get any sunlight, particularly those in nursing homes. The consequences are joint pain and lack of bone strength and density.

Osteoporosis

Vitamin D supplementation alone and in combination with calcium has been shown to reduce osteoporosis and hip fractures. In one study using vitamin D_3 alone it was shown that supplementation with 700 IU daily reduced the annual rate of hip fracture from 1.3 percent to 0.5 percent—nearly a 60 percent reduction. In another study, 400 IU of vitamin D_3 increased bone density by 1.9 percent in the left hip and 2.6 percent in the right hip. In comparison, the placebo group demonstrated decreases of 0.3 percent in the left hip and 1.4 percent in the right hip. Studies that combined vitamin D with calcium produced slightly better results in increasing bone density and reducing hip fractures. The studies imply that vitamin D is most helpful in elderly people living in nursing homes, people living farther away from the equator, and those who do not regularly get outside in the sunlight.

Available Forms

There are two major dietary forms of vitamin D, vitamin D_2 (ergocalciferol) and vitamin D_3 (cholecalciferol). Vitamin D_2 is the form most often added to milk and other foods as well as the form most often used in nutritional supplements. Vitamin D_3 in nutritional supplements is most often derived from fish liver oil or sheep's wool.

Cautions and Warnings

If you are taking digoxin (Lanoxin) or a thiazide diuretic, consult a physician before using vitamin D. These drugs decrease calcium loss in the urine, possibly leading to elevated blood and tissue calcium levels.

Possible Side Effects

Vitamin D is generally well tolerated with no side effects at the recommended dosages.

Drug Interactions

The drugs cholestyramine (Questran), colestipol (Colestid), phenytoin (Dilantin), phenobarbital, and orlistat (Xenical), as well as mineral oil, all interfere with the absorption and/or metabolism of vitamin D. Corticosteroids such as prednisone increase the need for vitamin D. Vitamin D supplementation must be used with caution when using digoxin (Lanoxin) and thiazide diuretics. Consult a physician before using vitamin D if you are taking any of these drugs.

Food and Nutrient Interactions

Vitamin D is intricately involved in calcium metabolism. Olestra (a fat substitute) as well as sources of dietary fiber (psyllium, pectin, guar gum, etc.) may decrease the absorption of vitamin D.

Usual Dosage

The RDA for vitamin D is 200 to 400 IU daily. For elderly people who are not exposed to sunlight or who live in the northern latitudes, a daily intake of 400 to 800 IU is recommended. Supplementation greater than 400 IU per day in most adults, young children, and adolescents appears to be unwarranted.

Overdosage

Vitamin D has the potential to cause toxicity. Dosages greater than 1,000 IU per day are certainly not recommended. Toxicity is characterized by increased blood concentration of calcium (a potentially serious situation), deposition of calcium into internal organs, and kidney stones.

Special Populations

Pregnant/breast-feeding women
As vitamin D is a fat-soluble vitamin, it should not be taken during pregnancy and lactation at greater than recommended levels.

Children
The recommended dosage for infants less than 6 months of age is 300 IU daily. For children over the age of one year the dosage recommendation is 400 IU—the same as adults.

Seniors
No special precautions are known.

Vitamin E

Used For

Alzheimer's disease prevention
Effectiveness: B   Safety: A

Cancer prevention
Effectiveness: B+   Safety: A

Diabetes
Effectiveness: B+   Safety: A

Fibrocystic breast disease
Effectiveness: B   Safety: A

Heart disease and stroke prevention
Effectiveness: B+   Safety: A

Intermittent claudication
Effectiveness: B+   Safety: A

Low immunity and immune support
Effectiveness: B+   Safety: A

Tardive dyskinesia
Effectiveness: B+   Safety: A

General Information

Vitamin E functions primarily as an antioxidant, protecting against damage to the cell membranes. Without vitamin E, the cells of the body would be quite susceptible to damage. Severe vitamin E deficiency is quite rare, but there are four major groups among whom low levels of vitamin E are common: (1) people with a fat malabsorption syndrome, such as celiac disease, cystic fibrosis, and postgastrectomy syndrome; (2) premature infants; (3) people with hereditary disorders of red blood cells such as sickle cell disease and thalassemia; and (4) hemodialysis patients.

Symptoms of vitamin E deficiency in adults include nerve damage, muscle weakness, poor coordination, involuntary movement of the eyes, and breaking of red blood cells leading to anemia (hemolytic anemia). In premature infants, vitamin E deficiency is characterized by hemolytic anemia and a severe eye disorder known as retrolental fibroplasia.

Alzheimer's disease prevention

There is considerable evidence that oxidative damage plays a major role in the development and progression of Alzheimer's disease. A two-year double blind study of 341 individuals with Alzheimer's disease of moderate severity found that 2,000 IU per day of vitamin E extended the time patients were able to care for themselves (such as bathing, dressing, and carrying out other necessary daily functions) compared with patients taking a placebo.

Cancer prevention

As with other antioxidants, population studies have shown that a high vitamin E intake appears to offer significant protection against cancer. Over a dozen population-based studies have shown that low vitamin E levels (especially if combined with low selenium levels) increases the risk of certain types of cancer, particularly cancers of the gastrointestinal tract, breast, prostate, and lung. Whether vitamin E supplementation reduces the risk of cancer, however, has not been sufficiently studied. Studies evaluating vitamin E's ability to prevent lung cancer in smokers failed to show a significant protective effect.

Diabetes

Diabetics appear to have an increased requirement for vitamin E for a number of reasons, but primarily because oxidative stress is a major factor in diabetes. Vitamin E also improves insulin action, and it exerts a number of beneficial effects that may aid in preventing the long-term complications of diabetes especially cardiovascular disease. Several double-blind studies have shown vitamin E supplementation is not only helpful in improving glucose metabolism and insulin action, but also that it improves diabetic neuropathy (nerve disease).

Fibrocystic breast disease

Fibrocystic breast disease (FBD) is a mildly uncomfortable to severely painful benign cystic swelling of the breasts. Several double-blind clinical studies have shown vitamin E to relieve the symptoms of fibrocystic breast disease.

Heart disease and stroke prevention

A substantial body of scientific documentation indicates that vitamin E supplementation may be helpful in protecting against heart disease and strokes. The primary protective effect is an ability to reduce oxidative damage to LDL cholesterol. When LDL cholesterol becomes damaged, it in turn damages the lining of an artery, thereby initiating the process of atherosclerosis. Several large populations have demonstrated that vitamin E levels may be more predictive of developing a heart attack or stroke than total cholesterol levels. Of all the antioxidants, vitamin E appears to produce the greatest protection against the oxidation of LDL cholesterol because of its ability to be easily incorporated into the LDL molecule.

A couple of large-scale studies with relatively low dosages of vitamin E supplements have shown a significant reduction in the risk of dying of a heart attack or a stroke. One study that looked at 87,245 nurses concluded that those who took 100 IU of vitamin E daily for more than two years had a 41 percent lower risk of heart disease compared to nonusers of vitamin E supplements. Another study involved 39,910 male health care professionals. The results were similar: A 37 percent lower risk of heart disease was associated with the intake of more than 30 IU of supplemental vitamin E daily. In patients with existing heart disease, one study found that vitamin E supplementation at a dosage of either 400 or 800 IU daily produced a more than 70 percent reduction in the number of heart attacks compared to a placebo group. However, another study using a dosage of only 400 IU found no protective effect.

Intermittent claudication

Intermittent claudication is a vascular disease characterized by pain in the calf while walking.

Vitamin E supplementation has been shown in double-blind studies to help increase blood flow through the arteries of the lower legs. However, it appears that a minimum of four to six months of vitamin E supplementation is necessary before significant improvement can be seen.

Low immunity and immune support

A vitamin E deficiency results in significant impairment of immune function. Even without signs of vitamin E deficiency, supplementation with vitamin E has been shown to exert a number of positive effects on immune function in double-blind studies. The benefits of vitamin E are especially helpful in enhancing immune function in the elderly.

Tardive dyskinesia

Several double-blind studies have shown vitamin E (800 to 1,600 IU daily) to be effective in improving tardive dyskinesia, a syndrome that is characterized by involuntary movements of the face and mouth and is most often caused by a reaction to drugs used in the treatment of schizophrenia, such as haloperidol (Haldol). Vitamin E is most effective when administered to patients who have taken the antipsychotic drugs for less than five years. When the drugs have been used for more than five years the level of improvement is about half that observed in patients who have been taking the drugs for less than five years.

Available Forms

Vitamin E is available in many different forms in tablets and capsules. Natural forms of vitamin E are designated *d-,* as in d-alpha-tocopherol, while synthetic forms are designated *dl-,* as in dl-alpha-tocopherol. The letters *d* and *l* represent mirror images of the vitamin E molecule. In the human body, only the *d* form can be utilized. Although the *l* form has antioxidant activity, it may actually inhibit the *d* form from entering cell membranes.

Cautions and Warnings

Vitamin E may increase bleeding tendencies. Do not use for at least one week prior to any elective surgery.

Vitamin E may potentiate the effects of the blood-thinning drug warfarin (Coumadin) as well as enhance the antiplatelet effects of drugs such as aspirin and ticlopidine (Ticlid).

Possible Side Effects

Vitamin E is not associated with any significant side effects. Although vitamin E is a fat-soluble vitamin, it has an excellent safety record. Doses as high as 3,200 IU daily for periods of up to two years have not shown any unfavorable side effects. Detailed safety assessments have also shown that vitamin E supplementation is extremely safe.

Drug Interactions

Vitamin E may potentiate the effects of the blood-thinning drug warfarin (Coumadin) as well as enhance the antiplatelet effects of drugs such as aspirin and ticlopidine (Ticlid).

The drugs cholestyramine (Questran), colestipol (Colestid), phenytoin (Dilantin), phenobarbital, and orlistat (Xenical), as well as mineral oil, all interfere with the absorption and/or metabolism of vitamin E.

Food and Nutrient Interactions

Vitamin E interacts extensively with other antioxidant nutrients, especially vitamin C and selenium. Vitamin E also improves the use of vitamin A, may be necessary in the conversion of vitamin B_{12} to its most active form, and protects essential fatty acids from becoming damaged. Olestra (a fat substitute) as well as sources of dietary fiber (psyllium, pectin, guar gum, etc.) may decrease the absorption of vitamin E.

Usual Dosage

The typical dosage for vitamin E for general and therapeutic purposes is 100–800 IU per day.

Overdosage

None known.

Special Populations

Pregnant/breast-feeding women

Vitamin E supplementation is generally regarded as safe during pregnancy and lactation.

Children

Infants less than six months can safely take 5 to 30 IU daily. Children between the ages of one and three years can take 30 to 200 IU; children four to eight years, 30 to 300 IU; and children nine to thirteen years, 30 to 600 IU.

Seniors

No special precautions are known.

Vitamin K

Hemorrhagic disease of the newborn
Effectiveness: A   Safety: A

Osteoporosis
Effectiveness: B   Safety: A

General Information

Vitamin K is an often neglected vitamin because deficiency is quite rare—there are good dietary sources, and gut bacteria can produce a form of vitamin K. Rich sources of vitamin K are dark green leafy vegetables, broccoli, lettuce, cabbage, spinach, and green tea. Good sources are asparagus, oats, whole wheat, and fresh green peas.

Vitamin K's most famous role is in the manufacture of clotting factors. However, recent studies have shown that vitamin K is also necessary for building healthy bones and may play a role in treating and preventing osteoporosis.

Hemorrhagic disease of the newborn
Since 1961 vitamin K_1 injections have been given to all newborn babies to prevent hemorrhagic disease of the newborn. This condition occurs because of a lack of vitamin K. When a baby is born the intestinal tract is sterile. Since a major source of vitamin K (in the form of K_2) is synthesized from gut bacteria and most women do not have high concentrations of vitamin K_1 in their breast milk, the baby

must rely on the amount of vitamin K delivered through the placenta before birth until the gut microflora get established.

Osteoporosis

Vitamin K_1 plays an important role in bone health, as it is responsible for converting the inactive form of the bone protein osteocalcin to its active form. Osteocalcin is the major noncollagen protein found in our bones that anchors calcium into place within the bone. Low intake of vitamin K_1 is linked to osteoporosis and hip fractures. Since vitamin K_1 is found in green leafy vegetables, it may be one of the reasons a vegetarian diet seems to be protective against osteoporosis.

Available Forms

There are three major forms of vitamin K. Natural vitamin K from plants is termed vitamin K_1, or phylloquinone. Vitamin K_2, or menaquinone, is derived from bacteria in the gut, and vitamin K_3, or menadione, is a synthetic derivative. Vitamin K is available in capsules and tablets.

Cautions and Warnings

If you are taking anticoagulant drugs such as warfarin (Coumadin), consult your physician before taking any supplement with vitamin K.

Possible Side Effects

There are no known side effects or toxicity with the administration of vitamin K_1.

Drug Interactions

Vitamin K administration may counteract the anticoagulant actions of drugs such as warfarin (Coumadin) that work to prevent clot formation by blocking vitamin K's activation of clotting factor. Aspirin, certain antibiotics, and the antiseizure drug phenytoin (Dilantin) also antagonize vitamin K action.

Food and Nutrient Interactions

High dosages of vitamin E (e.g., greater than 600 IU) may antagonize vitamin K's action on blood clotting.

Usual Dosage

Generally vitamin K is recommended at a dosage of 150 to 500 mcg in supplement form.

Overdosage

None known.

Special Populations

Pregnant/breast-feeding women
Considered safe during pregnancy and lactation.

Children
Suitable for children at one-half the adult dosage.

Seniors
No special precautions are known.

PART II
Minerals

The human body utilizes minerals for the proper composition of bone and blood, and for maintenance of normal cell function. Together with vitamins, they are essential components in enzymes and coenzymes. If an enzyme is lacking an essential mineral, it cannot function properly no matter how much of the vitamin is available. For example, zinc is necessary for the enzyme that activates vitamin A in the visual process. Without zinc in the enzyme, vitamin A cannot be converted to its active form. This deficiency can result in what is known as night blindness. By supplying the enzyme with both zinc and vitamin A, the enzyme is able to perform its vital function.

The minerals that play a role in human nutrition are classified into two categories: major and minor. The categories refer to the *amount* of a mineral required, not to its importance to good health. A mineral required at a level greater than 100 mg per day is classified as major.

Major minerals
Calcium
Chloride
Magnesium
Phosphorus
Potassium
Sodium
Sulfur

Minor (trace) minerals
Boron
Chromium
Copper
Iodine
Iron
Manganese
Molybdenum
Selenium
Silicon
Vanadium
Zinc

Nonessential minerals

Minerals not listed above have *not* been shown to be important in human nutrition. In fact, many of them are considered toxic. However, some manufacturers of trace mineral products (particularly those in "colloidal" liquid form) feature nonessential minerals such as silver, gold, tin, and nickel as a key benefit. In reality, products containing these and other nonessential minerals are best avoided.

Keep in mind that the ratings on effectiveness and safety refer to the following:

Effectiveness
A = Excellent results in multiple double-blind studies

B+ = Very good results in a small number of double-blind studies

B = Some clinical evidence of effectiveness

B– = Some clinical evidence of effectiveness but also some studies showing no effect

C = Strong historical use or scientific rationale but no clinical trials to show effectiveness in humans

D = No significant documentation of historical use or scientific rationale, or majority of clinical studies show no effect

F = Documentation that it is *not* effective

Safety

A = Excellent safety profile

B = Good safety profile

C = Generally regarded as safe at recommended levels

D = Generally regarded as safe at recommended levels but must be used with caution

F = Potentially dangerous, should not be used

Boron

Used For

Arthritis
Effectiveness: B+   Safety: B

Osteoporosis prevention and treatment
Effectiveness: B+   Safety: B

General Information

Boron is a trace mineral. Although not officially listed as an essential nutrient, recent studies indicate that boron may be essential in maintaining healthy bone and joint function.

Fruits and vegetables are the main dietary sources of boron. However, the level of boron in these foods is dependent upon adequate levels of boron in the soil. It is estimated that the average boron intake of Americans is somewhere between 1.7 and 7 mg per day. As the minimum amount required by humans to maintain health has not been determined, it is not known whether these amounts are optimal. Research suggests that they are not.

Boron deficiency may be associated with an increased risk for postmenopausal bone loss. Boron appears to be necessary for the action of vitamin D, the vitamin that stimulates the absorption and utilization of calcium. Supplementing the diet of postmenopausal women with 3 mg of boron per day reduced urinary calcium excretion by 44 percent. However, in a study in younger women, boron had no effect on calcium absorption.

Boron may also play a role in joint health. Preliminary studies have shown that patients with osteoarthritis, juvenile arthritis, and rheumatoid arthritis may see some improvement by taking 6–9 mg of boron (as sodium tetraborate decahydrate) daily.

Available Forms

There are several different forms of boron on the marketplace in capsules and tablets. For general health and osteoporosis, sodium borate or boron chelates are suitable. For the treatment of arthritis, sodium tetraborate decahydrate may be the best form.

Cautions and Warnings

Do not take more than 9 mg of boron daily, as no long-term safety studies have been performed.

Possible Side Effects

Orally administered boron is extremely safe when it is taken at recommended levels (3 to 9 mg/day). Problems, such as nausea, vomiting, and diarrhea, occur only at extremely high doses (greater than 500 mg/day).

Drug Interactions

Boron supplementation may increase the level of active estrogen in women taking Premarin or other forms of estrogen after menopause, but it did not raise estrogen levels in postmenopausal women not taking estrogen or in men and younger women. The significance of this effect has not been determined, but results imply that women taking estrogens may

need a lower dosage of estrogens if they are also
taking boron.

Food and Nutrient Interactions

There are no known interactions between boron and
any food. Boron appears to work with vitamin D in
calcium metabolism.

Usual Dosage

Typical dosage is 3 to 9 mg.

Overdosage

Problems such as nausea, vomiting, and diarrhea
occur only at extremely high doses (greater than 500
mg/day).

Special Populations

Pregnant/breast-feeding women
Considered safe during pregnancy and lactation.

Children
Suitable for children at one-half the adult dosage.

Seniors
No special precautions are known.

Calcium

Used For

Colon cancer prevention
Effectiveness: B   Safety: A

High blood pressure
Effectiveness: B+   Safety: A

Osteoporosis treatment and prevention
Effectiveness: A   Safety: A

Premenstrual syndrome
Effectiveness: B+   Safety: A

General Information

Calcium is the most abundant mineral in the body. It constitutes 1.5 to 2 percent of the total body weight, with more than 99 percent of the calcium being present in the bones. In addition to its major function in building and maintaining bones and teeth, calcium is also important in the activity of many enzymes in the body. The contraction of muscles, release of neurotransmitters, regulation of heartbeat, and clotting of blood are all dependent on calcium.

Colon cancer prevention

Calcium supplementation has been shown to reduce the risk of colon cancer as well as to reduce the formation of polyps (precancerous lesions). It is thought that calcium binds to bile acids in the gut and neutralizes their cancer-causing effects.

High blood pressure (hypertension)

Population studies have suggested a link between high blood pressure and a low dietary intake of calcium. Several clinical studies have demonstrated that calcium supplementation can lower blood pressure in hypertension, but the results have been inconsistent. It appears that calcium supplementation (1–1.5 g per day) is most likely to produce effective reductions in blood pressure in blacks, people who are salt sensitive, and elderly patients. Typical reductions in blood pressure reported in these groups with calcium supplementation are around 10 mm Hg and 5 mg Hg for the systolic and diastolic readings respectively.

Another condition associated with high blood pressure that may respond to or be prevented by calcium supplementation is preeclampsia (a serious condition of pregnancy associated with elevations in blood pressure, fluid retention, and loss of protein in the urine). Early studies in pregnant women suggested that low calcium intake was a major risk factor for hypertension and preeclampsia during pregnancy. The results from clinical studies have now demonstrated that pregnant women who receive calcium supplementation during pregnancy have a reduced risk of hypertension and preeclampsia.

Osteoporosis treatment and prevention

The body works very hard at maintaining blood levels of calcium. Even though the calcium in the blood represents only a small percentage of the total calcium in the body, it is critical to life that blood levels be maintained within a very narrow normal range. In addition to their structural role, the bones serve as a calcium reserve. Bone is constantly remodeling (breaking down and rebuilding) in order to maintain blood levels of calcium within the normal range. If a person does not get enough calcium from the diet or through supplementation, the body automatically takes calcium from the bones. If the body continues to tear down more bone than it replaces over a period of years in order to maintain blood calcium levels, it can lead to the crippling bone disease called osteoporosis. Approximately twenty-five million American women have some degree of osteoporosis; the disease will affect one-third to one-half of postmenopausal women. About five million American men suffer from osteoporosis as well.

Supplementation of calcium has been shown to be effective in both preventing and treating osteoporosis. Building bone density through calcium supplementation before menopause can help delay osteoporosis later in life, as there is a strong correlation between premenopausal bone density and the risk of osteoporosis. That being the case, building strong bones should be a lifelong goal beginning in childhood. However, most women probably are not concerned about osteoporosis until a few years before menopause. Fortunately, calcium supplementation does improve bone density in the time just before menopause (the perimenopause). In a two-year study, 214 perimenopausal women received either 1,000 or 2,000 mg of calcium. While the control group actually lost 3.2 percent of their spinal bone density, the calcium-treated groups increased their density by 1.6 percent (there was no difference between the two calcium groups). These results highlight the importance of calcium supplementation prior to menopause in the battle against osteoporosis. In postmenopausal women, although calcium supplementation by itself does not completely halt calcium loss, long-term studies have demonstrated that calcium supplementation does slow the rate

down by at least 30 to 50 percent and offers significant protection against hip fractures.

Premenstrual syndrome

Numerous early studies suggested that disturbances in calcium regulation may underlie the hormonal disturbances characteristic of premenstrual
syndrome and that calcium supplementation may
be an effective therapeutic approach. Recently a
well-designed double-blind, placebo-controlled
study in nearly five hundred women with PMS
demonstrated that supplementation with 1,200 mg
of calcium (as calcium carbonate) over a three-
month period was very effective in reducing seventeen core symptoms and four symptom factors
(negative affect, water retention, food cravings, and
pain). By the third month of use calcium effectively
resulted in an overall 48 percent reduction in total
symptoms compared with a 30 percent reduction
achieved by placebo.

Available Forms

Calcium supplements are available in capsules,
tablets, chewable wafers, and liquids. The most
widely used form is calcium carbonate. This form of
calcium appears suitable for most people, with the
possible exception of those who do not produce
enough stomach acid. But even in these people it
appears that taking the calcium carbonate with food
overcomes the problem.

Calcium bound to citrate and other Krebs cycle intermediates such as fumarate, malate, succinate,
and aspartate as well as lactate are probably the
overall best forms of calcium. These substances
have advantages over other forms of calcium in that
they are (1) easily ionized, (2) almost completely

roken down and utilized by the body, (3) virtually
nontoxic, and (4) able to increase the absorption of
not only calcium but other minerals as well. The
problem with calcium supplements bound to these
compounds is their bulk—it basically requires three
to four times as many capsules or tablets to provide
the same level of calcium compared to calcium carbonate sources.

Brand names available include Caltrate, Citracal,
OsCal, and Tums.

Advantages and Disadvantages of the Various Forms of Calcium

Form	Disadvantages	Advantages
Calcium carbonate	May not be adequately absorbed in people with insufficient output of stomach acid. Should be taken with foods for maximal absorption.	Inexpensive. Easier to take because it is not as bulky as other forms.
Calcium citrate, calcium fumarate, calcium malate, calcium succinate, calcium aspartate, calcium gluconate, calcium lactate	Molecules are larger than calcium carbonate, thus requiring more tablets/capsules to achieve the same dosage.	Easily aborbed regardless of the output of stomach acid.

Calcium phosphate	Poorly absorbed compared to other forms. Has a greater effect in blocking the absorption of iron and other minerals.	Least likely to cause constipation.
Oyster shell calcium, dolomite, bone meal	May contain high levels of lead and other impurities.	None.
Micro-crystalline calcium hydroxyap-atite	Poorly absorbed compared to other forms. More expensive.	May exert additional benefits in bone health due to other components.

Cautions and Warnings

Patients with hyperparathyroidism and cancer should not take calcium unless under the direct supervision of a physician.

Possible Side Effects

Calcium supplements are generally well tolerated at dosages less than 2,000 mg. Higher dosages may increase the risk for kidney stones and soft-tissue calcification; however, neither of these two conditions has been conclusively linked to calcium supplementation.

Drug Interactions

Aluminum-containing antacids are known to ultimately lead to an increase in bone breakdown and
calcium excretion. Antiulcer drugs such as cimetidine (Tagamet), ranitidine (Zantac), famotidine
(Pepcid), omeprazole (Prilosec), and others can decrease calcium absorption because they block the
output of hydrochloric acid.

The bone-building drugs alendronate (Fosamax),
etidronate (Didronel), and risedronate (Actonel) as
well as tetracycline antibiotics and thyroid hormones (e.g., levothyroxine, [Levoxyl, Synthroid])
should not be taken within two hours of calcium
supplements, as the calcium may decrease their absorption and effectiveness. Calcium supplementation may also reduce the effectiveness of gallium
nitrate (Ganite) and phenytoin (Dilantin). If you are
taking one of these drugs, please consult your
physician before taking a calcium supplement.

Food and Nutrient Interactions

Absorption of calcium carbonate is enhanced when
taken with food. Calcium interacts with many nutrients, especially vitamin D, vitamin K, and magnesium. Calcium absorption is negatively affected by
high dosages of magnesium, zinc, fiber, and oxalates. Calcium excretion is increased by caffeine, alcohol, phosphates, protein, sodium, and sugar.

Usual Dosage

The dosage range used for supplementation generally reflects the recommended dietary allowance
(RDA) for calcium. In the treatment of osteoporosis,

the effectiveness of calcium supplementation at a
particular dosage is ultimately dependent upon diet
and lifestyle. Bone health and osteoporosis treat-
ment/prevention involve much more than calcium.
That being said, an effective dosage for supplemental calcium is 600 to 1,200 mg per day for most
women. If there is significant bone loss, the dosage
may need to be in the range of 1,000 to 1,500 mg per
day. For other applications such as colon cancer prevention and high blood pressure, a dosage of 1,000
to 1,500 mg per day is usual.

Recommended Dietary Allowance for Calcium

Infants	
Birth–6 months	**400 mg**
6 months–1 year	**600 mg**
Children	
1–3 years	**800 mg**
4–6 years	**800 mg**
7–10 years	**800 mg**
Young Adults and Adults	
Males 11–24 years	**1,200 mg**
Males 25+ years	**800 mg**
Females 11–24 years	**1,200 mg**
Females 25+ years	**800 mg**
Pregnant women	**1,200 mg**
Lactating women	**1,200 mg**

Overdosage

Acute overdosage is rare. Excessive intake over several days or weeks may produce signs and symptoms related to overdosage. Early signs of an overdose are constipation (severe), dryness of mouth, headache (continuing), increased thirst, irritability, loss of appetite, mental depression, metallic taste, and unusual tiredness or weakness. Later signs of an overdose can include confusion, drowsiness (severe), high blood pressure, increased sensitivity of eyes or skin to light, unusually large amount of urine or increased frequency of urination, and irregular, fast, or slow heartbeat.

Special Populations

Pregnant/breast-feeding women

It is especially important that pregnant and lactating women receive enough calcium. Calcium supplementation is considered safe during pregnancy and lactation at dosages up to the RDA.

Children

Proper calcium intake is very important during childhood. Calcium supplements are suitable for children at dosages up to the RDA.

Seniors

No special precautions are known.

Chromium

Used For

Diabetes
Effectiveness: B   Safety: B

Elevated blood cholesterol and triglyceride levels
Effectiveness: B–   Safety: B

Hypoglycemia
Effectiveness: B   Safety: B

Weight loss
Effectiveness: B–   Safety: B

General Information

Chromium functions in the body as a key constituent of the glucose tolerance factor. Chromium works closely with insulin in facilitating the uptake of glucose into cells. Without chromium, insulin's action is blocked and blood sugar levels are elevated. Chromium's key beneficial effect is to help insulin work properly.

Diabetes

Nearly twenty controlled studies have demonstrated a positive effect for chromium in the treatment of diabetes. Most of the studies were performed in patients with type 2, or non-insulin-dependent, diabetes mellitus (NIDDM), a condition characterized by elevated insulin levels due to a loss of sensitivity to insulin by the cells of the body, otherwise known as insulin resistance. In clinical studies in NIDDM patients, supplementing the diet with chromium has been shown to decrease fasting glu-cose levels, improve glucose tolerance, lower in-sulin levels, and decrease total cholesterol and triglyceride levels while increasing HDL cholesterol levels.

Elevated blood cholesterol and triglyceride levels

Although there are studies showing that chromium supplementation can reduce elevated blood cholesterol and triglyceride levels, it appears that unless initial body chromium levels are very low, the degree of change produced by chromium supplementation will not be that meaningful. In pa-tients who do respond to chromium supplementa-tion, the changes can be significant (e.g., 10 percent reduction in total cholesterol and triglycerides and a 12 percent increase in HDL).

Hypoglycemia

Hypoglycemia is low blood sugar. Normally the body maintains blood sugar levels within a narrow range through the coordinated effort of several glands and their hormones. If these control mecha-nisms are disrupted, hypoglycemia (low blood sugar) or diabetes (high blood sugar) may result. There is some evidence that correcting a chromium deficiency through chromium supplementation can improve hypoglycemia.

Weight loss

The most popular use of chromium is as a weight loss aid. Results from clinical studies are mixed. As with studies in other applications, results with chromium supplementation are going to be most obvious in those individuals with low body stores of chromium. Chromium supplementation has been shown to increase lean body mass while decreasing fat stores. These positive results were most apparent in elderly subjects and in men who took 400 mcg daily versus 200 mcg daily.

Available Forms

Popular forms of chromium on the market include chromium picolinate, chromium polynicotinate; and chromium-enriched yeast. Although each of these forms is touted by their respective suppliers to provide the greatest benefit, there is no firm evidence to indicate that one is a significantly better choice than another. Any one of these forms does, however, appear to be better absorbed and utilized compared to inorganic forms of chromium such as chromium chloride.

Cautions and Warnings

Individuals with diabetes need to be aware that chromium supplementation may alter insulin or drug requirements. Consult a physician to discuss proper monitoring of blood sugar levels before taking chromium.

Possible Side Effects

There have been no reports of any significant side effects or toxicity reactions with chromium supplementation in double-blind studies. There is one case report of anemia, liver dysfunction, and other problems appearing after taking 1,200–2,400 mcg of chromium picolinate per day for four to five months. It is therefore important not to exceed the recommended dosage.

Drug Interactions

Calcium carbonate and antacids may reduce chromium absorption. Chromium supplementation may increase the effectiveness of insulin and drugs that lower blood sugar levels. Consult a physician to discuss proper monitoring of blood sugar levels before taking a chromium supplement.

Food and Nutrient Interactions

Chromium levels can be depleted by refined sugars, white flour products, and lack of exercise. Vitamin C increases chromium absorption.

Usual Dosage

The typical dosage recommendation for chromium is 200 to 600 mcg per day.

Overdosage

Unknown.

Special Populations

Pregnant/breast-feeding women
Considered safe during pregnancy and lactation.

Children
Suitable for children at one-half the adult dosage.

Seniors
No special precautions are known.

Copper

Used For

Heart disease (atherosclerosis) prevention
Effectiveness: B   Safety: D

General Information

Copper is the third most abundant essential trace mineral in the human body after iron and zinc. The highest concentration of copper is found in the brain and liver. Copper is required for proper iron absorption and utilization; therefore a copper deficiency results in iron deficiency anemia. Copper is also required for the proper function of an enzyme (lysyl oxidase) that is required in the cross-linking of collagen and elastin to give connective tissue its integrity. Copper deficiency manifests itself in rupture of blood vessels, osteoporosis, and bone and joint abnormalities. Other symptoms of copper deficiency are brain disturbances, elevated LDL cholesterol and reduced HDL cholesterol levels, and impaired immune function.

Copper supplementation is most often recommended to prevent copper deficiency and in the prevention of heart disease.

CAUSES OF COPPER DEFICIENCY
Decreased intake
Low-copper infant formulas Total parenteral nutrition without added copper Malnutrition

Decreased absorption

High dosage of supplemental zinc
High dosage of supplemental vitamin C
Chronic antacid intake
Chronic diarrhea
Malabsorptive states (e.g., celiac disease, Crohn's
disease, etc.)

Increased loss

Nephrotic syndrome
Chelation therapy
Burns

Increased requirement

Pregnancy
Lactation
Prematurity in infants

Available Forms

Copper supplements are available in many different
forms (e.g., complexed with sulfate, picolinate, gluconate, and amino acids). However, there is little data to
support any claim that one form is better than another.

Cautions and Warnings

People with Wilson's disease (a rare genetic disorder characterized by elevated copper levels) should
never take copper.

Possible Side Effects

At recommended levels copper supplements are well tolerated. At higher dosages copper supplementation can produce nausea (see "Overdosage," below).

Drug Interactions

The drug penicillamine is used to reduce toxic copper deposits in people with Wilson's disease—a rare genetic disorder characterized by elevated copper levels. Penicillamine binds to copper (and iron) and ushers it out of the body. The drug is also used in the treatment of rheumatoid arthritis and cystinuria. People taking penicillamine should avoid copper supplements.

Food and Nutrient Interactions

A high intake of vitamin C, zinc, iron, and other minerals may decrease the absorption of copper.

Usual Dosage

The estimated safe and adequate intake of copper for adults is 1.5 to 3 mg daily. Since nutrients such as zinc and vitamin C interfere with copper absorption, a popular dosage recommendation for copper is based on zinc intake. It has been proposed that the optimal ratio of zinc to copper is 10:1. This ratio would mean that if zinc is being supplemented at a dosage of 30 mg per day, a dosage of 3 mg of copper is required. However, when using zinc supplementation for specific treatment at dosages between 30 and 90 mg, I usually do not recommend copper at a level greater than 3 mg. When using long-term high-dose zinc therapy (>45 mg/day) it is a good idea to monitor LDL and HDL cholesterol levels. If significant alterations occur, the dosage of zinc should be reduced or the dosage of copper should be increased.

Overdosage

Copper is an emetic. As little as 10 mg will usually produce nausea, and 60 mg will usually produce vomiting. The lethal dose for copper is thought to be as low as 3.5 g. Copper supplements should be kept away from children.

Special Populations

Pregnant/breast-feeding women
Considered safe during pregnancy and lactation.

Children
Suitable for children at the following dosage levels:

Infants

Birth–6 months	0.4–0.6 mg
6 months–1 year	0.6–0.7 mg

Children

1–3 years	0.7–1.0 mg
4–6 years	1.0–1.5 mg
7–10 years	1.5–2.5 mg

Young Adults and Adults

11+ years	1.5–3.0 mg

Seniors
No special precautions are known.

Iodine

Used For

Iodine deficiency
Effectiveness: A   Safety: A

General Information

Iodine is a trace element required in the manufacture of thyroid hormone. Specifically, the thyroid gland adds iodine to the amino acid tyrosine to create thyroid hormone. A deficiency of iodine results in a wide spectrum of conditions collectively termed iodine deficiency disorders. They include goiter, impaired mental and physical development, increased risk of early and late miscarriage, neonatal hypothyroidism, and increased infant mortality. Iodine deficiency can occur at any age, but it is particularly harmful in pregnant women, the developing fetus, and the newborn.

Iodine deficiency is now quite rare in the United States and other industrialized countries because of the addition of iodine to table salt (in the United States, 70 mcg of iodine per g of salt). Sea salt, in comparison, has little iodine. Because most Americans have a high salt intake, the average intake of iodine in the United States is estimated to be over 600 mcg per day.

Available Forms

Iodine is generally available as a salt such as potassium iodide, or derived from kelp.

Cautions and Warnings

Too much iodine can inhibit synthesis of thyroid hormone. Keep dietary or supplementation levels of iodine below 500 mcg per day.

Possible Side Effects

Taking too much iodine (i.e., usually dosages in excess of 1,500 mcg per day) may inhibit thyroid hormone secretion, especially in individuals with hypothyroidism. Increased dietary intake of iodine is also associated with acnelike skin eruptions.

Drug Interactions

None known.

Food and Nutrient Interactions

Certain foods, such as turnips, cabbage, mustard, cassava root, soybean, peanuts, pine nuts, and millet, block the utilization of iodine. These foods are known as goitrogens. Fortunately, cooking usually inactivates the problematic substances in goitrogens.

Usual Dosage

The recommended dosage for iodine is based upon the recommended dietary allowance (RDA).

Recommended Dietary Allowance for Iodine

Infants

Birth–6 months	40 mcg
6 months–1 year	50 mcg

Children

1–3 years	70 mcg
4–6 years	90 mcg
7–10 years	120 mcg

Young Adults and Adults

11+ years	150 mcg
Pregnant women	175 mcg
Lactating women	200 mcg

Overdosage

Do the following in case of accidental overdose: If the victim is unconscious or having convulsions, call for an ambulance immediately. If you take the victim to an emergency room, be sure to bring the bottle or container with you. If the victim is conscious, call your local poison control center or a health care professional. The poison control center may suggest inducing vomiting with ipecac syrup (available without a prescription at any pharmacy). *Do not* induce vomiting unless specifically instructed to do so.

Special Populations

Pregnant/breast-feeding women
Considered safe during pregnancy and lactation at recommended levels.

Children
Suitable for children at the appropriate dosage level (see RDAs above).

Seniors
No special precautions are known.

Iron

Used For

Iron deficiency
Effectiveness: A   Safety: A

Restless legs syndrome
Effectiveness: A   Safety: A

General Information

Iron is critical to human life. It plays the central role in the hemoglobin molecule of red blood cells (RBCs), where it functions to transport oxygen from the lungs to the body's tissues and transport carbon dioxide from the tissues to the lungs. Iron also functions in several key enzymes involved in energy production and metabolism, including DNA synthesis.

Iron deficiency

Iron deficiency is the most common nutrient deficiency in the United States. The groups at highest risk for iron deficiency are infants under two years of age, teenage girls, pregnant women, and the elderly. Studies have found evidence of iron deficiency in as many as 30–50 percent of individuals in these groups.

Iron deficiency may be due to an increased iron requirement, decreased dietary intake, diminished iron absorption or utilization, blood loss, or a combination of factors. Increased requirements for iron occur during the growth spurts of infancy and adolescents, and during pregnancy and lactation. Currently the vast majority of pregnant women are routinely given iron supplements during pregnancy, as the dramatically increased need for iron during this time cannot usually be met through diet alone.

Iron deficiency is the most common cause of anemia (deficiency of red blood cells); however, it must be pointed out that anemia is the last stage of iron deficiency. Iron-dependent enzymes involved in energy production and metabolism are the first to be affected by low iron levels. Serum ferritin is the best laboratory test for determining body iron stores.

Restless legs syndrome

Low serum ferritin levels have been found in patients with so-called restless legs syndrome (RLS)—a syndrome characterized by an irresistible urge to move the legs. In individuals with RLS and low serum ferritin levels, iron supplementation has been shown to significantly improve symptoms.

Available Forms

There are two forms of dietary iron, heme iron and non-heme iron. Heme iron is iron bound to hemoglobin and myoglobin. It is the most efficiently absorbed form of iron. The absorption rate of non-heme iron supplements such as ferrous sulfate and ferrous fumarate is 2.9 percent on an empty stomach and 0.9 percent with food—much less than the absorption rate of heme iron, as found in liver, which is as high as 35 percent. In addition, heme iron lacks the side effects associated with non-heme sources of iron, such as nausea, flatulence, and diarrhea.

Unbound non-heme iron is also more likely than heme iron to spin off pro-oxidants and lead to the formation of free radicals. For this reason, many practitioners are electing to use heme iron over non-heme iron sources when iron supplementation is necessary.

Despite the superiority of heme iron, non-heme iron salts are the most popular iron supplements. One reason is that even though heme iron is better absorbed, it is easy to take higher quantities of non-heme iron salts so that the net amount of iron absorbed is about equal. In other words, if you take 3 mg of heme iron and 50 mg of non-heme iron, the net absorption for each will be about the same.

Cautions and Warnings

Keep all iron supplements out of the reach of children. Acute iron poisoning in infants can result in serious consequences. Severe iron poisoning is characterized by damage to the intestinal lining, liver failure, nausea and vomiting, and shock.

Possible Side Effects

The most common side effects are mild gastrointestinal irritation, constipation or diarrhea, and nausea. Recent studies have suggested that elevated iron levels may lead to an increased risk of heart attack by spinning off free radicals in the blood and either damaging LDL cholesterol or the artery walls directly. For these reasons, many experts believe that it is best to reserve iron supplementation for people with iron deficiency, menstruating women, and pregnant and lactating women.

Drug Interactions

Anti-inflammatory drugs such as aspirin and ibuprofen, which sometimes cause gastrointestinal bleeding, may contribute to iron loss. Antacids (including calcium carbonate) and antiulcer drugs such as cimetidine (Tagamet), ranitidine (Zantac), famotidine (Pepcid), omeprazole (Prilosec), and others can decrease iron absorption.

The bone-building drugs alendronate (Fosamax), etidronate (Didronel), and risedronate (Actonel) as well as tetracycline and quinolone antibiotics, penicillamine, thyroid hormones (e.g., levothyroxine, [Levoxyl, Synthroid]) should not be taken within two hours of iron supplements, as the iron may decrease their absorption and effectiveness.

Food and Nutrient Interactions

High intakes of other minerals, particularly calcium, magnesium, and zinc, can interfere with iron absorption. Vitamin C enhances iron absorption.

Usual Dosage

For iron deficiency, the usual recommendation is 30 mg of elemental iron twice daily between meals. If this recommendation results in abdominal discomfort, take 30 mg with meals three times daily. An alternative recommendation is to take a high-quality liver extract at a level that provides a daily intake of 4–6 mg of heme iron. For general health purposes, the RDA should be used as supplementation guidelines.

Recommended Dietary Allowance for Iron

Infants	
Birth–6 months	6 mg
6 months–1 year	10 mg
Children	
1–10 years	10 mg
Young Adults and Adults	
Males 11–18 years	12 mg
Males 19+ years	10 mg
Females 11–50 years	15 mg
Females 51+ years	10 mg
Pregnant women	30 mg
Lactating women	15 mg

Overdosage

Severe iron poisoning is characterized by damage to the intestinal lining, liver failure, nausea and vomiting, and shock. Do the following in case of accidental overdose: If the victim is unconscious or having convulsions, call for an ambulance immediately. If you take the victim to an emergency room, be sure to bring the bottle or container with you. If the victim is conscious, call your local poison control center or a health care professional. The poison control center may suggest inducing vomiting with ipecac syrup (available without a prescription at any pharmacy). *Do not* induce vomiting unless specifically instructed to do so.

Special Populations

Pregnant/breast-feeding women
Considered safe during pregnancy and lactation.

Children
   Iron supplementation is suitable for children at the RDA level.

Seniors
   No special precautions are known.

Magnesium

Used For

Asthma and chronic obstructive pulmonary disease (COPD)
Effectiveness: B   Safety: A

Attention deficit disorder (ADD) with hyperactivity
Effectiveness: B   Safety: A

Cardiovascular disease

Angina
Effectiveness: B+   Safety: A

Cardiac arrhythmias
Effectiveness: A   Safety: A

Congestive heart failure
Effectiveness: A   Safety: A

High blood pressure
Effectiveness: B   Safety: A

Diabetes
Effectiveness: B   Safety: A

Fatigue
Effectiveness: B   Safety: A

Fibromyalgia
Effectiveness: B+   Safety: A

Kidney stones
Effectiveness: A   Safety: A

Migraine and tension headaches
Effectiveness: B+   Safety: A

Pregnancy complications
Effectiveness: B+   Safety: D

Premenstrual syndrome and dysmenorrhea
Effectiveness: B+   Safety: A

General Information

Magnesium is second only to potassium in terms of concentration within the individual cells of the body. The functions of magnesium primarily revolve around its ability to activate many enzymes.

Magnesium deficiency is extremely common in Americans, particularly in the geriatric population and in women during the premenstrual period. Deficiency is often secondary to factors that reduce absorption or increase secretion of magnesium, such as high calcium intake, alcoholism, surgery, diuretics, liver disease, kidney disease, and oral contraceptive use.

Signs and symptoms of magnesium deficiency include fatigue, mental confusion, irritability, weakness, heart disturbances, problems in nerve conduction and muscle contraction, muscle cramps, loss of appetite, insomnia, and a predisposition to stress.

Asthma and chronic obstructive pulmonary disease (COPD)

Magnesium promotes relaxation of the bronchial smooth muscles; as a result, airways open and breathing is made easier. Intravenous magnesium is a well-proven and clinically accepted measure to halt an acute asthma attack as well as acute flare-ups of COPD. Unfortunately, long-term oral magnesium supplementation has not been fully evaluated in the treatment of asthma or COPD.

Attention deficit disorder (ADD) with hyperactivity

Magnesium deficiency may play a role in ADD, as research indicates many children with ADD have lower levels of magnesium. In a preliminary study, magnesium reduced hyperactivity in children with ADD with hyperactivity. In the study, fifty ADD children with low magnesium (as determined by red blood cell, hair, and serum levels of magnesium) were given 200 mg of magnesium per day for six months. Compared with twenty-five other magnesium-deficient ADD children, those given magnesium supplementation had a significant decrease in hyperactive behavior.

Cardiovascular disease

Magnesium is absolutely essential in the proper functioning of the heart. Magnesium's role in preventing heart disease and strokes is generally well accepted. In addition, there is a substantial body of knowledge demonstrating that magnesium supplementation is effective in treating a wide range of cardiovascular diseases.

Angina

Magnesium supplementation (most studies have used intravenous administration) has been shown to be helpful in angina that is due to either a spasm of the coronary artery or atherosclerosis. The beneficial effects of magnesium in angina relate to its ability to improve energy production within the heart; dilate the coronary arteries, resulting in improved delivery of oxygen to the heart; reduce peripheral vascular resistance, resulting in reduced demand on the heart; inhibit platelets from aggregating and forming blood clots; and normalize heart rate.

Cardiac arrhythmias

Magnesium was first shown to be of value in the treatment of cardiac arrhythmias in 1935. More than sixty years later, there are now numerous double-blind studies showing magnesium to be of benefit for many types of arrhythmias, including atrial fibrillation, ventricular premature contractions, ventricular tachycardia, and severe ventricular arrhythmias.

Congestive heart failure

Congestive heart failure (CHF) refers to an inability of the heart to effectively pump blood. CHF is most often due to long-term effects of high blood pressure, disorder of a heart valve, or cardiomyopathy. Magnesium levels appear to correlate directly with survival rates. In one study, CHF patients with normal levels of magnesium had one- and two-year survival rates of 71 percent and 61 percent, respectively, compared to rates of 45 percent and 42 percent for patients with lower magnesium levels. In addition to providing benefits of its own in CHF, magnesium supplementation also prevents the magnesium depletion caused by the conventional drug therapy for CHF—digitalis, diuretics, and vasodilators (beta-blockers, calcium channel blockers, etc.).

High blood pressure

There is considerable evidence from population studies that a high intake of magnesium is associated with lower blood pressure. Because of this evidence, researchers began investigating the effect of magnesium supplementation in the treatment of high blood pressure. The results from double-blind studies have been mixed. Some of the studies have shown a very good blood-pressure-lowering effect, while others have not. Magnesium appears most helpful if an individual is taking a diuretic or has a high level of renin—an enzyme released by the kidneys that eventually leads to the formation of angiotensin and the release of aldosterone. These compounds cause the blood vessels to constrict and the blood pressure to increase. The degree of blood pressure reduction with magnesium is generally modest (i.e., less than 10 mm Hg for both systolic and diastolic measures).

Diabetes

Magnesium is known to play a central role in the secretion and action of insulin. Several studies in patients with diabetes or impaired glucose tolerance have shown magnesium to be of value. Magnesium supplementation (usually 400 to 500 mg per day) improves insulin response and action, glucose tolerance, and the fluidity of the red blood cell membrane. In addition, magnesium levels are usually low in diabetics and lowest in those with severe retinopathy. Diabetics appear to have higher magnesium requirements.

Fatigue

An underlying magnesium deficiency can result in symptoms similar to those of chronic fatigue syndrome (CFS). Low red blood cell magnesium levels, a more accurate measure of magnesium status than routine blood analysis, have been found in many patients with chronic fatigue and CFS. Double-blind studies in people with CFS have shown that magnesium supplementation significantly improved energy levels, emotional state, and pain. These more recent studies support the results from clinical trials during the 1960s on patients suffering from chronic fatigue. The earlier studies utilized oral magnesium and potassium aspartate and found that between 75 and 91 percent of the nearly three thousand patients studied experienced relief of fatigue during treatment. In contrast, the number of patients responding to a placebo was between 9 and 26 percent. The beneficial effect was usually noted after only four or

five days, but sometimes ten days were required.
Patients usually continued treatment for four to six
weeks.

Fibromyalgia

Fibromyalgia is a recently recognized disorder regarded as a common cause of chronic musculoskeletal pain and fatigue. One study demonstrated
that a daily supplement of 300 to 600 mg of magnesium (as magnesium malate) resulted in tremendous improvements in the number and severity of
tender points.

Kidney stones

Magnesium increases the solubility of calcium in
the urine, thereby preventing kidney stone formation. Supplementing magnesium in the diet has
demonstrated significant effect in preventing recurrences of kidney stones. However, when used in
conjunction with vitamin B_6 (pyridoxine), an even
greater effect is noted.

Migraine and tension headaches

There is considerable evidence that low magnesium levels trigger both migraine and tension
headaches. In individuals with low magnesium levels, magnesium supplementation has been shown
to produce excellent results in double-blind studies.

Pregnancy complications

Magnesium needs increase during pregnancy, as
reflected in an increase in the RDA from 280 mg for
adults to 350 mg per day for pregnant women.
Magnesium deficiency during pregnancy has been
linked to preeclampsia (a serious condition of pregnancy associated with elevations in blood pressure,
fluid retention, and loss of protein in the urine),

preterm delivery, and fetal growth retardation. In contrast, supplementing the diet of pregnant women with additional oral magnesium has been shown to significantly decrease the incidence of these complications.

Premenstrual syndrome

Magnesium deficiency has been suggested as a causative factor in premenstrual syndrome. While magnesium has been shown to be effective on its own, even better results may be achieved by combining it with vitamin B_6 and other nutrients. Several studies have shown that when PMS patients are given a multivitamin-mineral supplement containing high doses of magnesium and vitamin B_6, they experience a better reduction in PMS symptoms compared to the results seen in studies with magnesium alone.

Available Forms

Magnesium is available in several different forms. Absorption studies indicate that magnesium is easily absorbed orally, especially when it is bound to citrate (and presumably aspartate and other intermediates in the Krebs cycle such as malate, succinate, and fumarate). Inorganic forms of magnesium such as magnesium chloride, magnesium oxide, or magnesium carbonate are generally well absorbed but are more likely to cause diarrhea at higher dosages.

Cautions and Warnings

If you suffer from a serious kidney disorder or are on hemodialysis, do not take magnesium supplements unless directed to do so by a physician.

People with severe heart disease (such as high-grade atrioventricular block) should not take magnesium (or potassium) unless under the direct advice of a physician.

Possible Side Effects

In general, magnesium is very well tolerated. Magnesium supplementation can sometimes cause a looser stool, particularly magnesium sulfate (Epsom salts), magnesium hydroxide, or magnesium chloride.

Drug Interactions

There are many drugs that appear to adversely affect magnesium status. Most notable are many diuretics, antacids and ulcer medications, insulin, and digitalis. Likewise, magnesium may interfere with the absorption of the bone-building drugs alendronate (Fosamax), etidronate (Didronel), and risedronate (Actonel) as well as tetracycline and quinolone antibiotics. Magnesium supplements should not be taken within two hours of these drugs.

Food and Nutrient Interactions

There is extensive interaction between magnesium and calcium, potassium, and other minerals. High dosages of other minerals will reduce the absorption of magnesium and vice versa. A high calcium intake and a high intake of dairy foods fortified with vitamin D result in decreased magnesium absorption. Vitamin B_6 works together with magnesium in many enzyme systems and also increases its absorption and utilization.

Usual Dosage

The usual recommendation for magnesium is supplementation at the level of the Recommended Dietary Allowance (RDA): 350 mg per day for adult males and 280 mg per day for adult females. Many nutritional experts feel the ideal intake for magnesium should be based on body weight (6 mg per kg [2.2 pounds] body weight). For a 110-pound person the recommendation would be 300 mg, for a 154-pound person 420 mg, and for a 200-pound person 540 mg.

Overdosage

Usually overdosage would result in diarrhea. Do the following in case of accidental overdose: If the victim is unconscious or having convulsions, call for an ambulance immediately. If you take the victim to an emergency room, be sure to bring the bottle or container with you. If the victim is conscious, call your local poison control center or a health care professional. The poison control center may suggest inducing vomiting with ipecac syrup (available without a prescription at any pharmacy). *Do not* induce vomiting unless specifically instructed to do so.

Special Populations

Pregnant/breast-feeding women

Considered safe during pregnancy and lactation at the Recommended Dietary Allowance level of 350 mg daily.

Children
Suitable for children at the level of the Recommended Dietary Allowance:

Infants
Birth–6 months   40 mg
6 months–1 year   60 mg

Children
1–3 years   80 mg
4–6 years   120 mg
7–10 years   170 mg

Seniors
No special precautions are known.

Manganese

Used For

Diabetes
Effectiveness: C   Safety: C

Epilepsy
Effectiveness: C   Safety: C

Strains, sprains, and inflammation
Effectiveness: C   Safety: C

General Information

Manganese functions in many enzyme systems, including enzymes involved in blood sugar control, energy metabolism, and thyroid hormone function. Manganese also functions in the antioxidant enzyme superoxide dismutase (SOD). This enzyme is responsible for preventing the superoxide free radical from destroying cellular components. Without SOD, cells are quite susceptible to damage and inflammation. Manganese supplementation has been shown to increase SOD activity, indicating increased antioxidant activity.

The principal uses of manganese supplementation are in the support of diabetes, epilepsy, and strains, sprains, and inflammation.

Diabetes

Manganese is an important cofactor in the key enzymes of glucose metabolism. Diabetics have been shown to have just one-half the manganese of normal individuals. However, the only report in the medical literature on manganese supplementation (3–5 mg daily) in human diabetics was a single case report showing a positive effect in a patient who was not responding to insulin therapy alone.

Epilepsy

Low whole blood and hair manganese levels have been found in epileptics, with those with the lowest levels typically having the highest seizure activity. However, there are no clinical studies that evaluate any therapeutic role for manganese in epilepsy.

Strains, sprains, and inflammation

Manganese has become a popular nutritional recommendation for strains, sprains, and inflammation, presumably due to the belief that manganese supplementation may increase the level of activity of manganese-containing SOD.

Available Forms

Manganese is available commercially in various forms. Manganese salts such as manganese sulfate or manganese chloride are generally thought to be not as well absorbed as manganese bound to picolinate, gluconate, or other chelates, although there is no data to prove this assumption.

Cautions and Warnings

None known.

Possible Side Effects

None known.

Drug Interactions

Antacids and antiulcer drugs such as ranitidine (Zantac), cimetidine (Tagamet), famotidine (Pepcid), and omeprazole (Prilosec) may inhibit the absorption of manganese.

Food and Nutrient Interactions

High intakes of magnesium, calcium, iron, copper, and zinc may inhibit the absorption of manganese. Zinc and copper work together with manganese in the antioxidant enzyme SOD.

Usual Dosage

Although there is no specific RDA for manganese, it is estimated that most people require between 2 and 5 mg per day. For specific purposes, the typical dosage ranges are as follows:

Sprains, strains, inflammation: first two weeks, 15–30 mg daily; thereafter, 5–15 mg daily
Epilepsy: 5–15 mg daily
Diabetes: 5–15 mg daily

Overdosage

There have been no reports of overdosage due to manganese-containing nutritional supplements. However, manganese toxicity as a result of environmental pollution or mining of manganese is a serious health problem. In its most severe forms, manganese toxicity can result in a syndrome called manganese madness, characterized by severe psychiatric symptoms such as hallucinations, violent acts, and hyperirritability.

Special Populations

Pregnant/breast-feeding women

As the effects of manganese during pregnancy and lactation have not been sufficiently evaluated, dosages greater than 5 mg should not be used during these times.

Children

Suitable for children at the Estimated Safe and Adequate Ranges:

Infants

Birth–6 months	**0.3–0.6 mg**
6 months–1 year	**0.6–1.0 mg**

Children

1–3 years	**1.0–1.5 mg**
4–6 years	**1.5–2.0 mg**
7–10 years	**2.0–3.0 mg**

Young Adults and Adults

11+ years	**2.5–5.0 mg**

Seniors
  No special precautions are known.

Molybdenum

Used For:

Cancer prevention
Effectiveness: C   Safety: C

Prevention of cavities
Effectiveness: C   Safety: C

Sulfite sensitivity
Effectiveness: C   Safety: C

General Information

Molybdenum is a trace mineral that functions as a component in several enzymes, including those involved in alcohol detoxification, uric acid formation, and sulfur metabolism. Molybdenum has three primary possible (although largely speculative) applications: sulfite sensitivity, cancer prevention, and prevention of cavities.

Cancer prevention

There is evidence from population studies that low molybdenum levels may be a factor in some forms of cancer. In the United States, there is a 30 percent higher rate of esophageal cancer in areas where there is no molybdenum in the drinking water. Presumably the anticancer effects of molybdenum are the result of its role in the detoxification of cancer-causing chemicals.

Prevention of cavities

Several population studies have shown that areas where the molybdenum intake is high are associated with a low rate of tooth decay. Conversely, areas where molybdenum levels are low are associated with higher rates of tooth decay. Molybdenum might enhance the effect of fluoride, as the combined administration of molybdenum (25 or 50 ppm) and fluoride (50 ppm) was more effective in reducing dental cavities than water containing only fluoride (50 ppm).

Sulfite sensitivity

Low molybdenum levels may lead to increased allergic reactions to sulfites, which are often added to foods and wine to prevent spoilage. The link between low molybdenum and sulfite sensitivity was discovered when subjects receiving total parenteral (intravenous) nutrition manifested an inability to detoxify sulfites. Molybdenum supplementation brought about complete resolution of symptoms of

sulfite toxicity, such as increased heart rate, shortness of breath, headache, disorientation, nausea,
and vomiting.

Available Forms

Molybdenum is most often available commercially
as sodium molybdate.

Cautions and Warnings

None known.

Possible Side Effects

None known.

Drug Interactions

None known.

Food and Nutrient Interactions

None known.

Usual Dosage

The typical dosage range for molybdenum supplementation in adults is 100 to 250 mcg. Higher dosages,
under the advice of a licensed physician, may be
required in the adjunctive therapy of Wilson's disease.

Overdosage

Molybdenum is relatively nontoxic. In order to produce toxicity, a dosage of more than 100 mg per kg
(2.2 pounds) body weight would have to be in-

gested. A daily intake of 10 to 15 mg may produce in some people goutlike symptoms due to enhanced production of uric acid.

Special Populations

Pregnant/breast-feeding women
Considered safe during pregnancy and lactation at the recommended dosage levels.

Children
Suitable for children at the Estimated Safe and Adequate Ranges:

Infants

Birth–6 months	15–30 mcg
6 months–1 year	20–40 mcg

Children

1–3 years	25–50 mcg
4–6 years	30–75 mcg
7–10 years	50–150 mcg

Young Adults and Adults

11+ years	75–250 mcg

Seniors
No special precautions are known.

Potassium

Used For

Deficiency of potassium
Effectiveness: A   Safety: A

High blood pressure
Effectiveness: A   Safety: A

General Information

Potassium is an extremely important electrolyte for the maintenance of many body functions. It plays a key role in the regulation of water balance and distribution, acid-base balance, and the function of the heart, the kidneys and adrenal glands, and muscle and nerve cells.

Potassium supplementation is most often used to overcome potassium depletion and to lower blood pressure.

Deficiency of potassium

Potassium deficiency most often occurs whenever the rate of loss of potassium through urinary excretion, sweat, or the gastrointestinal tract (vomiting or diarrhea) exceeds the rate of potassium intake. Severe potassium deficiency is most often the result of the use of certain diuretics but can also occur as a result of extended diarrhea or vomiting. Because severe potassium deficiency can have serious consequences, it is best to consult a physician if you suspect you may be suffering from potassium depletion.

A potassium deficiency is characterized by muscle

weakness, fatigue, mental confusion, irritability, weakness, heart disturbances, and problems in nerve conduction and muscle contraction. Dietary potassium deficiency is less common than deficiency due to excessive fluid loss (sweating, diarrhea, or urination) or the use of diuretics, laxatives, aspirin, and other drugs. Dietary potassium deficiency is typically caused by a diet low in fresh fruits and vegetables but high in sodium. It is more common to see dietary potassium deficiency in the elderly.

High blood pressure

Many double-blind studies have shown that potassium supplementation alone can produce significant reductions in blood pressure in people with high blood pressure. Typically these studies have utilized dosages ranging from 2.5 to 5 g of potassium per day. Significant drops in both systolic and diastolic values have been achieved, typically in the range of 12 mm Hg for the systolic measure and 16 mm Hg for the diastolic measure. Potassium supplementation appears to be especially useful in the treatment of high blood pressure in persons over the age of sixty-five.

Available Forms

Potassium supplements that are available in health food stores are either potassium salts (potassium chloride, potassium bicarbonate), potassium bound to various mineral chelates (e.g., potassium aspartate, potassium citrate), or food-based potassium sources. The FDA restricts the amount of potassium available in non-food-based forms to a mere 99 mg per dose. Potassium chloride preparations are also available by prescription in a vast array of formulations (timed-release tablets, liquids, powders, and effervescent tablets).

Cautions and Warnings

If you suffer from a serious kidney disorder or are on hemodialysis, do not take potassium supplements unless directed to do so by a physician.

Possible Side Effects

Generally potassium supplementation is well tolerated. The FDA restricts the level of potassium in nutritional supplements at 99 mg because higher doses of potassium given in pill form can cause nausea, vomiting, diarrhea, and ulcers.

Drug Interactions

Potassium supplementation (unless supervised by a physician) is contraindicated in patients taking a number of prescription medications, including digoxin (Lanoxin); potassium-sparing diuretics such as spironolactone (Aldactone), triamterene (Dyrenium), and amiloride (Midamor); the angiotensin-converting-enzyme (ACE) inhibitor class of blood-pressure-lowering drugs, such as enalapril (Vasotec), lisinopril (Zestril), captopril (Capoten), and benazepril (Lotensin); and the trimethoprim/sulfamethoxazole class of antibiotics (e.g., Bactrim, Cotrim, Septra, Uroplus). Use of these drugs with potassium supplementation can lead to potassium toxicity.

Food and Nutrient Interactions

An increased intake of high-potassium foods or salt substitutes can increase the risk of serious side effects in people with impaired kidney function or those who are taking potassium-sparing diuretics or ACE inhibitors (see "Drug Interactions," above).

Usual Dosage

The estimated safe and adequate daily dietary intake of potassium, as set by the Committee on Recommended Daily Allowances, is 1.9 to 5.6 g. If body potassium requirements are not being met through diet, supplementation is essential. The amount allowed in supplements is 99 mg per tablet or capsule, making it difficult to achieve necessary levels, yet so-called salt substitutes such as Morton's Salt Substitute, NoSalt, and Nu-Salt are in fact potassium chloride and provide 530 mg of potassium per 1/6 teaspoon, and a banana typically provides 500 mg of potassium. When potassium needs are not adequately being met by diet alone, potassium salts are commonly prescribed by physicians in the dosage range of 1.5 to 3.0 g per day.

Overdosage

Most people can handle any excess of potassium. The exception is people with kidney disease. These people do not handle potassium in the normal way and are likely to experience heart disturbances and other consequences of potassium toxicity. Individuals with kidney disorders usually need to restrict their potassium intake and follow the dietary recommendations of their physicians. Because potassium overdosage in these patients can be life-threatening, do the following in case of accidental overdose: If the victim is unconscious or having convulsions, call for an ambulance immediately. If you take the victim to an emergency room, be sure to bring the bottle or

container with you. If the victim is conscious, call
your local poison control center or a health care professional. The poison control center may suggest inducing vomiting with ipecac syrup (available without
a prescription at any pharmacy). *Do not* induce vomiting unless specifically instructed to do so.

Special Populations

Pregnant/breast-feeding women
Potassium supplementation during pregnancy
and lactation is recommended only under the direction of a physician.

Children
Potassium supplementation in children is recommended only under the direction of a physician.

Seniors
No special precautions are known.

Selenium

Used For

Antioxidant support
Effectiveness: A   Safety: D

Cancer prevention
Effectiveness: B+   Safety: D

Cataract prevention
Effectiveness: B+   Safety: D

Heart disease (atherosclerosis) prevention
Effectiveness: B+   Safety: D

Inflammatory conditions
Effectiveness: B   Safety: D

Low immunity and immune support
Effectiveness: A   Safety: D

Pregnancy nutrition
Effectiveness: A   Safety: D

General Information

The trace mineral selenium functions primarily as a component of the antioxidant enzyme glutathione peroxidase, which works with vitamin E in preventing free-radical damage to cell membranes. Low levels of selenium have been linked to a higher risk for cancer, cardiovascular disease, inflammatory diseases, and other conditions associated with increased free-radical damage, including premature aging and cataract formation.

Severe selenium deficiency is associated with Keshan disease, a serious heart disorder that affects primarily children and women of childbearing age in some areas of China where selenium levels in the soil are very low. However, severe selenium deficiency states are extremely rare in North America. More common is the chronically low selenium intake that is associated with an increased risk for cancer, an increased risk of heart disease, and low immune function.

Cancer prevention

A large body of scientific evidence indicates that cancer rates go up when dietary intake of selenium is low.

For example, a ten-year cancer prevention trial found that selenium supplementation appears to significantly lower the incidence of lung, colon, and prostate cancers in people with a history of skin cancer. The study began in 1983 and included a total of 1,312 skin cancer patients. Although there was no effect on skin cancer with selenium supplementation (200 mcg per day), total cancer incidence was significantly lower in the selenium group than in the placebo group (77 cases versus 119), as was the incidence of the specific cancers named above. The results also showed that overall mortality was 17 percent less in the selenium versus the control group (108 versus 129), with this difference largely due to a 50 percent reduction in cancer deaths (29 versus 57). There was no significant difference between the two groups for other causes of death.

Cataract prevention

Maintaining proper selenium levels appears to be important in protecting against cataract formation. Studies have shown the selenium content in the human lens with a cataract is only 15 percent of normal levels, and levels of free radicals are up to twenty-five times normal in the aqueous humor (eye fluid) of patients with cataracts.

Heart disease (atherosclerosis) prevention

Selenium appears to offer protection against heart disease and stroke, as rates for heart disease are highest where selenium intake is the lowest, although the association is not as strong as it is in cancer. Selenium supplementation has been shown to help prevent heart attacks. In one double-blind study, eighty-one patients who had a heart attack were randomly assigned to receive 100 mcg of selenium (from selenium-rich yeast) or a placebo. After six months, there were four fatal heart attacks and two nonfatal heart attacks in the placebo group compared to no deaths and one nonfatal heart attack in the selenium group.

Inflammatory conditions

Selenium levels have been shown to be low in patients with rheumatoid arthritis, eczema, and psoriasis. Clinical studies have not yet clearly demonstrated that selenium supplementation alone improves inflammatory conditions. For example, a study with selenium alone showed no benefit for rheumatoid arthritis. However, one clinical study of rheumatoid arthritis patients indicated that selenium combined with vitamin E did provide some benefit. Supplementing the diet with 50 to 200 mcg of selenium and 200 to 400 IU of vitamin E appears to be appropriate in inflammatory conditions due to an increased need, the low selenium levels typically seen in inflammatory conditions, and selenium's and vitamin E's synergistic effects as antioxidants.

Low immunity and immune support

Selenium affects all components of the immune system, including the development and expression of all white blood cells. Selenium deficiency has been shown to inhibit resistance to infection as a result of impaired white blood cell and thymus function, while selenium supplementation (200 mcg/day) has been shown to stimulate white blood cell and thymus function.

The ability of selenium supplementation to enhance immune function goes well beyond simply restoring selenium levels in selenium-deficient individuals. For example, in one study selenium supplementation (200 mcg/day) in individuals with normal selenium concentrations in their blood resulted in a 118 percent increase in the ability of white blood cells to kill tumor cells and an 82.3 percent increase in the activity of a type of white blood cell known as a natural killer cell because of its powerful ability to kill cancer cells and microorganisms.

Pregnancy nutrition

There is substantial evidence that selenium is essential for proper fetal growth and development. Selenium requirements appear to be increased during pregnancy, as selenium concentrations in the blood tend to be lower during pregnancy, particularly during the later stages. Selenium levels tend to be very low in low-birth-weight babies.

Available Forms

Popular forms of selenium on the market include sodium selenite, selenomethionine, and yeast-derived selenium. Several studies have shown that inorganic salts, such as sodium selenite, are less effectively absorbed and not as biologically active compared to organic forms of selenium such as selenomethionine and selenium-rich yeast.

Cautions and Warnings

Do not take selenium at levels greater than those recommended, as significant toxicity can occur at higher intake levels.

Possible Side Effects

The human body requires just a small amount of selenium. Dosages as low as 900 mcg per day over prolonged periods of time can produce signs of selenium toxicity in some people. Signs and symptoms related to chronic toxicity include depression, nervousness, emotional instability, nausea and vomiting, a garlic odor of the breath and sweat, and, in extreme cases, loss of hair and fingernails.

Drug Interactions

Selenium may increase the effectiveness of the chemotherapy drug cisplatin (Platinol-AQ).

Food and Nutrient Interactions

Selenium absorption is adversely affected by high dosages of vitamin C (this affects sodium selenite more than organic forms of selenium) and by high intakes of other trace minerals, particularly zinc. Selenium works closely with vitamin E in antioxidant mechanisms.

Usual Dosage

Although there is no specific RDA for selenium, for adults a daily intake of 50 to 200 mcg is often recommended. At high intake levels (daily intake in excess of 900 mcg for several months), selenium can produce toxicity (see "Possible Side Effects").

Overdosage

Do the following in case of accidental overdose: If the victim is unconscious or having convulsions, call for an ambulance immediately. If you take the victim to an emergency room, be sure to bring the bottle or container with you. If the victim is conscious, call your local poison control center or a health care professional. The poison control center may suggest inducing vomiting with ipecac syrup (available without a prescription at any pharmacy). *Do not* induce vomiting unless specifically instructed to do so.

Special Populations

Pregnant/breast-feeding women
Selenium supplementation is suitable during pregnancy and lactation at recommended levels.

Children
Selenium is suitable for use in children at appropriate levels. For children, a good dosage recommendation for selenium supplementation is 1.5 mcg per pound of body weight.

Seniors
No special precautions are known.

Silicon

Used For

Osteoporosis
Effectiveness: C   Safety: C

Strengthening nails
Effectiveness: B   Safety: C

General Information

Crystalline silicon (quartz) is the most abundant mineral in the earth's crust. Although the exact biological role of silicon has not been determined, it appears to be required for proper integrity of the skin, ligaments, tendons, and bone. Silicon appears to be required for the proper functioning of an enzyme (prolyhydroxylase) that is involved in the formation of collagen in bone, cartilage, and other connective tissues. It also appears that silicon may be important in bone calcification, as high concentrations of silicon have been found at the calcification sites of growing bones. The highest concentrations of silicon, however, are found in the skin and hair.

One of the few studies on the benefits of silicon featured the use of oral and topical colloidal silicic acid. A total of fifty women with signs of aging of their facial skin, thin hair, and brittle nails were enrolled in an open, uncontrolled ninety-day study. The women took a once-daily oral dose of 10 ml of colloidal silicic acid and applied colloidal silicic acid twice daily to the face. Statistically significant improvements were noted in the thickness of the skin, strength of the skin, wrinkles, and health of the hair and nails. Ultrasound examination revealed that silicon supplementation increased the thickness of the dermis—the connective-tissue support structure that lies just below the surface of the skin.

There have been no studies on the use of silicon for osteoporosis.

Available Forms

Silicon is available in several different forms: silicon-rich horsetail (the plant *Equisetum arvense),* sodium metasilicate, and colloidal silicic acid. There is no clear-cut advantage to any of these forms.

Cautions and Warnings

None known.

Possible Side Effects

None known.

Drug Interactions

None known.

Food and Nutrient Interactions

None known.

Usual Dosage

There is no RDA for silicon. The daily requirement is generally thought to be in the range of 5 to 20 mg. Daily dosages should not exceed this range until more is learned about the role of and need for silicon.

Overdosage

None known. Silicon is generally regarded as being nontoxic. However, increased levels of silicon and aluminum complexes have been detected in the neurofibrillary tangles and plaques in the brains of people with Alzheimer's disease, suggesting a possible association. Until more is known, excessive intake of silicon should be avoided.

Special Populations

Pregnant/breast-feeding women
As the effects of silicon during pregnancy and lactation have not been sufficiently evaluated, it should not be used during these times.

Children
Suitable for children at one-half the adult dosage.

Seniors
No special precautions are known.

Sulfur (*see* MSM)

General Information
Sulfur is an important element for all cells and body tissues. It is an especially important nutrient for joint tissue, where it functions in the stabilization of the connective-tissue matrix of cartilage, tendons, and ligaments. Sulfur is most commonly used as a supplement in the form of methylsulfonylmethane (MSM).

Vanadium

Used For

Diabetes
Effectiveness: B   Safety: C

General Information

Vanadium was named after the Scandinavian goddess of beauty, youth, and luster. Although vanadium has been suggested to be an essential trace mineral, functioning in hormone, cholesterol, and blood sugar metabolism, no specific deficiency signs or symptoms in humans have been reported. Some researchers have speculated that a vanadium deficiency may contribute to elevated cholesterol levels and faulty blood sugar control manifesting as either diabetes or hypoglycemia.

Most of the research on vanadium has focused on its role in improving or mimicking insulin action. In animal studies high dosages of vanadium (most often as vanadyl sulfate) have led to improved glucose tolerance. Preliminary studies have confirmed a blood-sugar-lowering effect in non-insulin-dependent diabetes mellitus (NIDDM). However, the researchers of these studies caution that the long-term safety of such large doses of vanadium remains unknown.

Available Forms

Vanadium exists in five different forms, with the most biologically significant being either vanadyl or vanadate. Vanadyl sulfate and bis-maltolato-oxo-vanadium (BMOV) have become the most popular form of vanadium for nutritional supplementation. Brand names available include Super Vanadyl Fuel.

Cautions and Warnings

Individuals with diabetes need to be aware that vanadium supplementation may alter insulin or drug requirements. Consult a physician to discuss proper monitoring of blood sugar levels before taking vanadium.

Possible Side Effects

Generally, vanadyl sulfate and BMOV are well tolerated, with no known side effects at recommended levels.

Drug Interactions

Vanadium supplementation may increase the effectiveness of insulin and drugs that lower blood sugar levels. Consult a physician to discuss proper monitoring of blood sugar levels before taking a vanadium supplement.

Food and Nutrient Interactions

None known.

Usual Dosage

The usual dosage for vanadyl sulfate is 10 to 100 mg. For BMOV the dosage range is 1 to 5 mg.

Overdosage

Toxic effects of vanadium observed in animal studies include elevation of blood pressure and interference with cellular energy production. However, a couple of distinctions need to be made: (1) the toxicity studies utilized vanadate, not vanadyl, and (2) human subjects appear to tolerate vanadium better than other species.

Special Populations

Pregnant/breast-feeding women
As the effects of vanadium supplements during pregnancy and lactation have not been sufficiently evaluated, it should not be used at levels above 100 mcg during these times.

Children
As the effects of vanadium supplements during childhood have not been sufficiently evaluated, it should not be used at levels above 100 mcg unless directed to do otherwise by a physician.

Seniors
No special precautions are known.

Zinc

Used For

Acne
Effectiveness: B   Safety: A

Alzheimer's disease
Effectiveness: B   Safety: A

Common cold
Effectiveness: B   Safety: A

Immune system enhancement
Effectiveness: B   Safety: A

Male sexual function
Effectiveness: B   Safety: A

Macular degeneration
Effectiveness: B   Safety: A

Pregnancy outcome
Effectiveness: B   Safety: A

Rheumatoid arthritis
Effectiveness: B   Safety: A

General Information

Zinc is a trace mineral that is found in virtually every cell in the body and is a component in over 200 enzymes. Enzymes are molecules involved in speeding up the chemical reactions necessary for body functions. Zinc functions in more enzymatic reactions than any other mineral; low zinc levels affect virtually every system of the body. Zinc is also required for proper action of many body hormones, including insulin, growth hormone, and sex hormones.

Adequate zinc levels are absolutely essential to good health. Zinc is especially important to proper immune function, wound healing, sensory functions, sexual function, and skin health.

Although severe zinc deficiency is very rare in developed countries, it is believed that many individuals in the United States have marginal zinc deficiency, especially in the elderly population. The zinc deficiency can be caused by decreased intake and/or utilization. Dietary surveys indicate that average zinc intakes range from only 47 percent to 67 percent of the RDA. Marginal zinc deficiency may be reflected by an increased susceptibility to infection, poor wound healing, a decreased sense of taste or smell, and a number of minor skin disorders including acne, eczema, and psoriasis. Other physical findings that often correlate with low zinc status include decreased ability to see at night or with poor lighting, growth retardation, testicular atrophy, mouth ulcers, a white coating on the tongue, and marked halitosis.

Acne

Several double-blind studies have demonstrated that zinc supplementation produces similar results to tetracycline (an antibiotic) in superficial acne and superior results in deeper acne. Although some people in these studies showed dramatic improvement immediately, the majority usually required twelve weeks of supplementation before good results were achieved.

Alzheimer's disease

Zinc deficiency is one of the most common nutrient deficiencies in the elderly and has been suggested to be a major factor in the development of Alzheimer's disease. Preliminary studies with zinc supplementation have shown some beneficial effects. In one small study, ten patients with Alzheimer's disease were given 27 mg of zinc (as zinc aspartate) daily. Only two patients failed to show improvement in memory, understanding, communication, and social contact.

Common cold

Zinc possesses some direct antiviral activity, including antiviral activity against several viruses that can cause the common cold. The use of zinc supplementation, particularly in the form of a lozenge, appears to be of value during a cold. However, out of eight double-blind studies, four found zinc lozenges to be effective, while the other four reported no difference between zinc and placebo therapy. This inconsistency is thought to be due to an ineffective lozenge formulation in the negative studies. It appears that, in order for zinc to be effective, it must be onized in saliva. The study showed that sucking on hard candy lozenges containing zinc gluconate and citric acid delivered an insignificant amount of ionized zinc. It was found that, in the presence of citric acid, saliva completely suppressed the ionization of zinc. It appears that in order for a zinc lozenge to be effective it must be free of sorbitol, mannitol, and citric acid.

In the positive double-blind studies, zinc-containing lozenges (Cold-Eeze) significantly reduced the average duration of common colds. The lozenges contained 23 mg of elemental zinc, which the patients were instructed to dissolve in their mouths every two waking hours after an initial double dose. In one study, after seven days, 86 percent of the thirty-seven zinc-treated subjects were symptom free, compared to 46 percent of the twenty-eight placebo-treated subjects.

Immune system enhancement

Zinc is involved in virtually every aspect of immune function. Zinc supplementation can reverse the low immune function characteristic of aging. In one study, the effect of low-dose zinc supplementation (20 mg/day) on nutritional and immune status was assessed in institutionalized elderly subjects. The most telling effect was that zinc supplementation produced a significant restoration of serum thymulin, an immune-enhancing hormone produced by the thymus gland that often decreases with age. Nutritional status was improved because both food intake and serum albumin levels were increased with zinc supplementation.

Male sexual function

Zinc is critical for male sexual function. It is involved in hormone metabolism, sperm formation, and sperm motility. Zinc deficiency is characterized by, among many other things, decreased testosterone levels and sperm counts. Zinc levels are typically much lower in infertile men with low sperm counts, indicating that a low zinc status may be a contributing factor to the infertility. Several double-blind studies have shown that zinc supplementation can improve sperm counts and motility. It is especially effective in boosting sperm counts in men with low testosterone levels.

Macular degeneration

Zinc has been shown to be beneficial in reducing vision loss in the treatment of macular degeneration.

Pregnancy outcome

Low zinc levels are linked to premature births, low birth weight, growth retardation, and preeclampsia—a serious condition of pregnancy associated with elevations in blood pressure, fluid retention, and loss of protein in the urine. Studies of zinc supplementation in pregnancy have shown that infants born to the zinc-supplemented mothers had greater body weight and head circumference compared to the placebo group. The zinc-supplemented mothers also had fewer complications of pregnancy.

Rheumatoid arthritis

Zinc has antioxidant effects as well as functions in the antioxidant enzyme superoxide dismutase (copper-zinc SOD). Zinc levels are typically reduced in patients with rheumatoid arthritis, and several studies of zinc in the treatment of rheumatoid arthritis have demonstrated a slight therapeutic effect. Most of the studies utilized zinc in the form of sulfate. Better results might have been produced by using a more absorbable form of zinc.

Available Forms

There are many forms of zinc to choose from. While most clinical studies have utilized zinc sulfate, several other forms of zinc have been shown to be better absorbed and utilized, including zinc bound to picolinate, acetate, citrate, glycerate, or monomethionine. Although manufacturers may claim superiority for their particular zinc chelate, there is data to support each of these forms as being very well absorbed.

Cautions and Warnings

Do not take more than recommended amounts, especially if pregnant or lactating.

Possible Side Effects

If taken on an empty stomach (particularly if taking zinc sulfate), zinc supplementation can result in gastrointestinal upset and nausea. Prolonged intake at levels greater than 90 mg per day may lead to anemia, reduced HDL-cholesterol levels, and depressed immune function.

Drug Interactions

Zinc may decrease the absorption of tetracycline (Achromycin, Sumycin) and ciprofloxacin (Cipro). Take any zinc supplement at least two hours before or after taking these antibiotics.

Use of the following drugs increases the loss of zinc from the body or interferes with absorption: aspirin; AZT (azidothymidine); zidovudine (Retrovir); captopril (Capoten); enalapril (Vasotec); estrogens (oral contraceptives and Premarin); penicillamine

(Cuprimine); and the thiazide class of diuretics including chlorothiazide (Diuril and others), chlorthalidone (Hygroton and others), hydrochlorothiazide (Esidrix, HCTZ, HydroDIURIL, Oretic, and others), and metolazone (Mykrox and Zaroxolyn). Supplementation may be required to maintain zinc status in people taking these drugs.

Food Interactions

Zinc supplements should be taken separately from high fiber foods for best absorption. High dosages of calcium or iron can adversely affect zinc absorption.

When using zinc-containing lozenges for the relief of a sore throat or common cold, do not eat or drink citrus fruits or juices 1/2 hour before or after; the citric acid will negate the effect of zinc.

Usual Dosage

The dosage range for zinc supplementation for general health support and during pregnancy or lactation is 15 to 20 mg. When zinc supplementation is being used to address specific health concerns, the dosage range for men is 30 to 45 mg; for women 20 to 30 mg.

For a common cold, use lozenges that supply 15 to 25 mg of elemental zinc and dissolve them in the mouth without chewing every two waking hours after an initial double dose. Continue for up to seven days. Because high doses of zinc can actually impair immune function, a daily intake of greater than 150 mg of zinc for longer than one week cannot be recommended.

Recommended Dietary Allowance of Zinc

Infants
Birth–1 year   5 mg

Children
1–10 years   10 mg

Young Adults and Adults
Males 11+ years   15 mg
Females 11+ years   12 mg
Pregnant women   15 mg
Lactating women   19 mg

Overdosage

Acute toxicity is quite rare, as the ingestion of amounts large enough to cause toxicity symptoms (2 g per kg body weight) will usually provoke vomiting. Do the following in case of accidental overdose: If the victim is unconscious or having convulsions, call for an ambulance immediately. If you take the victim to an emergency room, be sure to bring the bottle or container with you. If the victim is conscious, call your local poison control center or a health care professional. The poison control center may suggest inducing vomiting with ipecac syrup (available without a prescription at any pharmacy). DO NOT induce vomiting unless specifically instructed to do so.

Special Populations

Pregnant/breast-feeding women

Zinc supplementation at recommended levels is considered beneficial during pregnancy and lactation.

Children

Suitable for children at one-half the adult dosage. Note: Toddlers and infants can choke on zinc lozenges, and children often cannot avoid chewing them.

Seniors

Zinc requirements may increase with increasing age due to impaired absorption and utilization.

PART III
Accessory Nutrients and Other Natural Products

This section contains nutrients that are not considered essential in the same manner that vitamins and minerals are, as well as other natural products. Included in this section are amino acids and their derivatives, fatty acids and phospholipids, fiber sources, glandular preparations, probiotics (bacterial products such as lactobacillus preparations), vitaminlike compounds, and other natural products.

Amino Acids and Their Derivatives

Amino acids are the building blocks of protein. The human body can manufacture most of the amino acids it requires. However, nine amino acids, termed "essential" amino acids, cannot be manufactured by the body and must be obtained from our dietary intake. These essential amino acids are arginine, histadine, isoleucine, lysine, methionine, phenylalanine, threonine, tryptophan, and valine.

Some amino acids act as neurotransmitters, chemicals that play a vital role in transmitting messages within the neurons of the brain. Some are involved in detoxification reactions and as cofactors in the building of structural and metabolic components. Some derivatives of amino acids, such as melatonin, also exert hormonelike activity.

Bioflavonoids

Bioflavonoids are a group of plant pigments that are largely responsible for the colors of many fruits and flowers. Recent research suggests that bioflavonoids may be useful in the treatment and prevention of many health conditions. In fact, many of the medicinal actions of foods, juices, herbs, and bee pollen are now known to be directly related to their bioflavonoid content. Over four thousand bioflavonoid compounds have been characterized and classified according to chemical structure. The most commonly used bioflavonoids are **citrus bioflavonoids** (including **rutin** and **hesperidin), grape seed** and **pine bark extracts,** and **quercetin**. Soy isoflavones are also included in the bioflavonoid category.

Fatty Acids and Phospholipids

Some experts estimate that as much as 80 percent of the United States population consumes an insufficient quantity of essential fatty acids. This dietary insufficiency presents a serious health threat to Americans. Essential fatty acids are important for the regulation of a host of bodily functions, including: inflammation, pain, and swelling; blood pressure; heart function; gastrointestinal function and secretions; kidney function and fluid balance; blood clotting and platelet aggregation; allergic response; nerve transmission; and steroid production and hormone synthesis.

The signs and symptoms of essential fatty acid deficiency may be either quite obvious or somewhat hard to detect. Following is a list of the most common signs and symptoms of EFA deficiency (they may also be indicative of other conditions):

Signs and Symptoms Typical of EFA Deficiency

Aching, sore joints
Angina, chest pain
Arthritis
Cardiovascular disease
Constipation
Cracked nails
Depression
Dry mucous membranes (tear ducts, mouth, vagina)
Dry, lifeless hair
Dry skin
Fatigue, malaise, lack of energy
Forgetfulness
Frequent colds and other sicknesses
High blood pressure
Immune system weakness
Indigestion, gas, bloating
Lack of endurance
Lack of motivation

Fiber Sources

The term "dietary fiber" refers to the components of plant cell wall and non-nutritive residues. Fiber is divided into two general categories—water soluble and water insoluble. Water-insoluble fiber, such as wheat bran, is a good laxative but lacks some of the beneficial effects noted with the water-soluble fibers. In addition to the well-known use of dietary fiber as a bulk-forming laxative, the principal use of supplemental dietary fiber is in the treatment of irritable bowel syndrome and other functional disturbances of the colon, elevated cholesterol levels, and obesity. For these purposes, water-soluble fiber is best. Examples of water-soluble fiber sources are psyllium, guar gum, oat bran, glucomannan, gum karaya, chitosan, and pectin.

Glandular preparations

Historically, glandular therapy has been an important form of medicine. The basic concept underlying the medicinal use of glandular substances from animals is that "like heals like." For example, to strengthen the adrenal glands, a person would eat the adrenal glands from an animal.

Dietary supplements containing animal parts—for instance, dried and ground thymus gland or brain tissue—are marketed to support the function of related human tissues. Since the early '90s, supplement manufacturers have been alerted to potential contamination by bovine spongiform encephalopathy (BSE), or mad cow disease, by both the U.S. Department of Agriculture (USDA) and the FDA. In an alert published January 24, 2001, the FDA further asked manufacturers of cosmetic and dietary supplement products to "assure, with a high degree of certainty," that bovine materials they purchase do not come from countries where BSE outbreaks have been identified. In a survey of companies belonging to the National Nutritional Foods Association, all members who manufactured products from bovine tissue reported that they were in compliance with the FDA's directive regarding imports. They further reported that they required a BSE-free certificate of analysis of the raw materials even from approved sources. These manufacturers also typically screen for other unwanted ingredients, such as hormones and heavy metals.

Probiotics

Probiotics are products containing bacteria that are found in the human intestine that are considered beneficial to our health. At least four hundred different species of microflora colonize the human gastrointestinal tract. The types of bacteria and other organisms that colonize our intestinal tract play a major role in our health, as the intestinal flora are intimately involved in nutritional status and affect immune system function, the risk of cancer, cholesterol metabolism, toxin load, and aging. The most important healthful bacteria are certain species in the genera *Lactobacillus* and *Bifidobacterium.*

Vitaminlike Compounds

More and more research indicates that accessory nutrients play a major role in preventing and treating illness, although most are not considered essential in the same manner as vitamins and minerals. The compounds in this category are important for maintaining normal body functions and structures.

Other Natural Products

This category contains products that are of a natural origin that do not easily fall into one of the more recognized categories. It includes hormones like DHEA and androstenedione; bee products like propolis and royal jelly; medicinal mushrooms (e.g., reishi, shiitake, maitake); and other substances.

Format for Entries

The format of the entries in this section follows the outline as presented in "How to Use This Book."

Keep in mind that the ratings on effectiveness and safety refer to the following:

Effectiveness

A = Excellent results in multiple double-blind studies

B+ = Very good results in a small number of double-blind studies

B = Some clinical evidence of effectiveness

B– = Some clinical evidence of effectiveness, but also some studies showing no effect

C = Strong historical use or scientific rationale but no clinical trials to show effectiveness in humans

D = No significant documentation of historical use or scientific rationale, or majority of clinical studies show no effect

F = Documentation that it is *not* effective

Safety

A = Excellent safety profile

B = Good safety profile

C = Generally regarded as safe at recommended levels

D = Generally regarded as safe at recommended levels but must be used with caution

F = Potentially dangerous, should not be used

Adrenal Extracts

Used For

Whole adrenal extracts

Energy
Effectiveness: C   Safety: C

Stress
Effectiveness: C   Safety: C

Reduced resistance
Effectiveness: C   Safety: C

Adrenal cortex extracts

Allergies (e.g., asthma, eczema)
Effectiveness: C   Safety: C

Inflammatory conditions (psoriasis, rheumatoid arthritis)
Effectiveness: C   Safety: C

General Information

The adrenal glands are a pair of small glands that lie just above the kidneys. Adrenal extracts are derived from the adrenal glands from bovine (beef) sources. Commercially available adrenal extracts are made using the whole gland (whole or total adrenal extracts) or just the cortex or outer portion of the gland (adrenal cortex extracts).

Adrenal extracts have been used in medicine since 1931, yet there is little in the area of scientific documentation. The possible benefits in these applications are thought to be the result of a combination of supplying low levels of adrenal hormones and promoting improved adrenal function. The adrenal medulla secretes the hormones epinephrine (adrenaline) and norepinephrine (noradrenaline), while the adrenal cortex secretes an entirely different group of hormones called corticosteroids. Although all corticosteroids have similar chemical formulas, they differ in function. The three major types of corticosteroids are mineralcorticoids (e.g., aldosterone), glucocorticoids (cortisone), and 17-ketosteroids (e.g., DHEA). The use of adrenal extracts has declined with the increase in popularity of using isolated adrenal hormones such as **pregnenolone** and **DHEA**.

Whole adrenal extracts (usually in combination with essential nutrients required for proper adrenal function) are most often used in cases of low adrenal function presenting as fatigue, inability to cope with stress, and reduced resistance. Because extracts made from the adrenal cortex contain small amounts of corticosteroids, they are typically used as "natural" cortisone in severe cases of allergy and inflammation (asthma, eczema, psoriasis, rheumatoid arthritis, etc.). The effectiveness of adrenal extracts in these applications has not been sufficiently evaluated.

Available Forms

Adrenal extracts are available in capsules or tablets.

Cautions and Warnings

None known.

Possible Side Effects

Stomach irritation and/or nausea are a common side effect, especially with higher-potency products.

Other possible side effects include a general stimulatory effect that may manifest itself as anxiety, irritability, and/or insomnia.

Drug Interactions

None known.

Food and Nutrient Interactions

Generally recommended to be taken on an empty stomach.

Usual Dosage

The dosage of adrenal extract will depend upon the quality and potency of the product. Follow the recommendations given on the product label or those given by your health care provider.

Overdosage

Overdosage may produce signs and symptoms of corticosteroid excess similar to those experienced with the drug prednisone. However, serious side effects are more likely to occur when adrenal extracts are taken in high doses over a long period of time. The number and severity of side effects depend on dosage and length of treatment. With prednisone at lower doses (less than 10 mg per day) the most notable side effects are usually increased appetite, weight gain, retention of salt and water, and increased susceptibility to infection. These side effects are almost always expected with corticosteroids such as prednisone.

Common side effects of long-term corticosteroid use at higher dosage levels include depression and other mental/emotional disturbances (up to 57 percent of patients being treated with high doses of prednisone for long periods of time), high blood pressure, diabetes, peptic ulcers, acne, excessive facial hair in women, insomnia, muscle cramps and weakness, thinning and weakening of the skin, osteoporosis, and susceptibility to the formation of blood clots.

Special Populations

Pregnant/breast-feeding women
Since no safety data exist for use during pregnancy or breast-feeding, use of this product is not recommended.

Children
Suitable for children over the age of six years at one-half the adult dosage.

Seniors
Seniors tend to be more susceptible to the stomach irritation and nausea that may be caused by these products.

Androstenedione

Used For

Boosting testosterone levels
Effectiveness: B   Safety: F

Increasing strength and muscle growth
Effectiveness: B   Safety: F

General Information

Androstenedione is a natural prohormone, a substance that the body will change into a more active hormone. Androstenedione is a prohormone that can be converted into the hormones testosterone and estrogen. Androstenedione is found naturally in meats and even some plants.

Androstenedione, also called andro for short, was first seen in capsule form in the United States in the 1990s. However, the history of androstenedione goes back to at least 1935, when it was first synthesized. In 1936 it was shown that androstenedione exerted both androgenic (masculinizing) and anabolic (tissue-building) properties. The anabolic effects of androstenedione were ignored by the scientific community until 1962. At that time, two researchers conducted an experiment in which normal women were given either 100 mg of DHEA or 100 mg of androstenedione. The study found that both hormones led to elevated testosterone levels—but androstenedione increased testosterone levels twice as much as DHEA. In the women given DHEA, testosterone levels, normally less than 199 ng/dl, rose to 280 ng/dl within sixty minutes, while the group taking androstenedione had testosterone levels elevated as high as 660 mg/dl an hour later—a threefold increase above normal levels. Studies in men demonstrated that 50 mg of oral androstenedione can raise blood testosterone levels to 140–183 percent of normal.

While there is some evidence that androstenedione can raise testosterone levels in adult females and males, it should definitely not be used for this purpose in people below the age of thirty years, especially young men. When testosterone levels are already high, the body's normal metabolic pathways convert additional androstenedione into estrogen.

A 1999 article that appeared in the *Journal of the American Medical Association* clearly demonstrated that androstenedione should *not* be taken by young men and teenagers. It offers no benefit and carries with it significant health risks. The study, conducted at the University of Iowa, involved thirty healthy men age 19 to 29 with normal testosterone levels. Twenty of the men performed eight weeks of whole-body resistance training. During weeks one, two, four, five, seven, and eight, ten of the men were given 300 mg of androstenedione a day, and the others were given a placebo.

The researchers discovered that muscle strength did not differ between the placebo and androstenedione groups before training or after four and eight weeks of resistance training and supplementation. They also found that testosterone levels in the blood were not affected by the supplement intake, but that estrogen levels increased dramatically. There were also slightly higher levels of LDL ("bad") cholesterol and slightly lower levels of HDL ("good") cholesterol in the subjects who took androstenedione. The bottom line is that androstenedione provides no benefit to this age group but carries with it significant health risks.

Available Forms

Androstenedione is available in capsules and tablets as well as in a spray that is administered under the tongue (sublingually). There is also at least one androstenedione gum product. The sublingual administration of androstenedione may prove to be more advantageous. When androstenedione pills are swallowed, most of the active androstenedione gets metabolized in the liver. Only a small portion survives to add to the body's testosterone pool in the blood. In contrast, it is believed that a person would get much better absorption into the bloodstream by taking androstenedione as a sublingual spray or lozenge, which allows it to bypass the liver.

Cautions and Warnings

Androstenedione should not be used by children, adolescents, pregnant or lactating women, or anyone under the age of thirty unless under specific instructions from their physician.

Possible Side Effects

Women taking androstenedione may experience acne, increased facial and body hair, and a deepening of the voice due to the conversion of androstenedione to testosterone. Men typically do not experience any immediate or short-term side effects with androstenedione use. Most of the long-term health risks for androstenedione are not known. Currently available information suggests androstenedione would have the same long-term side effects noted for testosterone and estrogen. Perhaps the most worrisome of these long-term side effects is an increased risk of prostate cancer in men and an increased risk of breast cancer in women.

Drug Interactions

Androstenedione may interact with other sex hormones such as those in birth control pills, conjugated estrogens (such as Premarin), progesterone, and of course testosterone.

Food and Nutrient Interactions

Grapefruit consumption may further increase testosterone or estrogen levels if taken with androstenedione. Grapefruit contains high levels of a flavonoid (plant compound) called naringin. This substance reduces the activity of a group of enzymes that break down hormones and various drugs. If the hormones are not broken down, they remain in the body in higher concentrations. This effect may increase the risk of androstenedione use. Other citrus fruits are not a problem; they do not contain significant amounts of naringin but do have lots of other important nutrients and flavonoids.

Usual Dosage

For women, the typical recommendation is 25–50 mg of androstenedione three times per week. For men, the dosage is typically 50–100 mg taken at bedtime, or the same dose may be taken 30–60 minutes before exercise (purportedly for enhanced performance) or after completion of exercise (purportedly to enhance muscle recovery and growth).

Overdosage

The effects of an overdosage are unknown, but any overdose should definitely be avoided. Do the following in case of accidental overdose: If the victim is unconscious or having convulsions, call for an ambulance immediately. If you take the victim to an emergency room, be sure to bring the bottle or container with you. If the victim is conscious, call your local poison control center or a health care professional. The poison control center may suggest inducing vomiting with ipecac syrup (available without a prescription at any pharmacy). *Do not* induce vomiting unless specifically instructed to do so.

Special Populations

Pregnant/breast-feeding women
Must not be used during pregnancy and lactation.

Children
Must not be used by children or adolescents.

Seniors
Any man over the age of forty should have a prostate exam to rule out prostate cancer before beginning androstenedione use. Elevated levels of testosterone have been linked to an increase in prostate cancer risk.

Aortic Glycosaminoglycans

Used For

Disorders of the arteries

Cerebral vascular insufficiency
Effectiveness: A   Safety: A

Peripheral vascular insufficiency
Effectiveness: A   Safety: A

Disorders of the veins

Venous insufficiency and varicose veins
Effectiveness: A   Safety: A

Hemorrhoids
Effectiveness: A   Safety: A

General Information

The aorta is the main artery of the human body. It arises directly from the heart to supply oxygenated blood to all other arteries of the body. The structural support of the aorta is provided by the presence of molecules known as glycosaminoglycans (GAGs). These molecules act as skeletal components of the artery's ground substance, the intracellular cement that holds the tissue together.

Aortic GAGs as a nutritional supplement refers to a mixture of highly purified GAGs derived from bovine (beef) aortas. This product is composed of GAGs naturally present in the human aorta, including dermatan sulfate, heparan sulfate, hyaluronic acid, chondroitin sulfate, and related compounds. It has been shown to protect and promote normal artery and vein function.

Over fifty clinical studies have shown aortic GAGs to be effective in a number of vascular disorders, including cerebral vascular insufficiency, peripheral arterial insufficiency, venous insufficiency and varicose veins, and hemorrhoids. Significant improvements in both symptoms and blood flow have been noted.

Disorders of the arteries

GAGs are essential for maintaining the health of arteries. Supplementing the diet with aortic GAGs has been shown to increase the integrity and function of arteries throughout the body. In addition, aortic GAGs have many important effects that interfere with the process of atherosclerosis (hardening of the arteries), including preventing damage to the surface of the artery, formation of damaging blood clots, and formation of fat and cholesterol deposits. Aortic GAGs have also demonstrated a small effect on lowering total blood cholesterol levels while raising the level of protective HDL cholesterol.

Several clinical studies have demonstrated that supplementing the diet with aortic GAGs is effective in improving decreased blood flow. Symptoms of cerebral vascular insufficiency can include short-term memory loss, vertigo, headache, ringing in the ears, and depression. These symptoms are often referred to as symptoms of aging and are almost entirely the result of a reduced supply of blood and oxygen to the brain due to atherosclerosis. Symptoms of peripheral vascular disease can include coldness of hands or feet, pain, muscle cramps, and (in males) impotence.

Significant improvements in both symptoms and blood flow after use of aortic GAGs have been noted in these clinical studies.

Disorders of veins

GAGs provide the skeletal framework of the vein and are therefore essential in maintaining the structure and integrity of veins. Veins are fairly fragile structures. Without proper structural support provided by GAGs, the veins will eventually dilate, and valve damage will occur. When the valves become damaged, the increased pressure results in the bulging veins known as varicose veins. Hemorrhoids are varicose veins in the rectal area.

Aortic GAGs have demonstrated impressive clinical results in improving the function and structure of both veins and arteries. Individuals with poor vein function in the legs may have varicose veins and typically experience such symptoms as a sense of heaviness in the legs, a tingling sensation, fluid retention, itching, and painful cramps. These symptoms are reduced with aortic GAGs due to the substance's ability to improve the structure and function of the vein, thereby allowing improved blood flow. It has been suggested that aortic GAGs should be used as the drug of first choice in the treatment of hemorrhoids because double-blind studies have shown them to be superior to other natural products commonly used in treating hemorrhoids, such as flavonoids and flavonoid-rich extracts including bilberry extract.

Available Forms

Aortic GAGs are available in capsule form. Brands include Aorta-Glycan.

Cautions and Warnings

None known.

Possible Side Effects

None known.

Drug Interactions

None known.

Food and Nutrient Interactions

None known.

Usual Dosage

50 to 100 mg daily.

Overdosage

None known.

Special Populations

Pregnant/breast-feeding women
Considered safe during pregnancy and lactation.

Children
Suitable for children at one-half the adult dosage.

Seniors
No special precautions are known.

Arginine

Used For

Cardiovascular disease
Effectiveness: A   Safety: A

Erectile dysfunction
Effectiveness: B   Safety: A

Interstitial cystitis
Effectiveness: B   Safety: A

Male infertility
Effectiveness: B   Safety: A

Promotion of growth hormone secretion
Effectiveness: B   Safety: A

General Information

Arginine is an amino acid that plays an important role in wound healing, detoxification reactions, immune functions, and the secretion of several hormones, including insulin and growth hormone. Recently there has been a considerable amount of scientific investigation regarding arginine's role in the formation of nitric oxide. This compound exerts a relaxing effect on blood vessels, thereby improving blood flow. Normally the body makes enough arginine, even when the diet is lacking. However, in some instances the body may not be able to keep up with increased requirements, and supplementation may prove useful.

Cardiovascular disease
Arginine supplementation has been shown to be beneficial in a number of cardiovascular diseases including angina pectoris, congestive heart failure, high blood pressure, and peripheral vascular insufficiency (decreased blood flow to the legs or arms). Its beneficial effect in all of these disorders shares a common mechanism—increasing nitric oxide levels. Nitric oxide plays a central role in regulating blood flow. By increasing nitric oxide levels, arginine supplementation improves blood flow, reduces blood clot formation, and improves blood fluidity (the blood becomes less viscous and therefore flows through blood ves-

sels more easily). The degree of improvement offered by arginine supplementation in angina and other cardiovascular diseases can be quite significant.

Erectile dysfunction

Arginine, by raising the production of nitric oxide, may help improve erectile dysfunction by improving blood flow to erectile tissues. In a double-blind study a proprietary formula containing arginine (ArginMax) produced improvement in ability to maintain an erection during intercourse in 87.5 percent of subjects compared to only 22.2 percent in the placebo group.

Interstitial cystitis

Interstitial cystitis is characterized by symptoms typical of a urinary tract infection (pain or burning upon urination, sense of urgency, increased urinary frequency, etc.), but without evidence of an infection. Compared to people without interstitial cystitis, nitric oxide manufacture is decreased in patients with chronic interstitial cystitis. Nitric oxide plays a role in bladder function. Since arginine is the building block for nitric oxide manufacture, researchers have sought to find out if arginine supplementation could improve interstitial cystitis. In a pilot study, good results were observed after one month of use in ten patients receiving 1,500 mg of arginine daily. In a follow-up double-blind study, fifty-three interstitial cystitis patients were assigned to receive daily 1,500 mg arginine or placebo orally for three months. Results indicated that 48 percent of the patients receiving arginine compared to 24 percent of the placebo group experienced a decrease in pain intensity and a tendency toward improvement in urgency and frequency of pain. These results indicate that arginine is helpful in some interstitial cystitis patients. Further research is needed to help identify responders.

Male infertility

Arginine supplementation is often but not always an effective measure to improve male fertility. The critical factor appears to be the sperm count. If the sperm count is less than 20 million per ml, arginine supplementation is less likely to be of benefit. In order to be effective, it appears that the dosage of arginine needs to be at least 4 g a day for three months. In perhaps the most favorable study, 74 percent of 178 men with low sperm count had significant improvements in sperm count and motility. Arginine therapy should be reserved for use after other nutritional measures have been tried.

Promotion of growth hormone secretion

One of the more popular uses of arginine has been in the promotion of the secretion of growth hormone by the pituitary gland. Growth hormone is responsible for stimulating muscle and skeletal growth. Bodybuilders often utilize arginine supplementation in an attempt to boost the natural output of growth hormone. There appears to be some validation for this use. The effect of arginine increasing growth hormone output is well accepted. In fact, measuring growth hormone levels in the blood after arginine is administered intravenously is used to gauge whether a child or adult is secreting enough growth hormone. However, arginine supplementation does not appear to be able to enhance growth hormone release in older subjects.

Available Forms

Arginine is available as L-arginine in powder form as well as in capsules, tablets, and food bars. It is most often part of a combination formula rather than as a single entity. Brand names available include ArginMax.

Cautions and Warnings

Should not be used in dosages above 20 g daily or by patients with advanced kidney or liver disease unless under direct physician supervision.

Possible Side Effects

Arginine is one of the least toxic amino acids. Used at appropriate dosages, side effects are uncommon. Nausea, vomiting, flushing of the skin, and headache may be experienced at dosages beyond 30 g per day. Because the herpes virus utilizes arginine, supplementation of arginine in people harboring the herpes virus may lead to reactivation. For this reason, supplementation with an equal amount of **lysine** is often recommended to counteract this possibility.

Drug Interactions

Preliminary research indicates that arginine may increase the effects of various drugs used to lower blood pressure (e.g., enalapril and hydrochlorothiazide).

Food and Nutrient Interactions

None known.

Usual Dosage

The dosage of arginine is based upon its application.

Cardiovascular disease: Good results have been
   achieved with daily dosages in the 6–8 g/day
   range. However, better results have been shown
   with dosages in the 18–20 g/day range.
Interstitial cystitis: 1,500 mg/day
Male infertility: 4,000–6,000 mg/day
Promotion of growth hormone secretion: 5–10 g/day

Overdosage

Although there have been no reports of overdosage
with oral preparations, injection of arginine at dosages
greater than 3 g per kg (2.2 pounds) body weight can
be fatal. Achieving these dangerous levels with oral
supplementation is highly unlikely. Nonetheless, in
cases of suspected overdosage of arginine, the subject should be transported to an emergency room immediately.

Special Populations

Pregnant/breast-feeding women
   Considered safe during pregnancy and lactation.

Children
   Not suitable for children unless under the supervision of a health care professional.

Seniors
   No special precautions are known.

Aspergillus Enzymes

Used For

Food allergies
Effectiveness: C   Safety: C

Pancreatic insufficiency
Effectiveness: B   Safety: C

Peripheral vascular disease
Effectiveness: C   Safety: C

General Information

Aspergillus oryzae is a fungus that produces enzymes important in the production of fermented soy foods such as soy sauce, tamari, and miso. These same enzymes are also used for medicinal purposes similar to the applications of **pancreatin** and **bromelain**. The advantages of the enzymes derived from *A. oryzae* are that they possess an unusually high stability and activity under a broader range of pH conditions. These properties distinguish them from animal enzymes such as pepsin, pancreatin, trypsin, chymotrypsin, pancrelipase, and pancreatic amylase, which require pH conditions often not found in those with impaired health. For example, pepsin is active only below a pH of about 4.5, while pancreatin has digestive activity only in an alkaline medium. In contrast, some preparations of *A. oryzae* enzymes are stable and active at pH values of 2 through 12. The primary uses of *A. oryzae* enzyme preparations include pancreatic insufficiency.

Food allergies

It has been suggested that *A. oryzae* enzyme preparations may be helpful in dealing with food allergies as well as sensitivities to gluten (a substance found in wheat, rye, and other grains). However, these applications have not been evaluated in detailed clinical trials. In order for a food molecule to produce an allergic response, it must be fairly large. The concept behind the use of *A. oryzae* enzymes in food allergies is that they partially or fully break down the large food molecule into smaller, nonallergenic molecules.

Pancreatic insufficiency

Decreased output of pancreatic enzymes can lead to poor digestion and poor assimilation of protein and fat. Pancreatic insufficiency is characterized by impaired digestion, malabsorption, nutrient deficiencies, and abdominal discomfort. The most severe level of pancreatic insufficiency is seen in cystic fibrosis. Although cystic fibrosis is quite rare, mild pancreatic insufficiency is thought to be a relatively common condition, especially in the elderly. Enzyme preparations from *A. oryzae* have been shown to be highly effective in treating pancreatic insufficiency, evidenced by an improvement in the absorption of fat and the breakdown of protein as well as improvements in symptoms of indigestion. In fact, the fungal enzyme preparation was shown to be superior to pancreatin in head-to-head comparison studies.

Peripheral vascular disease

In peripheral vascular disease, arterial obstruction or narrowing causes a reduction in blood flow during exercise or at rest. In addition to experiencing cold hands or feet or a pins-and-needles sensation, many people with peripheral vascular disease experience pain upon exertion (intermittent claudication). The pain usually occurs in the calf and is described as a cramp, tightness, or severe fatigue. The pain of intermittent claudication is quite similar to the chest pain associated with angina. Numerous studies have confirmed the effectiveness of a proteolytic (protein-digesting) enzyme derived from *A. oryzae* in treating peripheral vascular disease and intermittent claudication. However, these studies used an intravenous preparation. It is not known whether oral supplementation would produce similar results.

Available Forms

Aspergillus oryzae enzyme preparations are available in capsule and tablet form.

Cautions and Warnings

Do not use if you suffer from gastritis or peptic ulcer. The enzymes can further irritate the stomach and tend to worsen symptoms.

Possible Side Effects

Generally well tolerated at recommended dosages.

Drug Interactions

None known.

Food and Nutrient Interactions

Generally, enzyme preparations are recommended on an empty stomach (for nondigestive purposes) or at the very beginning of a meal.

Usual Dosage

The dosage is based upon the activity of the various enzymes based upon either USP (United States Pharmacopoeia) or FCC (Food Chemicals Codex) methods. A dosage to be taken at the beginning of the meal should provide the following:

Protease	15,000–30,000 USP
Amylase	20,000–40,000 USP
Lipase	1,000–2,000 FCC lipase units

Overdosage

None known.

Special Populations

Pregnant/breast-feeding women
As the effects of aspergillus enzyme preparations during pregnancy and lactation have not been sufficiently evaluated, they should not be used during these times unless directed to do so by a physician.

Children
Suitable for children at one-half the adult dosage.

Seniors
No special precautions are known.

Bee Pollen

Used For

Allergies
Effectiveness: C   Safety: F

Boosting stamina and vitality
Effectiveness: C   Safety: D

General health tonic and source of nutrients
Effectiveness: C   Safety: D

General Information

Bee pollen comes from the male germ cell of flowering plants. The pollen is collected and brought to the hive, where the bees add enzymes and nectar to the pollen. Bee pollen is a complete protein (it typically is 10–35 percent total protein), as it contains all eight essential amino acids. Bee pollen also provides B vitamins, vitamin C, carotenes, at least twenty-eight minerals, DNA and RNA, numerous flavonoid molecules, and plant hormones. Bee pollen is used primarily as a general nutritional supplement and has been referred to as "nature's most perfect food."

Bee pollen needs to be differentiated from **propolis, royal jelly,** and **Cernilton** (flower pollen extract). While there are good scientific studies on these related products, there are insufficient scientific studies to evaluate any health-promoting effects of bee pollen. The studies that do exist are somewhat conflicting. For example, while there are studies that have shown bee pollen to exert energy-boosting effects in athletes, these studies were not very well designed. The bottom line is that the jury is still out on the health benefits of bee pollen.

Available Forms

Bee pollen is available in bulk as loose granules as well as in capsules and tablets.

Cautions and Warnings

Individuals with pollen-sensitive allergies such as asthma or hay fever should not use bee pollen. Although rare, severe and even fatal allergic reactions have been reported in people with asthma and hay fever who have taken bee pollen.

Possible Side Effects

Bee pollen is generally well tolerated with no side effects. Allergic reactions are rare but can include stomach upset, diarrhea, and asthma and hay-fever-like symptoms.

Drug Interactions

None known.

Food and Nutrient Interactions

None known.

Usual Dosage

Bee pollen is most commonly consumed as a food. Up to 1 tablespoon of bee pollen granules daily is the usual dosage. For other forms of bee pollen, follow the manufacturer's recommendation.

Overdosage

None known.

Special Populations

Pregnant/breast-feeding women
Considered safe during pregnancy and lactation.

Children
Suitable for children at one-half the adult dosage.

Seniors
No special precautions are known.

Beta-1,3-glucan

Used For

Enhancing immune function
Effectiveness: C   Safety: C

General Information

Beta-1,3-glucan is a sugar derived from the cell wall of baker's yeast. Numerous experimental studies in test tubes and animals have shown this substance to activate white blood cells. In fact, there have been over 1,600 research papers on beta-1,3-glucan since the 1960s. The research indicates that beta-1,3-glucan is very effective at activating a type of white blood cell known as macrophages. These cells compose the immune system's first line of defense against foreign invaders. A macrophage can recognize and kill tumor cells, remove cellular debris resulting from oxidative damage, speed up recovery of damaged tissue, and further activate other components of the immune system. Although the research in test tube and animal studies is positive, there still remain many questions about the effectiveness of beta-1,3-glucan as an oral supplement in humans. In short, most of the claims used to market beta-1,3-glucan are currently not substantiated by human research.

Available Forms

Beta-1,3-glucan is available in liquid form as well as in capsules and tablets.

Cautions and Warnings

None known.

Possible Side Effects

None known.

Drug Interactions

None known.

Food and Nutrient Interactions

Generally recommended to be taken on an empty stomach.

Usual Dosage

Beta-1,3-glucan is usually recommended in a dosage range of 50–100 mg daily, although some products contain as much as 500 mg per capsule.

Overdosage

None known.

Special Populations

Pregnant/breast-feeding women
Considered safe during pregnancy and lactation.

Children
Suitable for children at one-half the adult dosage.

Seniors
No special precautions are known.

Beta-sitosterol

Used For

Benign prostatic hyperplasia (prostate enlargement)
Effectiveness: B+   Safety: A

High cholesterol
Effectiveness: B–   Safety: A

General Information

Beta-sitosterol is a plant sterol, similar in structure to cholesterol, found naturally in corn, beans (especially soy), nuts, seeds, avocados, and vegetable oils. Since beta-sitosterol can block the absorption of cholesterol, most of the early research focused on its use in lowering cholesterol. Beta-sitosterol was shown in clinical trials to lower cholesterol levels by 9–20 percent when given in dosages ranging from 3 to 18 g daily. Beta-sitosterol is now rarely used to lower cholesterol levels. A similar compound, sitostanol, has replaced beta-sitosterol in this application and is now available in margarine products (e.g., Benecol). Sitostanol is effective at much lower dosages than beta-sitosterol.

Most of the recent interest in and use of beta-sitosterol has been in its ability to improve benign prostatic hyperplasia (BPH). In one of the better double-blind studies, two hundred men with BPH were given either beta-sitosterol (20 mg) or placebo three times daily. The beta-sitosterol group demonstrated significant improvements in maximum urine flow rate and the amount of urine left in the bladder after urination, both good indicators of bladder obstruction due to BPH. The daily dosage of 60 mg, however, can easily be achieved by dietary measures. For example, a 3½-ounce serving of soybeans, tofu, or other soy food provides approximately 90 mg of beta-sitosterol.

Available Forms

Beta-sitosterol is available in tablets and capsules.

Cautions and Warnings

If you suffer from a very rare genetic disorder known as familial hyper-beta-sitosterolemia (only a handful of cases have ever been reported) or suffer from xanthomas (yellowish fatty tumors of the skin, particularly around the eyes), avoid dietary and supplemental intake of beta-sitosterol.

Possible Side Effects

Side effects are very uncommon with beta-sitosterol. At dosages greater than 2,000 mg, beta-sitosterol may cause loose stools or diarrhea in some individuals.

Drug Interactions

None known.

Food and Nutrient Interactions

The absorption of beta-sitosterol is generally quite poor (less than 10 percent). Absorption may be increased by taking it with vegetable oils.

Usual Dosage

In the treatment of BPH, the typical dosage is 20 mg three times daily. For lowering cholesterol levels, dosages range from 3 to 18 g per day.

Overdosage

None known.

Special Populations

Pregnant/breast-feeding women
Considered safe during pregnancy and lactation.

Children
Suitable for use in children, but there is no real indication for use.

Seniors
No special precautions are known.

Betaine (Trimethylglycine)

Used For

Alcohol-induced fatty liver
Effectiveness: B   Safety: A

Homocysteine elevations
Effectiveness: B–   Safety: A

Liver support
Effectiveness: B   Safety: A

General Information

Betaine (trimethylglycine) works very closely with choline, folic acid, vitamin B_{12}, and a form of the amino acid methionine known as SAMe (S-adenosylmethionine). All of these compounds function as methyl donors—they carry and donate methyl molecules to facilitate necessary chemical reactions. The donation of methyl groups by betaine is very important to proper liver function, cellular replication, and detoxification reactions. Betaine also plays a role in the manufacture of carnitine and serves to protect the kidneys from damage.

Betaine has been reported to play a role in reducing blood levels of homocysteine, a toxic product of amino acid metabolism that is believed to promote atherosclerosis and osteoporosis. While the main nutrients involved in controlling homocysteine levels are folic acid, vitamin B_6, and vitamin B_{12}, betaine has been reported to be helpful in occasional individuals whose elevated homocysteine levels did not improve with these other nutrients as well as in certain rare genetic disorders involving cysteine metabolism. In normal situations, however, or with supplementation of the other methyl donors, betaine is not likely to produce any lowering effect on homocysteine levels. Its primary use as a nutritional supplement is in supporting proper liver function.

Betaine is often referred to as a lipotropic factor because of its ability to help the liver process fats (lipids). In animal studies, betaine supplementation has been shown to protect against chemical damage to the liver. The first stage of liver damage as a result of alcohol is the accumulation of fat in the liver (alcohol-induced fatty liver disease). Betaine, because of its lipotropic effects, has demonstrated significant benefits in animal models and human clinical studies. Betaine has been studied in clinical trials conducted in Germany, Italy, and France in the treatment of alcohol-related liver disease. Some success was noted in these studies, but the popularity of betaine for alcohol-related liver disease has been supplanted by SAMe and milk thistle extract. However, it has recently been suggested that betaine may be a more cost-effective method as a first-step therapy for alcohol-induced fatty liver disease.

Available Forms

Dietary sources of betaine include fish, beets, and legumes. Betaine is most widely available as betaine hydrochloride, but that form is used primarily as a source of hydrochloric acid for individuals with hypochlorhydria (low stomach acid). The forms used specifically to provide betaine are betaine citrate and betaine aspartate. These are the forms that have been used to improve liver function.

Cautions and Warnings

None known.

Possible Side Effects

No side effects with betaine at recommended levels have been noted. As a betaine-containing substance in the urine (glycine-betaine) reduced the effectiveness of antibiotic therapy of urinary tract infections, and compounds similar to betaine have been found to enhance the growth of certain bacteria that cause urinary tract infections, betaine supplementation may be contraindicated during an active urinary tract infection.

Drug Interactions

A betaine-containing substance in the urine (glycine-betaine) reduced the effectiveness of antibiotic therapy of urinary tract infections. Whether this interaction also occurs with betaine supplementation is not known.

Food and Nutrient Interactions

None known.

Usual Dosage

For betaine citrate or betaine aspartate the usual recommended level for supplementation in alcohol-induced fatty liver is 1,000 to 2,000 mg three times daily. Lower levels are often used as nutritional support for general liver health.

Overdosage

None known.

Special Populations

Pregnant/breast-feeding women
Considered safe during pregnancy and lactation.

Children
Suitable for children at one-half the adult dosage.

Seniors
No special precautions are known.

Betaine Hydrochloride

Used For

Hypochlorhydria (low output of stomach acid)
Effectiveness: C   Safety: C

General Information

Betaine hydrochloride is used in the treatment of hypochlorhydria (deficient secretion of gastric hydrochloric acid) and achlorhydria (complete absence of gastric acid secretion). There are many symptoms and signs that suggest impaired gastric acid secretion, including bloating, belching, burning, and flatulence immediately after meals; a sense of pressure or fullness after eating; and indigestion, diarrhea, or constipation. Betaine hydrochloride can bring significant relief in cases of these symptoms by acting as a digestive aid.

Available Forms

Betaine hydrochloride is available in capsules or tablets.

Cautions and Warnings

Betaine hydrochloride should not be used in people with current peptic ulcers unless under the direct advice of a health care professional.

Possible Side Effects

May cause ulcer formation, especially at higher dosages.

Drug Interactions

None known.

Food and Nutrient Interactions

Betaine hydrochloride is best used during or immediately after meals.

Usual Dosage

A popular technique for determining dosage is the following challenge method:

1. Begin by taking one tablet or capsule containing 10 grains (600 mg) of hydrochloric acid at your next large meal. If this does not aggravate your symptoms, at every meal after that of the same size take one more tablet or capsule (one at the next meal, two at the meal after that, then three at the next meal).
2. Continue to increase the dose until you reach seven tablets or when you feel warmth in your stomach, whichever occurs first. A feeling of warmth in the stomach means that you have taken too many tablets for that meal, and you need to take one less tablet for that meal size. It is a good idea to try the larger dose again at another meal to make sure that it was the hydrochloric acid that caused the warmth and not something else.
3. After you have found the largest dose that you can take at your large meals without feeling any warmth, maintain that dose at all meals of similar size. You will need to take less at smaller meals.
4. When taking a number of tablets or capsules, it is best to take them throughout the meal.
5. As your stomach begins to regain the ability to produce the amount of hydrochloric acid needed to properly digest your food, you will notice the warm feeling again and will have to cut down the dose level.

Overdosage

Do the following in case of accidental overdose: If the victim is unconscious or having convulsions, call for an ambulance immediately. If you take the victim to an emergency room, be sure to bring the bottle or container with you. If the victim is conscious, neutralize the acid by taking an antacid preparation according to label instructions.

Special Populations

Pregnant/breast-feeding women
Because the effects of betaine hydrochloride during pregnancy and lactation have not been sufficiently studied, it is generally advised that it not be taken by women who are planning a pregnancy or who are pregnant or breast-feeding.

Children
Suitable for children at one-half the adult dosage.

Seniors
No special precautions are known.

Bifidobacteria

Used For

Promotion of healthy gut flora
Effectiveness: B   Safety: C

General Information

Bifidobacterium bifidum is one of the important "friendly" bacteria that normally inhabits the human gastrointestinal tract. *B. bifidum* is especially important during infancy. It is first introduced through breast-feeding to the sterile gut of the infant, after which large numbers are soon observed in the feces. Later, other bacteria (including such beneficial strains as *Lactobacillus acidophilus* and *L. rhamnosus)* become established in the gut through contact with the world. The therapeutic use of *B. bifidum* is not as well studied as *Lactobacillus acidophilus,* but it is generally recommended to promote healthy gut flora, especially in infants.

Available Forms

B. bifidum products are available in powder, liquid, tablet, and capsule form. It is often combined with *L. acidophilus.* Brand names available include Baby Bifidus and Lifestart Infant Probiotic.

Cautions and Warnings

None known.

Possible Side Effects

None known.

Drug Interactions

B. bifidum is negatively affected by alcohol and antibiotics.

Food and Nutrient Interactions

Yogurt and other dairy products appear to promote the growth of *B. bifidum* when administered simultaneously with the bacteria. Fructooligosaccha-rides (FOS) promote the growth of *B. bifidum.*

Usual Dosage

The dosage is based upon the number of live organ-isms. The ingestion of 1 billion to 10 billion viable *B. bifidum* cells daily is a sufficient dosage for most people. Amounts exceeding this may induce mild gastroin-testinal disturbances, while smaller amounts may not be able to colonize the gastrointestinal tract.

Overdosage

None known.

Special Populations

Pregnant/breast-feeding women
Considered safe during pregnancy and lactation.

Children
Suitable for children at one-half the adult dosage.

Seniors
No special precautions are known.

Bioflavonoids

General Information

Bioflavonoids are a group of plant pigments that are largely responsible for the colors of many fruits and flowers. Recent research suggests that bioflavonoids may be useful in the treatment and prevention of many health conditions. In fact, many of the medicinal actions of foods, juices, herbs, and bee pollen are now known to be directly related to their bioflavonoid content. Over four thousand bioflavonoid compounds have been characterized and classified according to chemical structure. The most commonly used bioflavonoids are **citrus bioflavonoids** (including **rutin** and **hesperidin), grape seed** and **pine bark extracts,** and **quercetin.**

Bismuth Subcitrate

Used For

Diarrhea
Effectiveness: B+   Safety: D

Gastritis
Effectiveness: A   Safety: D

Heartburn
Effectiveness: A   Safety: D

Peptic ulcer
Effectiveness: A   Safety: D

General Information

Bismuth is a naturally occurring mineral that can act as an antacid as well as exert activity against *Helicobacter pylori*—a bacterium linked to peptic ulcer disease, gastritis, and stomach cancer. It has been shown that 90–100 percent of patients with duodenal ulcers, 70 percent with gastric ulcers, and about 50 percent of people over the age of fifty test positive for *H. pylori.* The presence of *H. pylori* is determined by determining the level of antibodies to *H. pylori* in the blood or saliva, or by culturing material collected during an endoscopic procedure.

Eradication of *H. pylori* with the use of antibiotics is emerging as a primary therapy of peptic ulcer disease. One of the key advantages of bismuth preparations over standard antibiotic approaches is that while *H. pylori* may develop resistance to various antibiotics, it is very unlikely to develop resistance to bismuth.

The best-known and most widely used bismuth preparation is bismuth subsalicylate (Pepto-Bismol). However, bismuth subcitrate has produced the best results against *H. pylori* and in the treatment of non-ulcer-related indigestion as well as peptic ulcers.

Available Forms

Bismuth subcitrate is available in liquid form and in capsules and tablets.

Cautions and Warnings

Bismuth preparations should not be used for more than two days to control diarrhea unless prescribed by a doctor, as most common causes of diarrhea resolve within twenty-four to forty-eight hours.

Bismuth subcitrate should not be used for more than eight weeks in the treatment of gastritis or peptic ulcers.

Bismuth subcitrate should not be taken by people with severe kidney disease.

Possible Side Effects

Bismuth preparations are extremely safe when taken at prescribed dosages for no longer than eight weeks. Bismuth subcitrate may cause a temporary and harmless darkening of the tongue and/or stool. Gastric upset with nausea and vomiting has also been reported.

Drug Interactions

Bismuth should not be taken at the same time as antacids or drugs that inhibit stomach acid output, such as famotidine (Pepcid), nizatidine (Axid), cimetidine (Tagamet), and ranitidine (Zantac).

Food and Nutrient Interactions

Should not be taken at the same time with milk or other dairy products. Generally recommended to be taken before meals.

Usual Dosage

The usual dosage for bismuth subcitrate is 240 mg twice daily before meals for a period of four weeks, extended to eight weeks if necessary. Maintenance therapy or long-term use of bismuth preparations is not appropriate.

Overdosage

Bismuth is essentially nontoxic in ordinary amounts, but prolonged or excessive use may lead to toxicity. Although there have been no reports of toxicity, long-term use or excessive dosages could cause mental confusion, memory loss, loss of coordination, slurred speech, joint pain, or muscle twitching and spasm.

Special Populations

Pregnant/breast-feeding women
Since there is insufficient data on its use during pregnancy and lactation, bismuth subcitrate should not be used.

Children
Suitable for children at one-half the adult dosage. Bismuth subsalicylate (Pepto-Bismol), because of its salicylate content (salicylate is an aspirinlike substance), should not be taken in children recovering from colds, the flu, chicken pox, or other viral infection, as it may mask the nausea and vomiting associated with Reye's syndrome, a rare but serious illness. This warning does not apply to bismuth subcitrate.

Seniors
No special precautions are known.

Black Currant Seed Oil (*see* Gamma-linolenic Acid)

General Information

Black currant seed oil is valued for its high content of polyunsaturated oils. It contains 17 percent gamma-linolenic acid, 13 percent alpha-linolenic acid, and 47 percent linoleic acid, making it an excellent source of essential fatty acids. It is available in liquid form and in capsules.

Borage Oil
(*see* Gamma-linolenic Acid)

General Information

Borage oil is valued for its high content of polyunsaturated oils. It contains 22 percent gamma-linolenic acid and 35 percent linoleic acid, making it an excellent source of essential fatty acids. It is available in liquid form and in capsules.

Bovine Colostrum

Used For

Boosting immune function
Effectiveness: B   Safety: C

Enhancing lean body weight
Effectiveness: B   Safety: C

Protection against ulcer formation
Effectiveness: B   Safety: C

General Information

Bovine colostrum is the liquid produced from the mammary glands of cows during the first twenty-four to forty-eight hours after giving birth. Bovine colostrum is rich in immunoglobulins (antibodies), growth factors, various proteins, and enzymes. Although various components of bovine colostrum theoretically may produce some benefits, there are few studies in which bovine colostrum in the forms that are commercially available has been given to humans.

Boosting immune function

There is absolutely no question that human colostrum transfers many important active immune-enhancing compounds to the human newborn. The question regarding bovine colostrum is if these factors meant for the calf exert any immune-enhancing effects in humans. The research studies used to support the claim that colostrum fights infections used colostrum derived from cows immunized in a way that caused them to produce unusually large amounts of a specific antibody in their colostrum. For example, in a double-blind study, children with diarrhea caused by a rotavirus were treated with immunoglobulins extracted from colostrum derived from cows immunized with rotavirus. Compared with the placebo, administration of the immunoglobulins significantly reduced the amount of diarrhea and the amount of oral rehydration solution required. In addition, the rotavirus was eliminated from the stool significantly more rapidly in the immunoglobulin group than in the placebo group (1.5 days versus 2.9 days).

In addition to a positive effect against acute rotavirus diarrhea, there is also evidence that specific

forms of colostrum (derived from specially immunized cows) are effective against diarrhea caused by
Cryptosporidium parvum, Helicobacter pylori, and
Clostridium difficile. However, it is not known
whether commercially available colostrum provides
significant amounts of the specific immunoglobulins that are active against these organisms. Furthermore, unless the immunoglobulins are present in
high enough concentrations, the preparation is not
likely to be effective, since there is evidence that the
majority of the antimicrobial effect of both bovine
colostrum and one of its chief antibiotic components
(lactoferrin) are destroyed by gastric secretions and
by the digestive enzyme trypsin.

Enhancing lean body weight

Bovine colostrum contains bovine versions of
many human growth factors, including insulinlike
growth factor, transforming growth factor, epithelial
growth factor, and even growth hormone, which are
capable of stimulating muscle growth. The concentration of bovine insulinlike growth factor 1 (ILGF-1)
in colostrum ranges from 200 to 2,000 mcg/L, compared with less than 10 mcg/L in normal cow's milk.
Thus, in theory, bovine colostrum might be able to
stimulate muscle growth in humans. However, although bovine ILGF-1 has been shown to be identical to human ILGF-1 in some analytical studies and
to be absorbed and transported into the circulation
in calves, the effect of bovine ILGF-1 and other
bovine growth substances in humans after oral administration has not been determined in clinical
trials.

In a preliminary study of male athletes, supplementation with 125 ml of colostrum per day for eight
days produced a statistically significant increase in
the serum concentration of insulinlike growth factor;

however, the magnitude of the increase was small, and the clinical significance of that change is not clear. Thus, claims that bovine colostrum can help burn fat and promote muscle growth by raising the level of ILGF-1 or other molecules must be considered premature.

Protection against ulcer formation

Bovine colostrum may be helpful in protecting against peptic ulcer formation caused by non-steroidal anti-inflammatory drugs such as aspirin, ibuprofen, and indomethacin. In a study in rats, pre-treatment with 0.5 or 1 ml of a colostrum preparation reduced indomethacin-induced gastric injury by 30 percent and 60 percent, respectively. Whether bovine colostrum exerts this effect in humans has not been determined.

Available Forms

Bovine colostrum is available in capsules, tablets, powdered drink mixes, liquid preparations, food bars, and skin care products.

Cautions and Warnings

None known.

Possible Side Effects

Side effects are uncommon. Allergic reactions are possible in people who are allergic to cow's milk.

Drug Interactions

None known.

Food and Nutrient Interactions

None known.

Usual Dosage

Most manufacturers recommend a daily dosage of 1,000 to 4,000 mg of freeze-dried colostrum.

Overdosage

None known.

Special Populations

Pregnant/breast-feeding women
Considered safe during pregnancy and lactation.

Children
Suitable for children at one-half the adult dosage.

Seniors
No special precautions are known.

Bovine Tracheal Cartilage

Used For

Cancer
Effectiveness: B   Safety: C

General Information

Bovine tracheal cartilage, like shark cartilage, is a popular nutritional supplement among cancer patients. The use of bovine tracheal cartilage predates shark cartilage. Much of the original research in the 1970s was conducted at the Massachusetts Institute of Technology under the direction of John F. Prudden, M.D., a Harvard-trained physician. In 1985 Dr. Prudden published case histories of thirty-one patients with a variety of malignancies including cancers of the ovary, colon, prostate, cervix, and thyroid, claiming that bovine tracheal cartilage produced an overall response rate of 90 percent. Therapy was usually started by injection and then continued with an oral dose of 3 grams every eight hours (9 grams per day).

In 1994, a group not associated with Dr. Prudden conducted a clinical trial of bovine tracheal cartilage in thirty-five patients with metastatic renal cell carcinoma (a very serious cancer of the kidneys). Of the twenty-two patients who completed three months of therapy and were available for evaluation for response, three patients were free from relapse of cancer after thirty months. While the response rate was not as good as that reported by Dr. Prudden, this independent confirmation indicates some potential value.

Although bovine tracheal cartilage has shown some benefit in preliminary studies, at this time it is not appropriate to substitute bovine cartilage for treatment of proven value where such treatment exists. Bovine tracheal cartilage can be used with conventional treatment, and some of the preliminary data suggest that it may be synergistic with certain chemotherapies and hormonal treatments, although this connection is far from firmly established.

It is thought that bovine cartilage works to slow the cell division within tumors (leading to slow tumor death) while also stimulating the body's immune system, especially macrophages (white blood cells that consume foreign or abnormal cells).

The chief component of bovine tracheal cartilage is **chondroitin sulfate,** indicating that it may also provide benefit in osteoarthritis as well.

Available Forms

Bovine tracheal cartilage is available in capsules, in tablets, and as a powder. Brand names available include Vita-Carte and Catrix.

Cautions and Warnings

None known.

Possible Side Effects

None known.

Drug Interactions

None known.

Food and Nutrient Interactions

Generally it is recommended that bovine tracheal cartilage be taken before meals or on an empty stomach.

Usual Dosage

The typical recommendation is 3,000 mg three times daily.

Overdosage

None known.

Special Populations

Pregnant/breast-feeding women

Because the effects of using bovine tracheal cartilage during pregnancy and lactation have not been
sufficiently studied, it is generally advised that it not
be taken by women who are planning a pregnancy
or who are pregnant or breast-feeding.

Children

Suitable for children at one-half the adult dosage.

Seniors

No special precautions are known.

Calcium D-glucarate

Used For

Cancer prevention and treatment

Effectiveness: B   Safety: A

General Information

Calcium D-glucarate is a natural substance used to
inhibit an enzyme, beta-glucuronidase, in certain
bacteria that reside in the gut. One of the key ways
in which the body gets rid of toxic chemicals as well
as hormones such as estrogen is by attaching glu-

curonic acid to them in the liver and then excreting this complex in the bile. Beta-glucuronidase is a bacterial enzyme that uncouples (breaks) the bond between the substance to be excreted and glucuronic acid. When beta-glucuronidase breaks the bond, the freed substance is available to be reabsorbed back into the body instead of being excreted. Elevated beta-glucuronidase activity is associated with an increased risk for various cancers, particularly hormone-dependent cancers such as breast and prostate cancer as well as colon cancer.

By taking calcium D-glucarate, beta-glucuronidase is inhibited. The body is then better able to get rid of various toxic chemicals and excess hormones that stimulate tumor formation, and as a result tumors tend to shrink. In particular, since most breast cancers are dependent upon estrogen, researchers at M. D. Anderson Cancer Center, Memorial Sloan-Kettering Cancer Center, and other major cancer centers began conducting research with calcium D-glucarate in the prevention and treatment of breast cancer. The preliminary results are quite encouraging. Currently, calcium D-glucarate is being studied at the National Cancer Institute in clinical trials as a preventive measure for breast cancer. Calcium D-glucarate may emerge as a better estrogen-blocking choice for women with a history of breast cancer than tamoxifen, which is associated with numerous side effects. In contrast, calcium D-glucarate is completely safe, and if preliminary results hold true, it may also be more effective.

Available Forms

Calcium D-glucarate is available in capsules and tablets.

Cautions and Warnings

Cancer is a serious disease. If you have cancer, do not self-medicate with calcium D-glucarate or any other substance without informing your supervising physician. Although preliminary research with calcium D-glucarate is promising, its real value has not been determined sufficiently at this time.

If you are taking any prescription medication, please consult your physician or pharmacist before taking calcium D-glucarate.

Possible Side Effects

None known.

Drug Interactions

Although there are no known drug interactions, many drugs (especially hormones) are detoxified in the liver by binding them to glucuronic acid, and so taking calcium D-glucarate could conceivably increase the elimination of the drug or hormone from the body, thereby reducing its effectiveness. If you are taking any prescription medication, please consult your physician or pharmacist before taking calcium D-glucarate.

Food and Nutrient Interactions

Dietary factors that can dramatically reduce the activity of beta-glucuronidase and are therefore useful in combination with calcium D-glucarate include the consumption of onion and garlic and foods high in glucaric acid such as apples, Brussels sprouts, broccoli, cabbage, and lettuce. The activity of glu-

:uronidase can also be reduced by establishing a proper bacterial flora; this can be achieved by supplementing the diet with the "friendly" bacteria *Lactobacillus acidophilus* and *Bifidobacterium bifidum*.

Usual Dosage

The recommended daily dosage for prevention is 200 to 400 mg. Higher dosages (i.e., 400 to 1,200 mg) may be necessary for individuals with existing breast cancer.

Overdosage

Not known.

Special Populations

Pregnant/breast-feeding women
Considered safe during pregnancy and lactation.

Children
Suitable for children at one-half the adult dosage.

Seniors
No special precautions are known.

Carnitine

Used For

Alzheimer's disease and age-related memory defects
Effectiveness: B+   Safety: B

Heart disease

   Angina pectoris
   Effectiveness: B+   Safety: B

   Congestive heart failure
   Effectiveness: B+   Safety: B

   Recovery from a heart attack
   Effectiveness: B+   Safety: B

Elevated cholesterol and triglyceride levels
Effectiveness: B+   Safety: B

Enhancing physical performance
Effectiveness: B+   Safety: B

Kidney disease and hemodialysis
Effectiveness: B+   Safety: B

Liver diseases
Effectiveness: B+   Safety: B

Low sperm count and decreased sperm motility
Effectiveness: B+   Safety: B

Peripheral vascular disease
Effectiveness: B+   Safety: B

General Information

Carnitine is a vitaminlike compound responsible for the transport of long-chain fatty acids into the energy producing units in cells—the mitochondria. Carnitine can be synthesized from the essential amino acid lysine, so it is not officially listed as a vitamin. Carnitine supplementation may improve the utilization of fat as an energy source. As a result, carnitine can exert a beneficial effect in the treatment of a wide variety of conditions associated with impaired fat utilization and energy production. Most clinical research, however, has revolved around its use in various cardiovascular diseases, enhancing physical performance, improving sperm count and motility, Alzheimer's disease and age-related senility, kidney disease, and hemodialysis.

Alzheimer's disease and age-related memory defects

A great deal of research has been conducted over the last decade with L-acetylcarnitine (LAC) in the treatment of Alzheimer's disease, senile depression, and age-related memory defects. LAC is a molecule composed of acetic acid and L-carnitine bound together. This reaction occurs naturally in the human brain, and so it is not exactly known how much greater an effect is noted with LAC versus L-carnitine. However, LAC is generally recommended over L-carnitine in conditions involving the brain.

LAC is structurally related to acetylcholine, a major neurotransmitter responsible for memory and proper brain function. In Alzheimer's disease, and to a lesser extent in the normal aging human brain, there is a defect in the utilization of acetylcholine. LAC mimics acetylcholine, and clinical studies have documented very well that it is of benefit not only in patients with early-stage Alzheimer's disease but also in elderly patients who are depressed or who have impaired memory. It has also been shown to act as a powerful antioxidant within the brain cell, stabilize cell membranes, and improve energy production within the brain cell.

Heart disease

Normal heart function is critically dependent on adequate concentrations of carnitine. Various heart diseases, including angina, congestive heart failure, and mitral valve prolapse, are characterized by impaired energy production and low carnitine concentrations. Supplementation of carnitine appears useful in these conditions due to its ability to improve oxygen utilization and energy metabolism in the heart muscle.

Angina pectoris

Numerous clinical trials have demonstrated that carnitine improves angina (the pressurelike pain in the upper chest that is often a harbinger of a heart attack). Improvements have been noted in the number of angina attacks, exercise tolerance, and heart function. Although all three commercial forms of carnitine have been shown to be effective, L-propionylcarnitine (LPC) may offer the greatest benefit in angina, as well as other cardiovascular diseases. LPC is taken up and utilized much more rapidly by the heart than other forms of carnitine. Dosages in these studies have typically been 1,500 to 2,000 mg daily in divided dosages.

Congestive heart failure

Congestive heart failure (CHF) refers to an inability of the heart to effectively pump enough blood. CHF is most often due to long-term effects of high blood pressure, previous heart attack, disorder of a heart valve or the heart muscle, or chronic lung diseases such as asthma and emphysema. Weakness, fatigue, and shortness of breath are the most common symptoms of CHF. Several double-blind clinical studies have shown that carnitine (again, LPC appears to be the most effective) improves heart function and leads to improvements in symptoms in patients with CHF.

Recovery from a heart attack

In several large clinical trials conducted in Italy, carnitine has been shown to be useful in helping individuals recover more quickly from a heart attack. Subjects taking carnitine showed significant improvements in heart rate, blood pressure, angina attacks, rhythm disturbances, and clinical signs of impaired heart function compared to the subjects taking placebo.

Elevated cholesterol and triglyceride levels

Carnitine exerts a beneficial effect on blood lipids by lowering triglycerides and total cholesterol levels while raising HDL cholesterol. Typical changes observed in clinical trials after four months of use are a 20 percent reduction for total cholesterol, a 28 percent decrease in triglycerides, and a 12 percent increase in HDL levels. These results compare quite favorably to prescription cholesterol-lowering drugs.

Enhancing physical performance

The ability to improve exercise tolerance and physical performance with carnitine has been demonstrated conclusively in patients with cardiovascular disease. Carnitine's ability to produce similar benefits in healthy subjects or athletes is not as well documented, as there are conflicting results from clinical trials. It appears that those most likely to benefit from carnitine supplementation are serious bodybuilders and individuals engaged in endurance-related events.

Kidney disease and hemodialysis

Carnitine supplementation is very much indicated in kidney disease because the kidney is a major site of carnitine manufacture in the body. Damage to the kidney or reduced kidney function can lead to low body stores of carnitine. It is also well established that patients undergoing hemodialysis suffer from carnitine deficiency due to the loss of considerable quantities of carnitine during dialysis as well as decreased manufacture because of impaired kidney function. Blood levels of carnitine drop nearly 80 percent during hemodialysis.

People with kidney disease, especially those on hemodialysis, benefit considerably from carnitine supplementation (1–2 g daily in divided dosages). Carnitine lowers blood cholesterol and triglyceride levels, leads to disappearance of angina pectoris and arrhythmias occurring during dialysis, reduces muscle symptoms including muscle cramps, increases muscle mass, and significantly improves the chronic anemia seen in these patients as demonstrated by an increased hematocrit, hemoglobin, and red blood cell count.

A major advancement in the treatment of the anemia associated with hemodialysis is genetically enineered human erythropoietin (EPO) therapy. EPO stimulates red blood cell manufacture considerably. However, this therapy is expensive and not without side effects. Taking carnitine (1 g daily) enhances the effectiveness of EPO and may significantly reduce the dosage of EPO needed.

Liver disease

Carnitine plays an extremely important role in the liver, as it is centrally involved in the metabolism of fat there. There is some evidence that carnitine deficiency within the liver promotes fatty infiltration (also known as steatosis or liver congestion). Alcohol consumption is a common cause of fatty infiltration of the liver. Carnitine supplementation at a dosage of 300 mg three times daily has been shown to significantly inhibit, and even reverse, alcohol-induced fatty liver disease, and it appears useful in other causes of fatty infiltration of the liver such as exposure to pesticides, herbicides, and other xenobiotics (man-made chemicals toxic to biological processes).

Low sperm count and decreased sperm motility

Low carnitine levels have been linked to low sperm count and abnormal motility. The lower a man's carnitine level, the more likely it is that he is infertile. Carnitine is very important in helping sperm produce enough energy for its important function. Carnitine supplementation (3,000 mg of L-carnitine daily for four months) has been shown to increase sperm counts and improve sperm motility. In one study, the number of ejaculated sperm increased by 20 billion; the percentage of motile sperm increased from 26.9 percent to 37.7 percent; the percentage of sperm with rapid linear progression increased from 10.8 percent to 18 percent; and the mean sperm velocity increased to 32.5 percent.

Peripheral vascular disease

Carnitine has been shown to be of benefit in the treatment of intermittent claudication, a peripheral vascular disease of the legs. Intermittent claudication is similar to angina pectoris, but instead of the pain occurring in the heart, it occurs usually in the calf muscle. Like angina, the pain is described as cramp or tightness. The cause of the pain is reduced oxygen delivery along with an increase in the production of toxic metabolites and free radicals. Carnitine's benefits in peripheral vascular disease are the result of improved energy production rather than any effect on blood flow. Nonetheless, good results have been obtained in intermittent claudication, as noted by improvements in walking distance. As much as a 75 percent increase in walking distance has been achieved after only three weeks of therapy.

Available Forms

Carnitine is available in several different forms, all of which are produced in capsules, tablets, and liquid. For Alzheimer's disease and brain effects, it appears that L-acetylcarnitine (LAC) is the best. For angina and other cardiovascular applications, L-propionyl carnitine (LPC) may be the best choice. However, L-carnitine is the most widely available, least expensive, and best-studied form of carnitine.

Cautions and Warnings

None known.

Possible Side Effects

Mild gastrointestinal irritation has been reported to occur at about the same frequency as that of a placebo.

Drug Interactions

There are no known adverse interactions between carnitine and any drug or nutrient. Carnitine has demonstrated an ability to protect against the toxicity to the heart caused by the chemotherapy drug adriamycin. Carnitine appears to potentiate the effectiveness of Epogen (genetically engineered erythropoietin) in the treatment of anemia in patients undergoing hemodialysis. Carnitine appears to work synergistically when combined with **coenzyme Q$_{10}$** and **pantethine** as well as drugs used in the treatment of arrhythmias (abnormal heart contraction rhythm).

Food and Nutrient Interactions

Carnitine manufacture in the body requires lysine, methionine, vitamin C, iron, niacin, and vitamin B$_6$.

Usual Dosage

The daily dosage of carnitine ranges from 900 to 6,000 mg daily in divided doses. Here are the dosage recommendations for the specific uses of carnitine:

Alzheimer's disease and age-related memory defects: 300–500 mg three times daily

Angina pectoris: 1,500–2,000 mg daily in divided doses

Congestive heart failure: 300–500 mg three times daily

Recovery from a heart attack: 4–6 g daily in divided doses

Elevated cholesterol and triglyceride levels: 300–500 mg three times daily

Enhancing physical performance: 2 g twice daily

Kidney disease and hemodialysis: 1–2 g daily in divided doses

Liver disease: 300 mg three times daily

Low sperm count and decreased sperm motility: 3 g daily in divided doses

Peripheral vascular disease: 2–4 g daily in divided doses

Overdosage

None known.

Special Populations

Pregnant/breast-feeding women
Considered safe during pregnancy and lactation.

Children
Suitable for children at one-half the adult dosage

Seniors
No special precautions are known.

Carnosine

Used For

Peptic ulcers
Effectiveness: B   Safety: B

General Information

Carnosine is a small protein composed of the amino acids histidine and alanine. It is found in relatively high concentrations in several body tissues, most notably in skeletal muscle, heart muscle, and the brain. The exact biological role of carnosine is still under investigation, but numerous animal studies have demonstrated that it possesses strong and specific antioxidant properties, protects against radiation damage, improves the function of the heart, and promotes wound healing. It has been suggested that carnosine is the water-soluble counterpart to vitamin E in protecting cell membranes from oxidative damage. Other suggested roles for carnosine include actions as a neurotransmitter, modulator of enzyme activity, and binder of heavy metals.

Many claims have been made regarding the therapeutic actions of carnosine, including exerting blood-pressure-lowering, immune-enhancing, wound-healing, and anticancer effects. Unfortunately, these claims, based primarily on preliminary Russian research, have not been convincingly documented nor subject to rigorous clinical evaluation. Furthermore, although carnosine is absorbed intact from the gastrointestinal tract, it is broken down extensively in the blood, especially in people who exercise regularly.

The well-documented application is in peptic ulcers. Experimental animal studies have shown that a zinc salt of carnosine exerts significant protection against ulcer formation as well as ulcer-healing properties. Clinical studies in humans demonstrate the same effects, including an ability to antagonize the bacterium (Helicobacter pylori) linked to indigestion (dyspepsia), peptic ulcer disease, and stomach cancer. When sixty patients suffering from dyspepsia with H. pylori infection were given either antibiotics alone or antibiotics plus zinc carnosine for seven days, better results were seen with the group getting zinc carnosine (94 percent success rate versus 77 percent).

Carnosine deficiency may occur in severe protein deficiency and in certain severe genetic disorders characterized by inborn errors in amino acid metabolism.

Available Forms

Dietary sources of preformed carnosine include meat, poultry, and fish.

Cautions and Warnings

None known.

Possible Side Effects

Due to the lack of human studies, side effects and interactions are not known.

Drug Interactions

The addition of zinc carnosine significantly improves the effectiveness of the antibiotics amoxycillin and clarithromycin used in treatment of peptic ulcers associated with *Helicobacter pylori*.

Food and Nutrient Interactions

None known.

Usual Dosage

In the treatment of peptic ulcers, the typical recommendation for zinc carnosine complex has been 150 mg twice daily. Due to the lack of human clinical trials, recommended levels for other applications are not known at this time.

Overdosage

None known.

Special Populations

Pregnant/breast-feeding women
As the effects of carnosine during pregnancy and lactation have not been sufficiently evaluated, it should not be used during these times.

Children
As the effects of carnosine in children have not been sufficiently evaluated, it should not be used in children unless under a physician's care.

Seniors
No special precautions are known.

Cell Forté with Ip6 (*see* Ip6 [Inositol Hexaphosphate])

General Information

Cell Forté with Ip6 is the combination of Ip6 (inositol hexaphosphate) and inositol developed by A. K. M. Shamsuddin, M.D., Ph.D., of the University of Maryland. This combination of compounds extracted from rice bran has demonstrated impressive anticancer and immune-enhancing effects in animal and test tube studies. Dr. Shamsuddin has demonstrated that the combination exerts much greater effect than Ip6 alone in animal models for breast cancer, lung cancer, colon cancer, and other cancers. It is very important to note that there are no human studies in cancer patients at this time, and the results in the animal and test tube studies should be viewed as preliminary studies.

Cetylmyristoleate (CMO)

Used For

Osteoarthritis
Effectiveness: B   Safety: B

Rheumatoid arthritis
Effectiveness: B   Safety: B

General Information

Cetylmyristoleate (CMO) is the common name for cis-9-cetylmyristoleate. CMO was discovered in 1972 by Harry W. Diehl, PhD., a researcher at the National Institutes of Health. At the time, Dr. Diehl was responsible for testing anti-inflammatory drugs on lab animals. In order for him to test the drugs, he first had to artificially induce arthritis in the animals by injecting a heat-killed bacterium called Freund's adjuvant. Dr. Diehl discovered that the Swiss albino mice did not get arthritis after injection of Freund's adjuvant. Eventually, he was able to determine that cetylmyristoleate was the factor present naturally in mice that was responsible for this protection. When CMO was injected into various strains of rats, it offered the same protection against arthritis. It has been proposed that CMO acts as a joint "lubricant" and anti-inflammatory agent. Patents were granted to Dr. Diehl for the use of CMO in both osteoarthritis and rheumatoid arthritis, based upon the animal studies and several case histories. In a double-blind study, 106 individuals with various types of arthritis that had failed to respond to non-steroidal anti-inflammatory drugs received cetylmyristoleate (540 mg per day orally for 30 days), while 226 other people received a placebo. These individuals also applied cetylmyristoleate or placebo topically, according to their perceived need. Some 63.5 percent of those receiving cetylmyristoleate improved, compared with only 14.5 percent of those receiving the placebo.

Available Forms

As a nutritional supplement it is found in a highly purified, refined form in capsules and tablets.

Cetylmyristoleate is also available for topical application in some creams and lotions.

Cautions and Warnings

None known.

Possible Side Effects

No side effects or drug interactions have been reported.

Drug Interactions

None known.

Food Interactions

None known.

Usual Dosage

Generally, CMO is given in one-month courses of 12 to 15 grams (i.e., 400 to 500 mg daily for 30 days).

Overdosage

None known.

Special Populations

Pregnant/breast-feeding women

As the effects of CMO during pregnancy and lactation have not been sufficiently evaluated, it should not be used during these times.

Children
As the effects of CMO in children have not been sufficiently evaluated, it should not be used unless under a physician's care.

Seniors
No special precautions are known.

Chitosan

Used For

Elevated cholesterol levels
Effectiveness: B   Safety: B

Weight loss
Effectiveness: B–   Safety: B

General Information

Chitosan is derived from the polysaccharide chitin, found in the shells of crustaceans such as crab, lobster, and shrimp. Similar in structure to cellulose (a dietary fiber), chitin is one of the most abundant of all polysaccharides found in the natural environment.

Elevated cholesterol levels
Like dietary fiber, chitosan may lower cholesterol by blocking the absorption of cholesterol, bile acids, and fat. Animal studies have confirmed an ability to lower cholesterol. Human studies have shown that 3–6 g per day of chitosan taken for two weeks resulted in a 6 percent drop in cholesterol and a 10

percent increase in HDL ("good") cholesterol. In people undergoing dialysis for kidney failure, the results were even more pronounced, as a preliminary study showed a 43 percent lowering of total cholesterol after a dosage of 4 g per day of chitosan for twelve weeks. This group also appeared to have improved kidney function and less severe anemia after chitosan treatment.

Weight loss

Chitosan is heavily promoted in the United States and other countries as an oral remedy to reduce fat absorption, and it has now been incorporated as a major constituent in over-the-counter weight loss formulas. There is some preliminary evidence that it may promote weight loss, but the most recent double-blind study in overweight subjects did not show any weight-loss-promoting effects with chitosan. After four weeks of treatment there were no differences in weight loss or blood levels of cholesterol and triglycerides in people receiving 1,000 mg of chitosan twice daily compared to those receiving a placebo. These results suggest that higher dosages may be required.

Available Forms

Chitosan is available in a variety of different grades and quality. Higher-quality products are those that are 90 percent deacetylated and are of lower molecular weight (30,000 to 70,000 daltons).

Cautions and Warnings

None known.

Possible Side Effects

As with other forms of dietary fiber, mild gastrointestinal discomfort and increased flatulence may be noted.

Drug Interactions

There are no known drug interactions with chitosan. However, because dietary fiber may decrease the absorption of any drug, most experts recommend taking any drug at least three hours before or after taking a bulk-forming laxative.

Food and Nutrient Interactions

Chitosan may reduce the absorption of minerals and fat-soluble vitamins.

Usual Dosage

Although chitosan is usually recommended at a dosage of 250 to 500 mg before meals, the results from clinical trials suggest that a dosage of 1–2 g three times per day before meals appears to be more likely to produce results.

Overdosage

None known.

Special Populations

Pregnant/breast-feeding women

Since chitosan may reduce the absorption of minerals and fat-soluble vitamins, it should not be used during pregnancy and lactation.

Children
   Since chitosan may reduce the absorption of minerals and fat-soluble vitamins, which are required for proper growth and development, it should not be used in children.

Seniors
   No special precautions are known.

Chlorella

Used For

Antioxidant support
Effectiveness: A   Safety: A

General Information

Chlorella is tiny, single-celled green algae (genus *Chlorella)* grown and harvested in special tanks and purified and processed by high-tech methods into a powder. Chlorella, like spirulina, is rich in nutrient content (56 percent protein and very high in minerals). It is also extremely rich in **chlorophyll** and **carotenes** and therefore a good antioxidant. It can also be used to promote healing of the gastrointestinal tract and as an internal deodorant, like chlorophyll.

Available Forms

Chlorella comes in a variety of forms, including capsules, tablets, granules, and soft gelatin capsules. Brands available include Sun-Chlorella.

Cautions and Warnings

If you are taking the drug warfarin (Coumadin), please consult with your doctor before taking this product, as it may contain vitamin K, which can counteract the effect of the drug.

Possible Side Effects

None known.

Drug Interactions

Because chlorella may contain vitamin K, it should not be used in people taking the anticoagulant drug warfarin (Coumadin) without the supervision of a physician.

Food and Nutrient Interactions

None known.

Usual Dosage

The dosage for chlorella ranges from 300 to 1,500 mg per day.

Overdosage

None known.

Special Populations

Pregnant/breast-feeding women

Considered safe during pregnancy and lactation.

Children
Suitable for children over the age of six months even at the adult dosage.

Seniors
No special precautions are known.

Chlorophyll

Used For

Reducing colostomy and fecal odor
Effectiveness: A   Safety: A

General Information

Chlorophyll is the green pigment of plants, found in the chloroplast (a compartment of plant cells), where electromagnetic energy (light) is converted to chemical energy in the process known as photosynthesis. The chlorophyll molecule is essential for this reaction to occur.

The natural chlorophyll found in green plants is fat soluble. The majority of the chlorophyll products found in health stores, however, contain water-soluble chlorophyll. In order to produce water-soluble chlorophyll, the natural chlorophyll molecule must be altered chemically. The fat-soluble form—the natural form of chlorophyll, as found in fresh juice—offers several advantages over water-soluble chlorophyll. This is particularly true regarding chlorophyll's ability to stimulate hemoglobin and red blood cell production and to relieve excessive menstrual blood flow. In fact, it is interesting to note that the chlorophyll molecule is very similar to the heme portion of the hemoglobin molecule of our red blood cells.

Because water-soluble chlorophyll is not absorbed from the gastrointestinal tract, its use is limited to soothing the gastrointestinal tract and reducing fecal odor. It is approved for use in reducing the fecal odor associated with a colostomy (removal of some or all of the colon and replacement with a small collection bag outside the body). The beneficial effect is largely due to its ability to attract water.

Available Forms

Chlorophyll is available primarily in liquid form.

Cautions and Warnings

None known.

Possible Side Effects

None known.

Drug Interactions

None known.

Food and Nutrient Interactions

None known.

Usual Dosage

Chlorophyll is usually taken in doses of 1 to 2 table-spoons daily.

Overdosage

None known.

Special Populations

Pregnant/breast-feeding women
Considered safe during pregnancy and lactation.

Children
Suitable for chidren at one-half the adult dosage.

Seniors
No special precautions are known.

Choline

Used For

Liver health
Effectiveness: B+   Safety: A

General Information

Choline is often referred to as an unofficial member of the B vitamin family. Although choline can be manufactured in the body from either the amino acid methionine or the amino acid serine, it has recently been designated an essential nutrient. Choline works very closely with other B vitamins in performing a vital function in the proper metabolism of fats. Without choline, fats become trapped in the liver, where they block metabolism. Specifically, it is required for the export of fat from the liver. Technically this is referred to as a lipotropic effect. Choline is also required to make the important neurotransmitter acetylcholine and main components of our cell membranes such as phosphatidylcholine (lecithin) and sphingomyelin. Dietary sources of choline (most commonly as phosphatidylcholine) include nuts, seeds, and legumes.

Available Forms

Choline is available in pill form (capsules or tablets) as a soluble salt in the form of choline bitartrate, choline citrate, or choline chloride. Choline is also available as **phosphatidylcholine**.

Cautions and Warnings

None known.

Possible Side Effects

None known.

Drug Interactions

Choline works together with folic acid, vitamin B_{12}, S-adenosylmethionine, and vitamin B_6, and it helps the body conserve carnitine and folic acid.

Food and Nutrient Interactions

None known.

Usual Dosage

50–300 mg per day.

Overdosage

Choline at high dosages (e.g., 20 g) will produce a fishy odor.

Special Populations

Pregnant/breast-feeding women
Considered safe during pregnancy and lactation.

Children
Suitable for children at one-half the adult dosage.

Seniors
No special precautions are known.

Chondroitin Sulfate

Used For

Osteoarthritis
Effectiveness: A   Safety: A

General Information

Chondroitin sulfate is a very large molecule composed of repeating units of glucosamine and glucuronic acid with sulfur molecules attached. It is a key component of joint cartilage, responsible for cartilage's gel-like nature and shock-absorbing qualities. The molecular weight of chondroitin sulfate ranges from 7,000 to over 30,000, making it very difficult for the body to absorb. Any clinical benefit from chondroitin sulfate is most likely due to the absorption of sulfur or smaller GAG molecules, which result when the chondroitin sulfate is broken down by the digestive tract.

There is some evidence that chondroitin sulfate stimulates the synthesis of cartilage components in the treatment of osteoarthritis—the most common form of arthritis, caused by degeneration of the cartilage. Several double-blind studies have shown that chondroitin sulfate reduces joint pain and improves joint function in osteoarthritis of the knees, hips, or hands. Typically results are apparent after three to four months of use and reach maximum benefit after six to twelve months of use. The beneficial effects gradually diminish over a period of three months when chondroitin sulfate is discontinued.

Available Forms

Chondroitin sulfate is available in powder, capsules, or tablets. It is usually derived from bovine (beef) sources.

Cautions and Warnings

None known.

Possible Side Effects

No adverse effects have been reported at recommended dosages.

Drug Interactions

None known.

Food and Nutrient Interactions

None known.

Usual Dosage

Most studies used a dosage of 400 mg three times daily.

Overdosage

Nausea may occur at intakes greater than 10 g per day.

Special Populations

Pregnant/breast-feeding women
    Considered safe during pregnancy and lactation.

Children
    Suitable for children at one-half the adult dosage.

Seniors
    No special precautions are known.

Citus Bioflavonoids

Used For

Capillary fragility
Effectiveness: A   Safety: A

Easy bruising
Effectiveness: A   Safety: A

Hemorrhoids
Effectiveness: A   Safety: A

Varicose veins
Effectiveness: A   Safety: A

General Information

Citrus bioflavonoid preparations contain rutin, hesperidin, and other bioflavonoids. Most of the clinical research on rutin and crude bioflavonoid complexes occurred before 1970. Since then, most of the clinical research has utilized a purified mixture of rutin derivatives known as hydroxyethylrutosides (HER). Impressive clinical results have been obtained with HER in the treatment of capillary permeability, easy bruising, hemorrhoids, and varicose veins (discussed below).

Citrus bioflavonoids display antioxidant activity and an ability to increase intracellular levels of vitamin C. They improve capillary permeability and blood flow, primarily via strengthening the cells that line the blood vessels and supporting the underlying collagen structures. Collagen, the most abundant protein in the body, is responsible for maintaining the integrity of ground substance—the matrix that holds cells together—as well as the integrity of tendons, ligaments, and cartilage.

In double-blind studies in patients with varicose veins, HER improved blood flow and clinical symptoms (pain, tired legs, night cramps, and restless legs) in 73 to 100 percent of patients. Several of the studies were performed in pregnant women, where HER was shown to be of great benefit in improving venous function as well as helping relieve hemorrhoidal signs and symptoms. In one study, 90 percent of the women given HER (1,000 mg daily for four weeks) had improved symptoms compared to only 12 percent in the placebo group. Similar results in hemorrhoids not associated with pregnancy have been reported.

Available Forms

Mixed preparations of citrus bioflavonoids are the most widely used and least expensive flavonoid sources. However, most commercially available sources of mixed citrus flavonoids only contain 50 percent flavonoids. Preparations containing pure rutin and hesperidin or those that clearly state the levels of rutin and hesperidin are better than products that do not quantify the amount of the individual flavonoid components.

Citrus bioflavonoids can be found in powders, capsules, and tablets.

Cautions and Warnings

None known.

Possible Side Effects

None known.

Drug Interactions

None known.

Food and Nutrient Interactions

Bioflavonoids work closely with vitamin C in the human body.

Usual Dosage

The dosage used for HER in double-blind clinical studies in varicose veins and hemorrhoids has ranged from 1,000 to 3,000 mg daily. This translates to a dosage of citrus bioflavonoids of 3,000 to 6,000 mg daily, or 1,000 to 3,000 mg daily for either rutin or hesperidin.

Overdosage

None known.

Special Populations

Pregnant/breast-feeding women
Considered safe during pregnancy and lactation at recommended dosages.

Children
Suitable for children at one-half the adult dosage.

Seniors
No special precautions are known.

Cod Liver Oil

Used For

Source of vitamins A and D, and EPA/DHA
Effectiveness: A   Safety: C

General Information

Cod liver oil is a light yellow oil found in the liver of the cod. As a natural source of vitamins A and D, it was once commonly prescribed to prevent deficiency diseases. Its use was somewhat replaced by the advent of vitamin A and D in tablets and capsules (much to the delight of many young children no longer required to swallow the not-so-pleasant oil). With the discovery of the health benefits of the fish oils EPA and DHA that are naturally present in cod liver oil and the development of more palatable forms, cod liver oil use is increasing. For more information on possible uses of cod liver oil, please see **vitamin A, vitamin D, eicosapentaenoic acid (EPA),** and **docosahexaenoic acid (DHA).**

Available Forms

Cod liver oil is available in liquid form (often flavored) and soft gelatin capsules.

Cautions and Warnings

Pregnant women and women of childbearing age who may possibly become pregnant should not take more than 5,000 IU of vitamin A daily due to the possible risk of birth defects with higher doses of vitamin A.

Possible Side Effects

Eructation (burping) of a disagreeable odor is a common side effect, especially if taken on a full stomach.

Drug Interactions

The drugs cholestyramine (Questran), colestipol (Colestid), neomycin (Neo-Fradin), and orlistat (Xenical), as well as mineral oil, all interfere with the absorption of vitamin A.

Using vitamin A at higher dosages in conjunction with synthetic vitamin A derivatives such as isotretinoin (Accutane) and etretinate (Tegison) can result in increased risk of toxicity.

Food and Nutrient Interactions

Vitamin E and zinc are particularly important to the proper function of vitamin A. Olestra (a fat substitute) as well as sources of dietary fiber (psyllium, pectin, guar gum, etc.) may decrease the absorption of vitamin A.

Usual Dosage

The usual dosage of a liquid preparation is 1 teaspoon daily (providing approximately 4,600 IU of vitamin A, 460 IU of vitamin D, 460 mg EPA, and 420 mg DHA). Dosage recommendations for capsules depend on the size of the capsule. Follow dosage recommendations on the label.

Overdosage

None known. See **vitamin A** for possible effects of overdosage.

Special Populations

Pregnant/breast-feeding women
  Pregnant women should not take more than 5,000 IU of vitamin A daily due to the possible risk of birth defects with higher doses of vitamin A. Dosages above 5,000 IU are also not recommended while lactating.

Children
  Suitable for children over the age of six months even at the adult dosage.

Seniors
  No special precautions are known.

Coenzyme Q₁₀

Used For

Antioxidant
Effectiveness: A   Safety: A

Cancer
Effectiveness: B   Safety: A

Diabetes
Effectiveness: B   Safety: A

Heart disease

Angina
Effectiveness: B+   Safety: A

Cardiomyopathy
Effectiveness: A   Safety: A

Congestive heart failure
Effectiveness: A   Safety: A

High blood pressure
Effectiveness: A   Safety: A

Muscular dystrophy
Effectiveness: A   Safety: A

Periodontal disease
Effectiveness: A   Safety: A

Weight loss
Effectiveness: B   Safety: A

General Information

Coenzyme Q$_{10}$ (CoQ$_{10}$), also known as ubiquinone, is an essential component of the mitochondria—the energy-producing unit of the cells of our body. CoQ$_{10}$ is involved in the manufacture of ATP, the energy currency of all body processes.

Although CoQ$_{10}$ can be synthesized within the body, deficiencies do exist as a result of impaired CoQ$_{10}$ synthesis or increased tissue needs. Examples of diseases that require increased tissue levels of CoQ$_{10}$ are cardiovascular diseases such as angina, high blood pressure, mitral valve prolapse, and congestive heart failure. In addition, the elderly in general may have increased CoQ$_{10}$ requirements, as CoQ$_{10}$ levels are known to decline with advancing age.

The therapeutic uses of CoQ$_{10}$ revolve around its ability to improve energy production and act as an antioxidant. As with other antioxidants, CoQ$_{10}$ supplementation may offer significant protection against atherosclerosis by preventing lipid peroxide formation and oxidation of LDL cholesterol (see **vitamin E** for further discussion).

Cancer

Use of CoQ$_{10}$ supplementation in cancer is based upon its immune-enhancing and antioxidant effects. Cells of the immune system require an adequate supply of CoQ$_{10}$ for optimal function. Several studies have documented an immune-enhancing effect of CoQ$_{10}$, including an ability to prevent or reverse age-related immune suppression.

Most of the studies in cancer patients given CoQ$_{10}$ have focused on CoQ$_{10}$'s ability to prevent damage to the heart done by chemotherapy drugs. Many potent chemotherapy drugs, such as adriamycin, are often of limited value because of the development of serious toxicity to the heart muscle after long-term treatment. CoQ$_{10}$ supplementation may help prevent this toxicity.

Diabetes

CoQ$_{10}$ appears to be beneficial in improving blood sugar control in patients with diabetes. The mechanism by which CoQ$_{10}$ accomplishes this is not known. It is likely more than simply correction of a CoQ$_{10}$ deficiency, since the percentage of positive responses is far greater (36–59 percent) than the incidence of CoQ$_{10}$ deficiency (8.3 percent).

Heart disease

The benefits of CoQ$_{10}$ in various types of heart disease have been clearly documented in both animal studies and human trials. CoQ$_{10}$ deficiency is common in people with heart disease of any kind. Clinical studies demonstrate that correcting a CoQ$_{10}$ deficiency can produce significant improvements.

CoQ$_{10}$ therapy is indicated in patients undergoing any cardiovascular surgery. Return of blood flow (reperfusion) after surgery results in oxidative damage to the lining of blood vessels and the muscle of the heart. CoQ$_{10}$ has been shown to prevent reperfusion injury in patients undergoing coronary artery bypass surgery; this is thought to significantly reduce the risk for a subsequent heart attack.

Angina

Angina is a squeezing or pressurelike pain in the chest that is caused by an insufficient supply of oxygen to the heart muscle. CoQ$_{10}$ has been shown to be effective in angina patients in several small studies. The results of these studies suggest that CoQ$_{10}$ may offer a safe and effective treatment for angina pectoris. However, these results need to be confirmed in larger studies.

Cardiomyopathy

Cardiomyopathy refers to any disease of the heart muscle that causes a reduction in the force of heart contraction and a resultant decrease in the efficiency of blood circulation. Cardiomyopathy may be the result of viral, metabolic, nutritional, toxic, autoimmune, degenerative, or genetic causes, or its cause may be unknown. Regardless of the cause, a deficiency of CoQ$_{10}$ has been found in the blood and myocardial tissue of most patients with cardiomyopathy.

In cases of cardiomyopathy, CoQ$_{10}$ supplementation can raise CoQ$_{10}$ levels and produce improvements in heart function as a result of improved energy production in the heart muscle. In one study in patients with very severe cardiomyopathy, of the eighty patients treated, 89 percent improved while on CoQ$_{10}$. The two most important findings were that the amount of blood pumped by each contraction of the heart (the mean ejection fraction) increased from about 25 percent to about 40 percent and that the two-year survival rate was 62 percent compared to less than 25 percent for a similar series of patients treated by conventional drug therapy alone. Individuals with cardiomyopathy will need to be on CoQ$_{10}$ indefinitely to maintain any real benefit from it.

Congestive heart failure

Congestive heart failure (CHF) refers to the inability of the heart to effectively pump blood. CHF is most often due to long-term effects of high blood pressure, disorder of a heart valve, or cardiomyopathy (see above). Numerous studies have shown CoQ$_{10}$ supplementation to be extremely effective in the treatment of CHF. Most of these studies utilized CoQ$_{10}$ along with conventional drug therapy. All together, the effectiveness and safety of CoQ$_{10}$ in these studies suggest that it is quite helpful in mild CHF when used as a sole therapy, and it can effectively reduce hospitalization and serious consequences when used along with conventional drug therapy in moderate to severe CHF.

High blood pressure

CoQ$_{10}$ deficiency occurs in roughly 40 percent of patients with high blood pressure. In several studies CoQ$_{10}$ has been shown to lower blood pressure in patients with hypertension; however, the effect is usually not seen until after four to twelve weeks of therapy. Typical reductions in both systolic and diastolic blood pressure with CoQ$_{10}$ therapy in patients with high blood pressure are in the 10 percent range. It is thought that CoQ$_{10}$ lowers blood pressure by lowering cholesterol levels and by stabilizing the vascular membrane via its antioxidant properties. As a result of these actions, peripheral resistance to blood flow is reduced and blood pressure drops accordingly.

Muscular dystrophy

Deficiency of CoQ$_{10}$ has been found in the muscles and heart of people with muscular dystrophy. Positive results have been demonstrated in patients with progressive muscular dystrophy (Duchenne's, Becker's, limb-girdle, and myotonic dystrophies; Charcot-Marie-Tooth disease; and Kugelberg-Welander disease). Significant improvements in heart function have been noted along with increased exercise tolerance, reduced leg pain, better control of leg function, and less fatigue. These results suggest that people with muscular dystrophy should take CoQ$_{10}$. Long-term use is required to maintain any benefit.

Periodontal disease

Published reports indicate that the frequency of CoQ$_{10}$ deficiency in gum tissue of patients with periodontal disease ranges from 60 to 96 percent. These studies have also shown CoQ$_{10}$ to be quite effective in improving gum health. Results of CoQ$_{10}$ therapy were evaluated according to criteria that included pocket depth, swelling, bleeding, redness, pain, exudate, and looseness of teeth. "Very impressive" and "extraordinary" were terms used to describe the degree of improvement and acceleration of healing produced by CoQ$_{10}$ therapy.

Weight loss

Since CoQ$_{10}$ is an essential cofactor for energy production, it is possible that CoQ$_{10}$ deficiency is a contributing cause in some cases of obesity. Low levels of CoQ$_{10}$ were found in 52 percent of the obese subjects tested in one study. Subjects with low CoQ$_{10}$ levels given 100 mg per day of CoQ$_{10}$ along with a 650-calorie diet lost an average of about thirty pounds after eight to nine weeks. In contrast, in the group with normal CoQ$_{10}$ levels, a 650-calorie diet for eight to nine weeks produced a weight loss of about thirteen pounds.

Available Forms

Coenzyme Q$_{10}$ is available primarily in tablet or capsules. Based on bioavailability studies, the best preparations are soft gelatin capsules, although taking any CoQ$_{10}$ preparation with meals greatly increases its absorption.

Cautions and Warnings

None known.

Possible Side Effects

Coenzyme Q_{10} is generally well tolerated, and no significant side effects have been reported with either short- or long-term use.

Drug Interactions

Many drugs appear to adversely affect CoQ_{10} levels. Conversely, CoQ_{10} is able to mitigate the side effects of many drugs. In addition to adriamycin (discussed above), many experts recommend supplementing CoQ_{10} at dosages ranging from 30 to 100 mg per day in people taking the following drugs, to prevent side effects or the depletion of CoQ_{10} in body tissues:

- *Cholesterol-lowering drugs* such as atorvastatin (Lipitor), gemfibrozil (Lopid), lovastatin (Mevacor), pravastatin (Pravachol), and simvastatin (Zocor).
- *Beta-blocker drugs* used in angina, high blood pressure, and heart arrhythmias, such as acebutolol (Sectral), atenolol (Tenormin), carteolol (Cartrol), metoprolol (Lopressor, Toprol XL), penbutolol (Levatol), propanolol (Inderal), and timolol (Blocarden).
- *Phenothiazine drugs* used in various psychiatric disorders, such as chlorpromazine (Thorazine), fluphenazine (Permitil, Prolixin), mesoridazine (Serentil), and trifluoperazine (Stelazine).
- *Tricyclic antidepressants,* such as amitriptyline (Elavil, Endep), desipramine (Norpramin, Pertofrane), doxepin (Adapin, Sinequan), imipramine (Imavate, Presamine, Tofranil), nortriptyline (Aventyl, Pamelor), and protriptyline (Vivactil).

There has been one case report where CoQ$_{10}$ interfered with warfarin (Coumadin). Individuals taking this drug should take CoQ$_{10}$ only with the guidance of their doctor.

Food and Nutrient Interactions

Taking CoQ$_{10}$ with food enhances its absorption. No other food interactions are known. CoQ$_{10}$ also works synergistically with **carnitine** and **pantethine**.

Usual Dosage

The usual dosage of CoQ$_{10}$ is 50 to 150 mg per day. Although most studies used a dosage of 100 mg per day, larger doses (up to 300 mg per day) may be needed in cases of severe heart disease. Perhaps a more accurate dosage recommendation is based upon the person's weight. Some of the studies used a dosage of 2 mg CoQ$_{10}$ per kg (2.2 pounds) body weight.

Overdosage

None known.

Special Populations

Pregnant/breast-feeding women

Safety during pregnancy and lactation has not been determined. CoQ$_{10}$ should not be used during these times unless the potential clinical benefit (as determined by a physician) outweighs the risks.

Children

Suitable for children at one-half the adult dosage.

Seniors
No special precautions are known.

Colloidal Silver

Used For

Infections
Effectiveness: F   Safety: F

General Information

Silver, like mercury, was used as a medicine in the late 1800s and early 1900s. Its primary application was as a topical antiseptic. Silver, in the form of silver nitrate solution, is still used today in newborns as topical eyedrops to prevent eye infections. In fact, in most states the law requires that newborns be treated with silver nitrate eyedrops.

In the early 1990s colloidal silver began appearing in the marketplace as a "nutritional supplement." The silver is suspended in water, hence the term *colloidal.* Tremendous claims and testimonials abound, yet the truth is that colloidal silver is of dubious effectiveness at best and potentially dangerous at worst.

Although silver is an effective antimicrobial agent, the concentrations of colloidal silver required for any sort of systemic effect are not likely to be obtained safely with oral administration. Yet colloidal silver is promoted as an alternative to antibiotics and as a "wonder substance" capable of treating virtually every infectious disease imaginable.

In response to the substance's growing popularity and these unsubstantiated claims, the FDA issued a Final Rule on August 17, 1999, that all over-the-counter (OTC) products containing colloidal silver or silver salts are not recognized as safe and effective and are misbranded. According to the Final Rule, any colloidal silver product for drug use will first have to be approved by the FDA under the new drug application procedures. The Final Rule classifies colloidal silver products as misbranded because adequate directions cannot be written so that the general public can use these drugs safely for their intended purposes. They are also misbranded when their labeling falsely suggests that there is substantial scientific evidence to establish that the drugs are safe and effective for their intended uses.

Despite this Final Ruling from the FDA, colloidal silver will likely continue to be sold as a trace mineral supplement without medical claims or claims of specific benefits even though its need in human nutrition is completely unsubstantiated.

Available Forms

Colloidal silver is found as a solution in bottles.

Cautions and Warnings

Overdosage can result in significant toxicity (see below).

Possible Side Effects

When taken in low dosages such as those recommended (e.g., 50 mcg daily) the body does appear to be able to efficiently excrete silver. However, any silver the body is unable to excrete accumulates in body tissues and can result in argyria—the depositing of silver in the internal organs, tissues, and skin.

Drug Interactions

None known.

Food and Nutrient Interactions

May interfere with the body's utilization of copper and selenium.

Usual Dosage

The typical recommendation is 1 teaspoon per day, with each teaspoon (5 ml) containing 10 ppm (50 mcg) of silver. This amount seems reasonable given the fact that the average amount of silver consumed from the food and water supply is roughly 350 mcg per day for most people. However, given the lack of long-term safety or even efficacy data for oral use, ingestion of colloidal silver cannot be recommended.

Overdosage

Excessive dosages, either acute or over time, can result in argyria, the depositing of silver in the internal organs, tissues, and skin. In argyria the skin turns gray or bluish gray and can turn dark on exposure to strong sunlight. This discoloration is permanent and there is no known effective treatment for it. In addition to argyria, the intake of very large doses (far in excess of the amount that causes discoloration of the skin) of silver can cause neurological and organ damage and arteriosclerosis.

The estimated accumulated dosage required over

a period of one year to produce argyria is estimated at 1 to 6 g of silver. This amount is very large compared to the 50 mcg typically recommended as a daily dosage of OTC colloidal silver products. Using the most conservative figure, 1 g of silver corresponds to the silver content in 100 l of 10 ppm colloidal silver, 50 l of 20 ppm colloidal silver, or 33.3 l of 30 ppm colloidal silver.

Special Populations

Pregnant/breast-feeding women
Should not be used during pregnancy and lactation.

Children
Should not be used by children.

Seniors
No special precautions are known, but the elderly may be at greater risk for problems with silver due to reduced ability to excrete silver.

Conjugated Linoleic Acid (CLA)

Used For

Cancer prevention
Effectiveness: C   Safety: C

Weight loss
Effectiveness: B   Safety: C

General Information

Conjugated linoleic acid (CLA) is a slightly altered form of the essential fatty acid linoleic acid. It occurs naturally in meat and dairy products. It was discovered in 1978 when researchers at the University of Wisconsin were seeking to find possible cancer-causing compounds in meat that are produced with cooking. Instead, they found what appears to be an anticancer compound—CLA. In preliminary animal and test tube studies, CLA has shown evidence that it might reduce the risk of breast, prostate, colorectal, lung, skin, and stomach cancers. Whether CLA will produce a similar protective effect in humans has yet to be determined.

Animal research also suggests that CLA supplementation might help prevent atherosclerosis and reduce body fat. In one human study at the University of Wisconsin involving 80 obese people, half took 3,000 mg of CLA daily, while the other half took a placebo. They were all put on a diet program and encouraged to exercise. Weight loss was about the same for both groups. However, of the people who regained the weight, people taking the placebo put it back on mainly as fat, while the people taking CLA put it back on primarily as lean muscle. Similar results were found in a study conducted at Lund University in Sweden.

Researchers believe that CLA interferes with a fat-storing enzyme known as lipoprotein lipase, as well as increasing the sensitivity of cells to insulin. CLA is also believed to help burn fat by revving up muscle metabolism and helping to increase lean muscle mass.

Available Forms

CLA is available primarily in soft gelatin capsules. Brand names available include CLA-One.

Cautions and Warnings

None known.

Possible Side Effects

None known.

Drug Interactions

None known.

Food and Nutrient Interactions

None known.

Usual Dosage

The recommended dosage given on the label of most CLA products is 1,000 to 3,000 mg daily.

Overdosage

None known.

Special Populations

Pregnant/breast-feeding women

As the effects of CLA during pregnancy and lactation have not been sufficiently evaluated, it should not be used during these times.

Children

As the effects of CLA in children have not been sufficiently evaluated, it should not be used in children unless under a physician's care.

Seniors

No special precautions are known.

Cordyceps (Cordyceps sinesis)

Used For

Low immunity and immune support
Effectiveness: C   Safety: B

General Information

Cordyceps is a mushroom that grows primarily on the Tibetan plateau at altitudes above 14,000 feet. It is a natural parasite on caterpillar larvae. The spores of cordyceps infect the larvae and the resulting mycelium grows, kills the larvae, and then blossoms into a dark, clublike mushroom. It takes five to seven years for the mushroom to complete its life cycle. Due to the scarcity and high price of cordyceps, its use was traditionally reserved exclusively for the emperor's palace, where it was used to restore energy and promote longevity. Cordyceps is now grown and harvested from large fermentation tanks, like other medicinal mushrooms.

In test tube and animal studies, cordyceps has been shown to enhance the function of white blood cells and increase the release of immune-enhancing substances. Studies in animals with cancer have also shown cordyceps to improve immune response, reduce tumor size, and lengthen survival time. Whether cordyceps will produce a similar protective effect in humans has yet to be determined.

Available Forms

Cordyceps is available in capsule, tablet, and powder form.

Cautions and Warnings

Since cordyceps may enhance immune function, it must not be used in people who have had organ transplants or who are taking drugs such as cyclophosphamide, cyclosporin, and aminoglycosides to purposely suppress the immune system.

Possible Side Effects

Allergic reactions are very rare but have been reported.

Drug Interactions

In animal studies, cordyceps was able to prevent some of the damage to the immune system caused by cyclosporin, a drug used to suppress the immune system after organ transplant. At this time, cordyceps should not be used by people who are taking drugs such as cyclophosphamide, cyclosporin, and aminoglycosides to purposely suppress the immune system.

Food and Nutrient Interactions

None known.

Usual Dosage

The usual recommended dosage is 1,000 to 3,000 mg daily.

Overdosage

None known.

Special Populations

Pregnant/breast-feeding women
As the efforts of cordyceps during pregnancy and lactation have not been sufficiently evaluated, it should not be used during these times.

Children
Suitable for children at one-half the adult dosage.

Seniors
No special precautions are known.

Cosamin DS

General Information

Cosamin DS is a patented combination of ingredients recommended for supporting cartilage manufacture in the treatment of osteoarthritis. Each capsule contains:

Glucosamine hydrochloride	**500 mg**
Chondroitin sulfate	**400 mg**
Ascorbate (as manganese ascorbate)	**66 mg**
Manganese (as manganese ascorbate)	**10 mg**

Although clinical studies have shown Cosamin DS to be effective in treating osteoarthritis, it is not known if the effectiveness is due to the combination of ingredients or the fact that it simply provides therapeutic levels of **glucosamine** and **chondroitin sulfate.** The dosage recommendation for adults weighing under 200 pounds is 3 capsules daily (2 in the morning, 1 at night), and for individuals weighing over 200 pounds it is 4 capsules daily (2 in the morning, 2 at night).

Creatine

Used For

Increasing lean body mass and strength
Effectiveness: A   Safety: B

General Information

Creatine monohydrate has become one of the most popular nutritional supplements for athletes and bodybuilders. It is used primarily to increase strength and lean body mass and has shown consistent results in promoting these effects in clinical studies. Creatine is used in muscle tissue for the production of phosphocreatine, an important factor in the formation of ATP, which is the source of energy for muscle contraction and many other functions in the body. Creatine supplementation works by increasing phosphocreatine levels in muscle.

Most, though not all, clinical studies have shown creatine supplementation to improve exercise performance and delay muscle fatigue during short-duration, high-intensity exercise such as sprinting and weight lifting. However, creatine supplementation does not appear to increase endurance performance and may actually impair it.

Available Forms

Because of the success of creatine monohydrate, several other forms of creatine have become available, including creatine phosphate and creatine citrate. These are claimed to produce similar results; however, creatine monohydrate is the only form studied to date, so the effectiveness of these other forms is unknown.

Brand names available include Creatine Fuel, Phosphagen, and Micro Pure.

Cautions and Warnings

If you suffer from any kidney or liver disease, please consult a physician before supplementing with creatine.

Possible Side Effects

Reported side effects from creatine supplementation include gastric disturbance, headaches, and an increased tendency toward muscle cramps. Little is known about the long-term side effects of creatine, but no consistent toxicity appears in most reports of creatine supplementation. One reported case history is a source of great concern: Interstitial nephritis, a serious kidney condition, developed in an otherwise healthy young man who had been taking 20 g of creatine per day. His kidney function improved after creatine was stopped. This case history is offset, however, by tremendous usage of creatine by so many people without side effects.

Drug Interactions

Caffeine appears to offset some of the effectiveness of creatine.

Food and Nutrient Interactions

The absorption of creatine is enhanced when it is taken with simple sugars.

Usual Dosage

There are two popular dosage recommendations. In the first, there is a loading phase followed by a maintenance phase. During the loading period (up to two weeks), 5 g are taken four times daily (20 g total). The dosage for maintenance is 3 to 5 g daily. In the other method, 3 g of creatine are taken daily. In this dosage method, muscle creatine levels rise more slowly, yet eventually reach levels similar to those achieved with the loading method.

Overdosage

Do the following in case of accidental overdose: If the victim is unconscious or having convulsions, call for an ambulance immediately. If you take the victim to an emergency room, be sure to bring the bottle or container with you. If the victim is conscious, call your local poison control center or a health care professional. The poison control center may suggest inducing vomiting with ipecac syrup (available without a prescription at any pharmacy). *Do not* induce vomiting unless specifically instructed to do so.

Special Populations

Pregnant/breast-feeding women

As the effects of creatine during pregnancy and lactation have not been sufficiently evaluated, it should not be used during these times.

Children

As the effects of creatine in children have not been sufficiently evaluated, it is recommended that it not be used by children under the age of eighteen years unless directed to do so by a physician.

Seniors

No special precautions are known.

Culturelle with Lactobacillus GG

General Information

Culturelle contains Lactobacillus GG (LGG), a patented strain of *Lactobacillus rhamnosus* bacteria that is the most extensively researched and clinically proven strain available. LGG takes its name from its discoverers, Drs. Sherwood Gorbach and Barry Goldin of Tufts University. Several studies have shown LGG to be better able to withstand stomach acid and colonize the large intestine than other lactobacillus varieties. Each capsule of Culturelle LGG contains a minimum of 10 billion live bacteria.

Daidzein (*see* Soy Isoflavones; *see also* Kudzu)

General Information

Daidzein is one of the principal phytoestrogens found in soy. It is also found in high concentrations in kudzu *(Pueraria species)*.

DHEA (Dehydroepiandrosterone)

Used For

Antiaging effects
Effectiveness: B+   Safety: C

Depression
Effectiveness: A   Safety: C

Erectile dysfunction
Effectiveness: B+   Safety: A

Systemic lupus erythematosus
Effectiveness: B+   Safety: A

General Information

Dehydroepiandrosterone (DHEA) is a hormone produced by the adrenal glands that acts as the building block for all other steroid hormones in the human body, including sex hormones and corticosteroids. Because DHEA levels tend to decline with age, it has been postulated that raising DHEA through supplementation may offer some protection against the effects of aging. In addition, over the last decade a number of studies have demonstrated that declining levels of DHEA are linked to such conditions as diabetes, obesity, elevated cholesterol levels, heart disease, arthritis, and autoimmune diseases.

Antiaging effects

The clinical studies evaluating DHEA supplementation in elderly patients have focused on enhancing memory and improving mental function as well as increasing muscle strength and lean body mass, enhancing immune function, and enhancing the quality of life. Most, but not all, studies show positive effects in all of these areas.

Depression

Researchers have reported that DHEA levels are lower in depressed patients. Clinical studies have shown that DHEA supplementation (usually 30 to 90 mg per day) significantly improves depression in elderly subjects after four weeks of use. In one study, 60 percent of the patients responded to DHEA at the end of the six-week treatment period compared with 20 percent on placebo. The symptoms that improved most significantly were loss of pleasure, loss of energy, lack of motivation, emotional numbness, sadness, inability to cope, and worry.

Erectile dysfunction

DHEA levels tend to be lower in men with erectile dysfunction (ED). One double-blind study demonstrated that DHEA supplementation produced a slight improvement in the ability to achieve or maintain an erection sufficient for satisfactory sexual performance.

Systemic lupus erythematosus

Defective manufacture of androgens (including testosterone and DHEA) has been proposed as a potential predisposing factor for systemic lupus erythematosus (lupus or SLE) as well as rheumatoid arthritis. Supplemental DHEA has shown moderate therapeutic benefits in patients with SLE in studies conducted at Stanford Medical Center. The results indicate that DHEA therapy, when added to conventional treatment for severe SLE, may produce some improvements in symptoms and appears to have a protective effect against corticosteroid-induced bone loss (osteopenia).

Available Forms

DHEA is available in tablet, capsule, liquid, and sublingual form.

Cautions and Warnings

The long-term safety of DHEA supplementation has not been determined. There is concern that higher DHEA levels may increase the risk of prostate or breast cancer.

If you have a history of a hormone-sensitive cancer such as breast or prostate cancer, do not use DHEA unless directed to do so by a physician.

Possible Side Effects

Side effects are rare at recommended levels, but at higher intakes (50–200 mg per day) DHEA can produce acne (in over 50 percent of people), increased facial hair (in 18 percent), and increased perspiration (in 8 percent). Other possible side effects include breast tenderness, weight gain, headache, oily skin, and menstrual irregularity.

Drug Interactions

None known.

Food and Nutrient Interactions

None known.

Usual Dosage

Many experts recommend using blood or saliva measurements to determine the dosage. Their recommendation is to not take DHEA unless there is confirmation that DHEA levels are in fact low. Nonetheless, the recommendations vary according to gender and age. For men age forty to fifty, the typical recommendation is 15 to 25 mg daily. For men over fifty, the recommendation is usually between 25 and 50 mg. For women, it is generally recommended that DHEA be used with caution and in low dosages ranging from 5 to 15 mg.

People with systemic lupus erythematosus and other autoimmune diseases appear to require high dosages (100–200 mg per day) of DHEA. Such high levels should never be taken without medical supervision.

Overdosage

None known.

Special Populations

Pregnant/breast-feeding women

DHEA supplementation should not be used during pregnancy and lactation unless under the advice of a physician.

Children

DHEA supplementation is not suitable for children.

Seniors

No special precautions are known.

D,L-phenylalanine (DLPA)

Used For

Depression
Effectiveness: B+   Safety: C

Pain
Effectiveness: B   Safety: C

General Information

D,L-phenylalanine (DLPA) is a mixture of the naturally occurring amino acid L-phenylalanine and its synthetic mirror image D-phenylalanine. L-phenylalanine can be converted to L-tyrosine (another amino acid) and subsequently to the neurotransmitters L-dopa, norepinephrine, and epinephrine. L-phenylalanine, besides being converted to tyrosine, can be converted to phenylethylamine (PEA); the same is true for D-phenylalanine. PEA has stimulant and antidepressant properties. Clinical studies have shown DLPA to be helpful in treating depression.

DLPA has also been used to treat chronic pain, such as that found in osteoarthritis and rheumatoid arthritis. However, both positive and negative results have been reported. DLPA has been used in amounts ranging from 75 to 1,500 mg per day.

Available Forms

DLPA is available in capsules and tablets.

Cautions and Warnings

None known.

Possible Side Effects

Generally without side effects; however, occasional nausea, heartburn, or transient headaches have been reported.

Drug Interactions

None known.

Food and Nutrient Interactions

DLPA is generally recommended to be taken on an empty stomach. L-phenylalanine competes with several other amino acids for transport sites into the brain. Therefore, it should not be taken with protein-containing foods.

Usual Dosage

The usual dosage is 200 to 400 mg per day.

Overdosage

None known.

Special Populations

Pregnant/breast-feeding women

As the effects of DLPA during pregnancy and lactation have not been sufficiently evaluated, it should not be used during these times.

Children
  As the effects of DLPA in children have not been sufficiently evaluated, it should not be used by children unless directed to do so by a physician.

Seniors
  No special precautions are known.

Docosahexaenoic Acid (DHA)

Used For

Brain and eye development
Effectiveness: A   Safety: B

Lowering triglycerides
Effectiveness: A   Safety: B

General Information

Docosahexaenoic acid (DHA) is an omega-3 long-chain polyunsaturated fatty acid found in fish and algae. In humans, DHA is required for proper mental and visual function, as it is the primary structural fatty acid in the gray matter of the brain and the retina of the eye.
  Adequate dietary intake of DHA is important for all ages but is particularly important for pregnant and nursing women. Significant brain and eye development occurs while the fetus is in the womb and continues during the first year after birth. Infants rely on their mothers to supply DHA for the developing brain and eyes, initially through the placenta and then through breast milk. DHA is the most abundant

omega-3 long-chain fatty acid in breast milk, and studies show that breast-fed babies have intelligence quotient (IQ) advantages over babies fed formula without DHA. But DHA levels in the breast milk of women in the United States are among the lowest in the world. Increasing DHA levels has been recommended by some experts for all pregnant or lactating women.

A child who is not breast-fed will very likely not get enough DHA for proper brain development. Although present in human milk, DHA is absent from artificial formulas in the United States (some European formulas contain supplemental DHA from algae). Since infants have limited ability to manufacture their own DHA, it is thought that using infant formulas instead of breast milk may lead to impaired mental function and a lower IQ. This hypothesis has been documented in several clinical studies.

DHA has been shown to reduce levels of blood triglycerides. The research indicates that DHA alone appears to be just as effective as fish oils (which contain both DHA and EPA) in beneficially lowering triglyceride levels in individuals at risk for heart disease.

Available Forms

DHA can be derived from algae or fish sources and is available in capsules, tablets, and even food bars. DHA is also found in **cod liver oil** and **fish oil supplements.** Brand names available include Neuromins.

Cautions and Warnings

None known.

Possible Side Effects

None known.

Drug Interactions

None known.

Food and Nutrient Interactions

DHA and other polyunsaturated fatty acids are easily damaged by oxygen, so the body's requirement for vitamin E, an antioxidant, increases as intake of polyunsaturated fatty acid increases.

Usual Dosage

For general health purposes, the recommended daily dosage is 200–500 mg.

Overdosage

None known.

Special Populations

Pregnant/breast-feeding women

Considered safe during pregnancy and lactation. For pregnant and lactating women the recommended daily dosage is 400–1,000 mg.

Children

Suitable for children at one-half the adult dosage.

Seniors

No special precautions are known.

DMAE
(2-dimethylaminoethanol)

Used For

Alzheimer's disease
Effectiveness: B–   Safety: C

Attention deficit disorder and hyperactivity
Effectiveness: B+   Safety: C

General Information

DMAE is naturally present in the human brain, and taking it as a supplement may increase DMAE levels in the brain as well as levels of the brain neurotransmitter acetylcholine; however, not all studies have confirmed these effects. In fact, there is some evidence that DMAE could actually reduce the availability of choline for acetylcholine manufacture. The role of DMAE in the brain is not known, but acetylcholine plays an important role in memory and behavior.

Alzheimer's disease
DMAE does not appear to be an effective treatment for Alzheimer's disease based on the results from most double-blind studies. Nor does it seem able to significantly improve mental function in elderly subjects.

Attention deficit disorder and hyperactivity
DMAE was shown to decrease hyperactivity, increase the capacity to learn, and reduce irritability in children between six and twelve years of age with attention deficit disorder in several double-blind

studies. In fact, DMAE was shown to be as effective as methylphenidate (Ritalin) in head-to-head trials.

Available Forms

DMAE is available in capsules, tablets, liquid, and even food bars.

Cautions and Warnings

The long-term side effects of DMAE are not known. There has been one case report where it appeared that long-term use (i.e., more than ten years) was associated with tardive dyskinesia (muscular trembling and inability to control muscular movement).

Possible Side Effects

When used at dosages up to 1,000 mg per day DMAE is usually not associated with side effects. At higher dosages DMAE may produce drowsiness, mental confusion, and signs of too much acetylcholine being produced, such as increased nasal secretions and excessive saliva production.

Drug Interactions

Certain antipsychotic drugs, such as phenothiazines, butyrophenones, and thioxanthenes, can produce a trembling disorder called tardive dyskinesia. Early research with DMAE suggested that it might be beneficial in relieving this disorder, although several controlled studies did not find the effects of DMAE any better than placebo.

Food and Nutrient Interactions
None known.

Usual Dosage
The dosage in adults is 1,000 mg daily. For children between six and twelve years of age the dosage is 500 mg daily.

Overdosage
None known.

Special Populations

Pregnant/breast-feeding women
DMAE use is not recommended during pregnancy and lactation.

Children
Suitable for children at one-half the adult dosage.

Seniors
No special precautions are known.

Eicosapentaenoic Acid (EPA) (*see* Fish Oils)

General Information
Eicosapentaenoic acid (EPA) is an omega-3 fatty acid that is a key component in fish oil supplements. EPA

plays a critical role in cell membranes and in other body functions and structures.

Evening Primrose Oil (*see* Gamma-linolenic Acid)

Fiber

Used For

Constipation
Effectiveness: A   Safety: A

Diabetes
Effectiveness: A   Safety: A

Hemorrhoids
Effectiveness: A   Safety: A

High cholesterol and triglycerides
Effectiveness: A   Safety: A

Irritable bowel syndrome
Effectiveness: A   Safety: A

Weight loss
Effectiveness: A   Safety: A

General Information

The term "dietary fiber" refers to the components of plant cell wall and non-nutritive residues. Fiber is divided into two general categories—water soluble and water insoluble. Insoluble fiber, such as wheat bran, is a good laxative but lacks some of the beneficial effects noted with the soluble fibers. In addition to the well-known use of dietary fiber as a bulk-forming laxative, the principal use of supplemental dietary fiber is in the treatment of irritable bowel syndrome and other functional disturbances of the colon, elevated cholesterol levels, and obesity. For these purposes, soluble fiber is best. Examples of soluble fiber sources are psyllium, guar gum, glucomannan, gum karaya, and pectin. These fiber sources are categorized together because of their similar effects and actions.

Constipation and hemorrhoids

Fiber has long been used in the treatment of constipation. Dietary fiber, particularly soluble fiber such as psyllium, increases stool weight as a result of its water-holding properties and is classified as a bulk-forming laxative. Of all types of laxatives, bulk-forming fiber is generally regarded as the most natural and the best. A larger, bulkier stool passes through the colon more easily, requiring less pressure to expel and subsequently less straining. As a result of less straining, bulk-forming laxatives are often recommended in the treatment of hemorrhoids. Bulk-forming laxatives generally help produce a bowel movement within twelve to twenty-four hours.

Diabetes

Double-blind studies have shown that supplementing the diet with soluble fiber before or with meals reduces after-meal increases in blood sugar levels. It accomplishes this effect largely by delaying the emptying of the stomach and thereby leading to a more gradual absorption of dietary sugar, as well as by increasing the tissues' sensitivity to insulin. The improvements noted in blood sugar levels in diabetics can be quite significant. For example, in one study, 23 non-insulin-dependent diabetics were given either 5 g of psyllium seed husk powder three times daily before meals or placebo for twelve weeks. In the patients receiving the psyllium there was a significant drop in fasting blood sugar levels from an initial level of 195 mg/dl down to 136 mg/dl. Diabetics must be aware, however, that many fiber supplements are loaded with sugar and thus must be avoided.

High cholesterol and triglycerides

The binding of bile acids and cholesterol to soluble fiber such as psyllium, pectin, and guar gum is very helpful in reducing blood cholesterol and triglyceride levels. Loss of cholesterol and bile salts through the feces is the major pathway for elimination of these compounds from the body. Dietary fiber also decreases cholesterol biosynthesis and increases the conversion of cholesterol to the bile acids. The typical reductions in total cholesterol levels with the more popular soluble fibers are as follows:

Soluble Fiber	Dosage	Decrease in Total Cholesterol
Guar gum	9–15 g	10 percent
Pectin	6–10 g	5 percent
Psyllium	10–20 g	10–20 percent

Irritable bowel syndrome

The treatment of irritable bowel syndrome (IBS) by increasing the intake of dietary fiber has a long history. The most effective fiber supplements are the soluble forms because of their ability to improve the function and tone of the large intestine (colon).

Weight loss

When taken with water before meals, soluble fiber binds to the water in the stomach to form a gelatinous mass that makes an individual feel full. As a result, he or she will be less likely to overeat. Fiber supplements have also been shown to reduce the number of calories absorbed by the intestines. In some of the clinical studies demonstrating weight loss, fiber supplements were shown to reduce the number of calories absorbed by 30 to 180 per day. Over the course of a year, this could result in a reduction of 3 to 18 pounds.

The most impressive results in weight loss studies have been achieved with guar gum, a soluble fiber obtained from the Indian cluster bean *(Cyamopsis tetragonolobra).* In several double-blind studies, 10 g of guar gum immediately before lunch and dinner promoted an average weight loss of 1 pound per week.

Available Forms

Fiber supplements are available in capsule, tablet, and powder form. Most often, because of the high dosage required, fiber supplements come in powder form to mix in water or juice. Brand names available include Metamucil, Konsyl, and Perdiem Fiber Therapy.

Cautions and Warnings

People with any disorder of the esophagus should not take any fiber supplement in a pill form, as the pill may expand in the esophagus and lead to obstruction.

Drink at least 8 ounces of water per dosage when taking any bulk-forming laxative.

If you have not had a bowel movement in seven days or are experiencing any abdominal pain, consult a physician before taking any bulk-forming laxative.

If you have rectal bleeding after using any bulk-forming laxative, consult a physician.

Possible Side Effects

Since soluble fiber is fermented by intestinal bacteria, a great deal of gas can be produced in individuals not used to a high fiber intake, leading to flatulence and abdominal discomfort. Allergic reactions to psyllium and other fiber sources have been reported.

Drug Interactions

Because taking any bulk-forming laxative may decrease the absorption of any drug, most experts recommend taking any drug at least three hours before or after taking a bulk-forming laxative.

Food and Nutrient Interactions

Since fiber reduces the absorption of most minerals, be sure to take mineral supplements at least forty-five minutes before or after taking a fiber supplement.

Usual Dosage

When using dietary fiber supplements, it is best to start out with a small dosage and increase gradually so that the intestines become used to the increased fiber intake; too rapid an increase can produce flatulence and abdominal discomfort. The recommended dosage as a laxative is generally 5 g at bedtime. For other purposes, it is generally recommended the dosage be started at 1 or 2 g before meals and at bedtime, gradually increasing the dosage to 5 g before meals and at bedtime.

Overdosage
None known.

Special Populations

Pregnant/breast-feeding women
Fiber supplements are generally regarded as safe during pregnancy and lactation.

Children
Suitable for children at one-half the adult dosage.

Seniors
No special precautions are known.

Fish Oils (Eicosapentaenoic Acid and Docosahexaenoic Acid)

Used For

Allergies, eczema, and asthma
Effectiveness: B   Safety: A

Cancer prevention
Effectiveness: B   Safety: A

Cardiovascular diseases

 Angina and arrhythmia
 Effectiveness: B+   Safety: A

 High blood pressure
 Effectiveness: B+   Safety: A

 High triglycerides
 Effectiveness: A   Safety: A

Crohn's disease
Effectiveness: B   Safety: A

Depression
Effectiveness: B   Safety: A

Psoriasis
Effectiveness: B+   Safety: A

Rheumatoid arthritis, lupus, and other autoimmune diseases
Effectiveness: B+   Safety: A

General Information

Fish oil supplements contain the omega-3 fatty acids EPA (eicosapentaenoic acid) and DHA (docosahexaenoic acid). A significant body of evidence now shows that consumption of fish oil may be beneficial to health, because of these important omega-3 fatty acids. Numerous studies have reported that diets rich in EPA and DHA reduce the risk of cardiovascular disease and various forms of cancer. Fish oil supplements have also been reported to be helpful in reducing the signs and symptoms of many diseases, especially those associated with inflammation and allergy such as psoriasis, eczema, and rheumatoid arthritis.

Omega-3 fatty acids play a critical role in cell membranes and in other body functions and structures. Especially important are the ways in which essential fatty acids are transformed into regulatory compounds known as prostaglandins. These compounds help control many body functions including blood pressure, immune function, allergic and inflammatory responses, and platelet stickiness (discussed below). It is through the effects of prostaglandins made from EPA and DHA as well as the effects that EPA and DHA have on cell membranes that fish oil supplements exert their beneficial effects.

Allergies, eczema, and asthma

Omega-3 fatty acids are important mediators of allergy and inflammation. Nutrition-oriented physicians believe that by altering the type of dietary oils consumed and stored in cell membranes, the prostaglandin metabolism involved in allergic reactions and inflammation can be manipulated. Preliminary studies and some double-blind studies indicate that fish oil supplementation may help reduce inflammation and allergic reactions in eczema, asthma, and other allergic disorders. Further research is required to verify these preliminary findings.

Cancer prevention

Numerous animal studies have demonstrated anticancer activity with fish oil supplementation, and there is considerable evidence from population-based studies that increased consumption of fish oils reduces the risk of many forms of cancer, especially breast cancer. However, most experts feel that it remains premature to recommend fish oil supplementation as an anticancer substance until there are more definitive clinical studies.

Cardiovascular diseases

The health benefits of fish oil were first investigated in Greenland Inuit, who consumed a diet that was high in saturated animal fat from seals, whales, and fish yet had very low rates of coronary heart disease. Later studies discovered that the Inuit diet contained large quantities of omega-3 fatty acids. Subsequently, fish oil supplementation has been studied in over three hundred clinical and scientific investigations, the majority of which involve looking at the protection fish oil consumption may provide against atherosclerosis-related diseases. One of the key effects of fish oils in the battle against hardening of the arteries appears to be its effect on platelets. While a high intake of saturated fat promotes platelet stickiness, a factor that leads to hardening of the arteries, heart disease, and strokes, fish oil consumption helps prevent platelets from sticking together. Fish oil supplementation has also been shown to reduce blood triglyceride levels, lower blood pressure, improve blood flow, and reduce inflammation. These effects are all significant goals in battling atherosclerosis.

Angina and arrhythmia

Fish oil supplementation has been shown to reduce the frequency of angina attacks and arrhythmias in double-blind studies. The improvement is thought to be the result of improved blood flow through coronary arteries, resulting in better delivery and use of oxygen by the heart muscle.

High blood pressure

There is evidence from over sixty double-blind studies that fish oil supplementation reduces blood pressure in patients with hypertension, but not in
subjects with normal blood pressure. The effect is
clearly dose-dependent—the higher the dosage, the
greater the reduction. It is thought that fish oils
lower blood pressure by helping to dilate the arteries as well as facilitate excretion of sodium and fluid
by the kidneys. However, it must be pointed out that
even at higher dosages, the blood-pressure-lowering effect of fish oil supplementation is generally in
the range of only 3 to 4 mm Hg for both the systolic
and diastolic measures.

High triglycerides

There is considerable evidence from over thirty
double-blind studies that fish oil supplementation
reduces blood triglyceride levels, especially in patients with severe elevations. Most, but not all, of
these double-blind studies have also shown fish oils
to lower blood cholesterol levels. The typical decrease in triglyceride levels with fish oil supplementation is 20 percent to 50 percent. Results are usually
apparent within the first month.

Crohn's disease

A special enteric-coated capsule (coated in a manner to prevent the pill from being broken down in
the stomach) containing highly purified EPA and
DHA has been shown to produce clinical improvement and reduce the relapse rate in individuals with
Crohn's disease. Apparently, the enteric-coated form

is better tolerated than the non-enteric-coated form in these patients, as it is does not cause the mild gastrointestinal symptoms often resulting from taking regular fish oil supplements (see "Possible Side Effects," below).

Depression

An insufficiency of omega-3 oils in the diet has been linked to depression, manic-depression, and schizophrenia. Preliminary evidence indicates that fish oil supplementation may help improve brain function, mood, and behavior in people suffering from these psychological disorders. These preliminary studies, however, need to be verified by larger well-designed studies. What is known is that omega-3 fatty acids are required for proper brain cell fluidity, neurotransmitter synthesis, signal transmission, uptake of serotonin and other neurotransmitters, neurotransmitter binding, and the activity of monoamine oxidase, the enzyme that breaks down serotonin and other monoamine neurotransmitters like epinephrine, dopamine, and norepinephrine. All of these factors have been implicated in depression and other psychological disturbances.

Psoriasis

In double-blind studies, patients with psoriasis have been successfully treated with fish oil. In one study, an impressive 77 percent of the patients reported either excellent, moderate, or mild improvement.

Rheumatoid arthritis, lupus, and other autoimmune diseases

Autoimmune disease such as rheumatoid arthritis, lupus (systemic lupus erythematosus), multiple sclerosis, and Raynaud's phenomenon are characterized by the immune system actually attacking the body's own tissue. The result is tremendous inflammation and tissue destruction in the area being attacked. There is mounting evidence that fish oil supplementation may beneficially influence the course of treatment in patients with these auto-immune diseases. The best-studied is rheumatoid arthritis, where double-blind studies have shown that fish oil supplementation is capable of producing significant clinical improvement in the number of painful joints, inflammation, and pain.

Available Forms

Most fish oil supplements are derived from herring, cod liver, salmon, and mackerel and usually contain 18 percent EPA and 12 percent DHA, or a total of 30 percent omega-3 fatty acids. However, some newer products contain higher percentages of total omega-3 oils and differing ratios of EPA and DHA. Fish oil supplements are available primarily in soft gelatin capsules. Cod liver oil contains large amounts of EPA and DHA but also contains high levels of vitamin A and D. Brand names available include MaxEPA and Ultimate Omega.

Cautions and Warnings

Be sure the product is fish oil, not fish liver oil. This distinction is important since fish liver oil contains fat soluble vitamins A and D, which if taken in excessive amounts have the potential to cause toxicity (see **cod liver oil**).

Individuals with diabetes must monitor blood sugar levels closely if electing to use fish oil supplements. Elevations in blood sugar and cholesterol levels have occurred in some diabetics taking fish oils.

Possible Side Effects

The most common side effect with fish oil supplementation is mild gastrointestinal upset. Some people who supplement with several grams of fish oil daily may burp up a "fishy" smell. Elevations in blood sugar and cholesterol levels may occur in some individuals who take fish oil.

Drug Interactions

Because fish oil supplementation may reduce platelet stickiness, it may also increase the risk of bleeding in patients taking anticoagulant drugs such as warfarin (Coumadin) and platelet-inhibiting drugs such as aspirin and ticlopidine (Ticlid).

Food and Nutrient Interactions

Polyunsaturated fatty acids are easily damaged by oxygen, so the body's requirement for vitamin E, an antioxidant, increases as intake of polyunsaturated fatty acids increases.

Usual Dosage

Most of the clinical research with fish oil has utilized a dosage of at least 1.8 g of EPA and 1.2 g of DHA daily—an amount that may require 10 g or more of fish oil. Because most fish oil supplements contain only 18 percent EPA and 12 percent DHA, that translates to roughly ten 1,000 mg capsules per day.

Overdosage

None known.

Special Populations

Pregnant/breast-feeding women
Fish oils, but not fish liver oil, are considered safe during pregnancy and lactation. *Note:* Due to its very high levels of vitamin A and vitamin D, cod liver oil should not be taken by women who are pregnant or who may become pregnant.

Children
Suitable for children at one-half the adult dosage.

Seniors
No special precautions are known.

Flaxseed Oil

Used For

Cancer prevention
Effectiveness: B   Safety: A

Essential fatty acid source
Effectiveness: A   Safety: A

Heart disease (atherosclerosis) prevention
Effectiveness: B   Safety: A

High blood pressure
Effectiveness: B   Safety: A

General Information

Flaxseed oil is unique because it contains two essential fatty acids—alpha-linolenic acid (an omega-3 fatty acid) and linoleic acid (an omega-6 fatty acid)—in high amounts. It contains roughly 58 percent alpha-linolenic acid (ALA), considerably more than other common vegetable oils. The body can convert ALA into EPA (eicosapentaenoic acid), an omega-3 oil found in **fish oils**. However, because the conversion from ALA to EPA is quite limited, some of the effects of fish oil (such as controlling triglycerides) do not occur when people supplement with flaxseed oil. The best utilization of flaxseed oil is as a source of essential fatty acids.

Cancer prevention

Alpha-linolenic acid has demonstrated some anti-cancer properties, especially against breast cancer. In addition to human studies suggesting a protective effect, animal models of mammary cancer have also shown that alpha-linolenic acid inhibits tumor growth.

As well as containing ALA, flaxseed oil contains lignans—special compounds that demonstrate some health benefits, including positive effects in relieving menopausal hot flashes as well as anti-cancer, antibacterial, antifungal, and antiviral activity. High-lignan flaxseed oil is produced by adding some of these lignans back to the oil.

Heart disease (atherosclerosis) prevention

Population studies have demonstrated that people who consume a diet rich in omega-3 oils from either fish or vegetable sources have a significantly reduced risk of developing heart disease (as well as strokes). In fact, in several studies the intake of ALA from vegetable sources had more of an effect than consumption of fish oils. Nonetheless, in clinical trials flaxseed oil typically produces less of an effect on cholesterol and triglyceride levels compared to fish oil.

High blood pressure

Increasing the intake of omega-3 fatty acids from either fish oil supplements or flaxseed oil can lower blood pressure. Although the fish oils typically have a more pronounced effect than flaxseed oil, one study indicated that along with reducing the intake of saturated fat, 1 tablespoon per day of flaxseed oil dropped both the systolic and diastolic readings by up to 9 mm Hg.

Available Forms

Flaxseed oil is available in liquid form in bottles and soft gelatin capsules.

Cautions and Warnings

Do not heat flaxseed oil. Heating leads to the production of harmful compounds (lipid peroxides) that display possible cancer-causing properties. Use as fresh as possible and be sure to check the expiration date.

Possible Side Effects

Since flaxseed oil is really simply a food source, side effects from supplementing with it are uncommon.

Drug Interactions

None known.

Food and Nutrient Interactions

Polyunsaturated fatty acids are easily damaged by oxygen, so the body's requirement for vitamin E, an antioxidant, rises as intake of polyunsaturated fatty acid increases.

Mixing flaxseed oil with another food—yogurt or cottage cheese, for example—helps to emulsify the oil (break up the oil globules into much smaller particles), aiding in optimal digestion, absorption, and utilization of the essential fatty acids.

Usual Dosage

A dosage of 1 tablespoon daily is often recommended.

Overdosage

None known.

Special Populations

Pregnant/breast-feeding women
Considered safe during pregnancy and lactation.

Children
Suitable for children at one-half the adult dosage.

Seniors
No special precautions are known.

Fructooligosaccharides

Used For

Diabetes
Effectiveness: B–   Safety: A

Elevated cholesterol and triglycerides
Effectiveness: B   Safety: A

Improving intestinal bacterial flora
Effectiveness: A   Safety: A

Irritable bowel syndrome
Effectiveness: F   Safety: A

General Information

The term *oligosaccharide* refers to a short chain of sugar molecules (oligo- means "few," *saccharide* means "sugar"). Fructooligosaccharides (FOS) and inulin, which are found in many vegetables, consist of short chains of fructose molecules. Galactooligosaccharides (GOS), which also occur naturally, consist of short chains of galactose molecules. These compounds can be only partially digested by humans. When oligosaccharides are consumed, the undigested portion serves as food for "friendly" bacteria such as bifidobacteria and lactobacilli. Clinical studies have shown that administering FOS, GOS, and inulin can increase the number of these friendly bacteria in the colon while simultaneously reducing the population of harmful bacteria. Other benefits noted with FOS, GOS, or inulin supplementation include increased production of beneficial short-chain fatty acids such as butyrate, increased absorption of calcium and magnesium, and improved elimination of toxic compounds.

Because FOS, GOS, and inulin improve colon function and increase the number of friendly bacteria, one might expect that these compounds would help relieve the symptoms of irritable bowel syndrome. However, a double-blind study found no clear benefit from FOS supplementation (2 g three times daily) in patients with this condition.

Several double-blind studies have looked at the ability of FOS or inulin to lower blood cholesterol and triglyceride levels. These studies have shown that in individuals with elevated total cholesterol or triglyceride levels, including people with non-insulin-dependent diabetes, FOS or inulin (in amounts ranging from 8 to 20 g daily) produced meaningful reductions in these blood lipids. But in individuals with normal or low cholesterol or triglyceride levels, FOS or inulin produced little effect.

FOS may help in lowering blood sugar levels in diabetes, but research into this area has produced conflicting results.

Available Forms

FOS and inulin are found naturally in Jerusalem artichokes, burdock, chicory, leeks, onions, and asparagus. FOS can be synthesized by enzymes of the fungus *Aspergillus niger* acting on sucrose. GOS is naturally found in soybeans and can be synthesized from lactose (milk sugar). FOS, GOS, and inulin are available as nutritional supplements in capsules, tablets, and as a powder.

Cautions and Warnings

Dosages greater than 40 g per day may produce diarrhea.

Possible Side Effects

Generally, oligosaccharides are well tolerated. Some individuals reported increased flatulence in some of the studies. At higher levels of intake, that is, in excess of 40 g per day, FOS and the other oligosaccharides may induce diarrhea.

Drug Interactions

None known.

Food and Nutrient Interactions

None known.

Usual Dosage

The average daily intake of oligosaccharides in the United States is estimated to be about 800 to 1,000 mg. For the promotion of healthy bacterial flora, the usual recommendation for FOS, GOS, or inulin is 2,000 to 3,000 mg per day with meals. In the studies involving diabetes and high blood lipids, amounts ranged from 8 to 20 g per day.

Overdosage

None known.

Special Populations

Pregnant/breast-feeding women
Considered safe during pregnancy and lactation.

Children
Suitable for children at one-half the adult dosage.

Seniors
No special precautions are known.

GABA
(Gamma-aminobutyric Acid)

Used For

Anxiety
Effectiveness: C   Safety: C

Epilepsy
Effectiveness: C   Safety: C

Insomnia
Effectiveness: C   Safety: C

Schizophrenia
Effectiveness: C   Safety: C

General Information

GABA is a natural calming and antiepileptic agent that the body manufactures from glucose and the amino acid glutamine. Some people with anxiety, insomnia, epilepsy, and other brain disorders may not manufacture sufficient levels of GABA. Since GABA does not cross the blood-brain barrier very well, virtually all of the GABA found in the brain is manufactured there. This fact implies that supplemental GABA would not increase levels of GABA in the brain. Nonetheless, GABA has been used with reported success in a variety of brain disorders, including anxiety, epilepsy, and schizophrenia, by two experts in amino acid therapy. However, these reports have not been substantiated with clinical trials.

High intake of GABA was shown to produce a significant elevation of plasma growth hormone levels (single administration of 5,000 mg of GABA) and prolactin (daily administration of 18,000 mg of GABA for four days) in one human study.

Available Forms

GABA is found as a nutritional supplement primarily in capsules and tablets.

Cautions and Warnings

Since benzodiazepine drugs such as diazepam (Valium) work by stimulating GABA receptors in the brain, GABA should not be used by individuals taking these drugs.

Possible Side Effects

The side effects of GABA are unknown, as it has not been sufficiently studied in humans.

Drug Interactions

GABA may potentiate drugs that stimulate GABA receptors in the brain, including benzodiapines such as diazepam (Valium).

Food and Nutrient Interactions

Usually GABA is given on an empty stomach.

Usual Dosage

GABA is usually recommended at a dosage of 200 mg four times daily.

Overdosage

None known.

Special Populations

Pregnant/breast-feeding women

As the effects of GABA during pregnancy and lactation have not been sufficiently evaluated, it should not be used during these times.

Children

As the effects of GABA in children have not been sufficiently evaluated, it should not be used in children unless under a physician's care.

Seniors

No special precautions are known.

Gamma-linolenic Acid (GLA)

Used For

Diabetic neuropathy
Effectiveness: B+   Safety: A

Eczema
Effectiveness: B–   Safety: A

Premenstrual syndrome
Effectiveness: D   Safety: A

Rheumatoid arthritis
Effectiveness: B   Safety: A

General Information

Evening primrose oil, black currant seed oil, and borage oil are vegetable oils that are somewhat unique in that they contain gamma-linolenic acid (GLA), an omega-6 fatty acid that the body converts to a hormonelike substance called prostaglandin E1 (PGE1), which has anti-inflammatory properties. Linoleic acid, a common fatty acid found in nuts, seeds, and most vegetable oils, should theoretically convert to PGE1, but it is thought by some that many things can interfere with this conversion, including various diseases including diabetes, the aging process, saturated fat, hydrogenated oils, blood sugar problems, and inadequate vitamin C, magnesium, zinc, and B vitamins. Supplements that provide GLA circumvent these conversion problems, leading to more predictable formation of PGE1. While these GLA supplements (i.e., black currant seed, borage, and evening primrose oils) are quite popular, their effect on those health conditions for which they are most commonly used is unknown.

FATTY ACID COMPOSITION OF SELECTED OILS
(% of total fat)

	SF	OA	LA	GLA	ALA
Evening primrose	10	9	72	9	0
Black currant	7	9	47	17	13
Borage	14	16	35	22	0
Flaxseed	9	19	14	0	58

SF = Saturated fats
OA = Oleic acid (a monounsaturated fat)
LA = Linoleic acid
GLA = Gamma-linolenic acid (an omega-6 oil)
ALA = Alpha-linolenic acid (an omega-3 oil)

Diabetic neuropathy

Diabetes is associated with a substantial disturbance in essential fatty acid (EFA) metabolism, including an impairment in the process of converting linoleic acid to gamma-linolenic acid (GLA). As a result, providing GLA in the form of borage, evening primrose, or black currant oil may offer a method to bypass some of this disturbance and possibly improve diabetic neuropathy. To test the hypothesis, in a double-blind study 111 patients with mild diabetic neuropathy took twelve capsules of evening primrose oil daily, with each capsule containing 40 mg of GLA. Sixteen different parameters were assessed, including conduction velocities, hot and cold thresholds, sensation, tendon reflexes, and muscle strength. After one year, all sixteen parameters improved. These results appear to support the use of GLA supplements in the treatment and prevention of diabetic neuropathy.

Eczema

Initially it was thought that patients with eczema might have decreased activity of the enzyme delta-6-desaturase, which converts linoleic acid to gamma-linolenic acid. If such a defect exists, supplementing the diet with a GLA source should prove helpful. Although preliminary double-blind studies using evening primrose oil showed benefit in improving the symptoms of eczema, the more recent studies do not support a significant therapeutic effect.

Premenstrual syndrome

Although evening primrose oil and other GLA supplements are quite popular for the treatment of PMS, three well-controlled double-blind studies on the use of GLA supplements (in the form of evening primrose oil) for PMS were largely negative in that they showed no greater benefit over a placebo.

Rheumatoid arthritis

Some studies have shown some benefit from GLA supplementation in cases of rheumatoid arthritis, but others have not. The key factor appears to be whether or not subjects are allowed to take their anti-inflammatory drugs. For example, in one double-blind study, thirty-seven patients with rheumatoid arthritis were given either GLA (1.4 g daily) or placebo for twenty-four weeks. GLA supplementation reduced the number of tender joints by 36 percent, tenderness by 45 percent, the number of swollen joints by 28 percent, and swelling by 41 percent. In contrast, no patients in the placebo group showed significant improvement in any measure. The superficial results of this study indicate that borage oil may be useful in reducing the inflammatory process of rheumatoid arthritis. However, in this study the subjects continued to take their anti-inflammatory drugs; this probably masked the detrimental effects on tissue arachidonic acid and EPA levels seen in other studies. Evening primrose oil supplementation increased arachidonic acid (pro-inflammatory) while reducing EPA (anti-inflammatory) within body tissues.

Available Forms

Evening primrose oil, black currant seed oil, and borage oil are available primarily in soft gelatin capsules.

Cautions and Warnings

None known.

Possible Side Effects

None known.

Drug Interactions

None known.

Food and Nutrient Interactions

Polyunsaturated fatty acids are easily damaged by oxygen, so the body's requirement for vitamin E, an antioxidant, rises as intake of polyunsaturated fatty acid increases.

Usual Dosage

The dosage used in most studies is much higher than most label recommendations. For example, in studies involving rheumatoid arthritis, researchers used a dosage of borage oil to provide 1.4 g of GLA. Since evening primrose oil is 9 percent GLA, this means that approximately thirty-one 500 mg capsules of evening primrose oil would have to be consumed each day to achieve this dosage. Studies with evening primrose oil typically involved subjects taking 3,000–6,000 mg per day (providing approximately 270–540 mg of GLA).

Overdosage

None known.

Special Populations

Pregnant/breast-feeding women
As the effects of GLA supplements during pregnancy and lactation have not been sufficiently evaluated, it should not be used during these times.

Children
Suitable for children at one-half the adult dosage.

Seniors
No special precautions are known.

Gamma-oryzanol

Used For

Elevated cholesterol levels
Effectiveness: B+   Safety: B

Enhancing physical performance
Effectiveness: B+   Safety: B

Menopause
Effectiveness: B+   Safety: B

General Information

Gamma-oryzanol (esters of ferulic acid) is a growth-promoting substance found in grains and isolated from rice bran oil. It has been used in Japan as a medicine since 1962. Initially it was used in the treatment of minor anxiety and later became approved in the treatment of menopause (1970) and elevated cholesterol and triglyceride levels (1986). It is also used by bodybuilders.

Elevated cholesterol levels

Gamma-oryzanol has been shown to be quite effective in lowering blood cholesterol and triglyceride levels in several double-blind studies lowering total cholesterol levels by 8–12 percent and triglycerides by 15 percent within the first four weeks. Gamma-oryzanol's cholesterol-lowering action appears to involve a combination of effects in that it increases the conversion of cholesterol to bile acids and inhibits the absorption of cholesterol.

Enhancing physical performance

Double-blind studies have shown gamma-oryzanol to increase lean body mass, increase strength, improve recovery from workouts, and reduce body fat and postexercise soreness.

Menopause

Gamma-oryzanol was first shown to be effective in menopausal symptoms, including hot flashes, in the early 1960s. Clinical studies demonstrated that 67 to 85 percent of the women had a 50 percent or greater reduction in their menopausal symptoms.

Available Forms

Gamma-oryzanol is available in capsules and tablets. It is also used as an antioxidant in cosmetic preparations.

Cautions and Warnings

None known.

Possible Side Effects

No significant side effects have ever been produced in experimental and clinical studies.

Drug Interactions

None known.

Food and Nutrient Interactions

None known.

Usual Dosage

The usual dosage of gamma-oryzanol for therapeutic purposes is 100 mg three times daily.

Overdosage

None known.

Special Populations

Pregnant/breast-feeding women

As the effects of gamma-oryzanol during pregnancy and lactation have not been sufficiently evaluated, it should not be used during these times.

Children

There does not appear to be any appropriate use of gamma-oryzanol in children.

Seniors

No special precautions are known.

Genistein (see Soy Isoflavones)

General Information

Genistein is one of the principal phytoestrogens found in soy.

Glucosamine

Used For

Osteoarthritis
Effectiveness: A   Safety: A

General Information

Glucosamine is a simple molecule that can be manufactured in the body. The main function of glucosamine on joints is to stimulate the manufacture of molecules known as glycosaminoglycans (GAGs) —key structural components of cartilage. It appears that as some people age, they lose the ability to manufacture sufficient levels of glucosamine. The result is that cartilage loses its ability to act as a shock absorber. The inability to manufacture glucosamine has been suggested to be the major factor leading to osteoarthritis, the most common form of arthritis, characterized by joint degeneration and loss of cartilage.

The most thoroughly researched form of glucosamine is glucosamine sulfate. This form has been the subject of over three hundred scientific investigations and over twenty double-blind studies. Glucosamine sulfate has been used by millions of people worldwide and is registered as a drug in the treatment of osteoarthritis in over seventy countries.

The more than twenty published clinical trials with glucosamine sulfate have demonstrated an overall success rate of 72 to 95 percent in various forms of osteoarthritis. In osteoarthritis of the knee the success rate is over 80 percent. In addition to being shown to be more effective than a placebo, in head-to-head double-blind studies comparing glucosamine sulfate to nonsteroidal anti-inflammatory drugs (NSAIDs), glucosamine sulfate was shown to produce better results than NSAIDs in relieving the pain and inflammation of osteoarthritis despite the fact that glucosamine sulfate exhibits very little direct anti-inflammatory effect and no direct analgesic (pain-relieving) effects. Glucosamine sulfate appears to address the cause of osteoarthritis. By treating the root of the problem through the promotion of cartilage synthesis, glucosamine sulfate not only improves the symptoms, including pain, but also helps the body repair damaged joints.

The double-blind studies indicate that with glucosamine sulfate supplementation, most people with osteoarthritis will experience significant improvement within four weeks. However, the longer it is used, the more obvious the results. The effects are cumulative and long-lasting.

Available Forms

Glucosamine sulfate is the preferred form of glucosamine. Other forms of glucosamine, such as N-acetyl-glucosamine or glucosamine hydrochloride, do not have the same level of scientific support. Glucosamine is often combined with chondroitin sulfate; however, most experts feel that the combination of glucosamine sulfate and chondroitin sulfate offers little, if any, benefit over glucosamine sulfate alone. Brands available include Dona.

Cautions and Warnings

Diabetics should monitor their blood sugar levels when using glucosamine sulfate. Although glucosamine sulfate has demonstrated no effect on blood sugar levels in humans, some animal studies have suggested that glucosamine sulfate may interfere with the utilization of insulin and raise blood sugar levels.

Possible Side Effects

Glucosamine sulfate has an excellent safety record in animal and human studies. Side effects, when they do appear, are generally limited to light to moderate gastrointestinal symptoms including stomach upset, heartburn, diarrhea, nausea, and indigestion. If these symptoms occur, it is recommended that glucosamine sulfate be taken with a meal.

People who are allergic to either sulfa drugs or sulfite-containing food additives may be concerned that they would also be allergic to glucosamine sulfate. This is unlikely to be the case, as the substances are very different chemically; the fact that they all contain sulfur is irrelevant, as it is impossible to be allergic to this essential mineral itself. The bottom line is that despite glucosamine sulfate's widespread use and popularity, there has only been one reported case of an allergic reaction.

Glucosamine sulfate appears to be safe for

diabetics as it has demonstrated no effect on blood sugar levels in humans. However, because glucosamine sulfate may theoretically interfere with the utilization of insulin and raise blood sugar levels, diabetics should monitor their blood sugar levels when using it.

Drug Interactions

There have been no reports of any adverse drug interactions with glucosamine sulfate. The only caveat is that individuals taking diuretics may need to take higher dosages (e.g., 20 mg per kg [2.2 pounds] body weight daily).

Food and Nutrient Interactions

None known.

Usual Dosage

The standard dosage for glucosamine sulfate is 500 mg three times per day. Individuals over 200 pounds may need higher dosages based on body weight (e.g., 20 mg per kg [2.2 pounds] body weight daily).

Overdosage

None known.

Special Populations

Pregnant/breast-feeding women
Considered safe during pregnancy and lactation.

Children
Suitable for children at one-half the adult dosage.

Seniors
No special precautions are known.

Glutamine

Used For

Crohn's disease and ulcerative colitis
Effectiveness: B   Safety: A

Enhancing athletic performance
Effectiveness: B   Safety: A

Improving immune function
Effectiveness: B+   Safety: A

Peptic ulcers
Effectiveness: B+   Safety: A

Prevention of chemotherapy side effects
Effectiveness: B+   Safety: A

General Information

Glutamine is the most abundant amino acid in the body (amino acids are the building blocks of protein) and is involved in more metabolic processes than any other amino acid. Glutamine is especially important as a source of fuel for cells lining the intestines and for the proper functioning of white blood cells. It is important to these cells because glutamine is utilized at higher rates by these cells and other rapidly dividing cells. Without glutamine, these cells do not divide properly. The importance of glutamine is becoming well appreciated in conventional medical circles, as it is an extremely important component of intravenous feeding mixes in hospitals; double-blind studies have shown it to dramatically increase survival in critically ill subjects.

Crohn's disease and ulcerative colitis

Crohn's disease and ulcerative colitis are characterized by inflammation and tissue destruction of the lining of the small and large intestine, respectively. Since the lining of the intestinal tract is so dependent upon adequate glutamine concentrations, researchers have studied glutamine supplementation in Crohn's disease and ulcerative colitis. Unfortunately, these preliminary studies failed to provide any clear-cut answers, and at this time the value of glutamine supplementation in Crohn's disease and ulcerative colitis is unknown.

Enhancing athletic performance

Glutamine is the most abundant amino acid in the blood and in the free amino acid pool of skeletal muscle. Glutamine stimulates the synthesis of proteins, inhibits their degradation, and is an energy source for muscle cell division. Glutamine is also a precursor for the synthesis of amino acids, proteins, nucleotides, glutathione, and other biologically important molecules. Glutamine has an anabolic effect on skeletal muscle.

There is some evidence that overtraining results in low glutamine levels and that glutamine supplementation can help prevent damage from overtraining in the first place as well as help an athlete recover from overtraining. Plasma glutamine concentrations increase during exercise. However, during the post-exercise recovery period, plasma concentrations decrease significantly. Several hours of recovery are required before plasma levels are restored to pre-exercise levels. If recovery between exercise bouts is inadequate, the acute effects of exercise on plasma glutamine concentrations can be cumulative, leading to very low levels of glutamine. This situation can have extremely detrimental effects on athletic performance and muscle growth. Glutamine supplementation has been shown to boost muscle levels of glutamine and promote muscle protein synthesis. However, it does not appear to enhance exercise performance in the absence of glutamine shortages in the body. The clearest benefit of glutamine supplementation in athletes is in prevention of infections (see "Improving Immune Function," below).

Improving immune function

Glutamine supplementation has been shown to boost immune function and fight infection. These effects have been best demonstrated in endurance athletes (extreme exercise suppresses the immune system) and critically ill subjects. It is not known if glutamine supplementation enhances immune function in healthy individuals.

Peptic ulcers

Glutamine promotes the healing of peptic ulcers. In a double-blind study of fifty-seven patients with peptic ulcers, twenty-four took 1.6 g of glutamine per day, and the rest used conventional therapy (antacids, antispasmodics, etc.). Glutamine proved to be the more effective treatment. Half of the glutamine patients showed complete healing (according to X-ray analysis) within two weeks, and twenty-two of the twenty-four showed complete relief and healing within four weeks.

Prevention of chemotherapy side effects

Glutamine, given its importance to the cells lining the gastrointestinal tract and immune system, has been shown to prevent the mouth ulcers (stomatitis), muscle and joint pain, and suppression of the immune system in cancer patients receiving some types of chemotherapy, most notably 5-fluorouracil and paclitaxel (Taxol).

Available Forms

Glutamine is available in capsules, tablets, and powder. Also, one of the best sources of glutamine is whey protein.

Cautions and Warnings

None known.

Possible Side Effects

No side effects have been reported at dosages as high as 21 g per day.

Drug Interactions

Glutamine may reduce some of the side effects of chemotherapy drugs on the gastrointestinal tract.

Food and Nutrient Interactions

None known.

Usual Dosage

The typical dosage of glutamine is 3 to 5 g daily. An alternative recommendation is 20 to 30 g of whey protein concentrate.

Overdosage

None known.

Special Populations

Pregnant/breast-feeding women
Because there is a lack of reliable information on its use during pregnancy and lactation, it is recommended that its use be avoided during these times.

Children
Suitable for children at one-half the adult dosage.

Seniors
No special precautions are known.

Glutathione

Used For

Antioxidant support
Effectiveness: D   Safety: C

General Information

Glutathione is a small protein composed of three amino acids—cysteine, glutamic acid, and glycine. Glutathione is an important antioxidant that is also involved in detoxification mechanisms. Glutathione binds to fat-soluble toxins such as heavy metals, solvents, and pesticides, transforming them into a water-soluble form, which allows more efficient excretion via the kidneys.

Studies using glutathione given intravenously have found it to be useful in preventing clot formation during operations, reducing the side effects and increasing the efficacy of chemotherapy drugs such as cisplatin, treating the symptoms of Parkinson's disease, and increasing sperm count in men with low sperm count. Whether oral preparations are effective is unknown at this time. While glutathione has been shown to be absorbed when given orally to rats, it may not be absorbed in humans. More important is the fact that taking extra glutathione may not raise blood glutathione levels. One study showed that oral supplements in single doses as high as 3,000 mg failed to increase glutathione levels in the blood. This result indicates that people should instead look to nutritional compounds that may help increase glutathione levels, including vitamin C, N-acetylcysteine (NAC), alpha-lipoic acid, glutamine, methionine, and whey protein. In one study, blood glutathione levels rose nearly 50 percent in healthy individuals taking 500 mg of vitamin C, which helps the body manufacture glutathione. In addition, to vitamin C, other nutrients required in the manufacture of glutathione are vitamin B_6, riboflavin, and selenium.

Available Forms

Glutathione is available as a dietary supplement in tablets and capsules, usually in a formula with other antioxidant compounds. Dietary glutathione is found in fresh fruits and vegetables, fish, and meat. Asparagus, avocado, and walnuts are particularly rich dietary sources of glutathione.

Cautions and Warnings

None known.

Possible Side Effects

None known.

Drug Interactions

None known.

Food and Nutrient Interactions

None known.

Usual Dosage

Effective oral dosages have not yet been established.

Overdosage

None known.

Special Populations

Pregnant/breast-feeding women
Safety is unknown, as there have been no safety studies during pregnancy and lactation.

Children
Safety and applications in children have not been established.

Seniors
No special precautions are known.

Guaifenesin

Used For

Bronchitis, coughs, respiratory congestion
Effectiveness: A   Safety: A

Fibromyalgia
Effectiveness: D   Safety: C

General Information

Guaifenesin (also known as glycerol guiacolate) is a derivative of a compound originally isolated from beech wood. Guaifenesin is an approved over-the-counter expectorant—a substance that helps thin mucus and loosens phlegm and bronchial secretions in cases of asthma, bronchitis, and other bronchial irritations. It is often combined with other compounds and included in cold and cough formulas.

Guaifenesin has also been suggested as helpful in fibromyalgia—a chronic condition associated with vague muscular pain, fatigue, and painful trigger points. The theory is that guaifenesin helps liberate toxins stored in muscle that are responsible for the fibromyalgia. There have been no studies to verify this effect.

Available Forms

Guaifenesin is available most often in liquid cough syrups but can also be found in tablets and capsules.

Cautions and Warnings

Persistent cough may indicate a serious condition. Consult your physician if cough persists for more than one week, recurs, or is accompanied by high fever, rash or persistent headache. If you are pregnant or nursing a baby, seek the advice of a physician before using this product.

Do not exceed recommended dosage.

Do not take guaifenesin if you are pregnant or lactating.

Possible Side Effects

Guaifenesin is generally well tolerated. When side effects do occur, the most common is mild gastrointestinal irritation and nausea. At dosages greater than the recommended level, guaifenesin can also induce vomiting.

Drug Interactions

None known.

Food and Nutrient Interactions

None known.

Usual Dosage

Adults and children twelve years of age and older: 200–400 mg every four hours. Do not take more than 2,400 mg in a twenty-four-hour period.

Overdosage

The effects of an overdosage of guaifenesin are unknown. Do the following in case of accidental overdose: If the victim is unconscious or having convulsions, call for an ambulance immediately. If you take the victim to an emergency room, be sure to bring the bottle or container with you. If the victim is conscious, call your local poison control center or a health care professional. The poison control center may suggest inducing vomiting with ipecac syrup (available without a prescription at any pharmacy). *Do not* induce vomiting unless specifically instructed to do so.

Special Populations

Pregnant/breast-feeding women

Animal studies have shown guaifenesin to be harmful to the fetus. Although these effects have not been confirmed in humans, it is recommended by most experts that guaifenesin not be used during pregnancy and lactation.

Children

The dosage for children age six to eleven years is 100–200 mg every four hours and no more than 1,200 mg in a twenty-four-hour period. For children age two to five years, the dosage is 50 to 100 mg every four hours and no more than 600 mg in twenty-four hours. Guaifenesin is not recommended for children under two years of age unless recommended by a physician, especially in cases of chronic cough such as chronic bronchitis and asthma.

Seniors

No special precautions are known.

Guar Gum (*see* Fiber)

General Information

Guar gum is a water-soluble, gel-forming fiber isolated from the legume *Cyamopsis tetragonolobus,* a plant cultivated in India for livestock feed. Guar gum is used in food processing as a protective stabilizer, emulsifier, and thickening agent in cheese, salad dressings, ice cream, soups, toothpaste, pharmaceutical jelly, lotion, skin cream, and tablets. Like other gel-forming fiber sources, guar gum is a laxative, lowers cholesterol levels, helps reduce fasting and after-meal glucose and insulin levels in both healthy and diabetic subjects, and has decreased body weight and hunger ratings when taken with meals by obese subjects.

Hesperidin (*see* Citrus Bioflavonoids)

General Information

Hesperidin is one of the chief citrus bioflavonoids.

HMB (beta-hydroxy-beta-methylbutyrate)

Used For

Promoting muscle growth
Effectiveness: B+   Safety: C

General Information

HMB (beta-hydroxy-beta-methylbutyrate) entered the marketplace at the end of 1995. The nutritional use of HMB was originally patented by the Iowa State University Research Foundation. HMB is a metabolite of the amino acid leucine. HMB decreases muscle protein turnover and minimizes muscle breakdown after exercise. In one human study conducted over a three-week period, 3 g per day of oral HMB supplementation was shown to decrease body fat, increase lean mass and strength, and reduce muscle damage in individuals beginning weight training exercises.

Available Forms

HMB is available primarily in capsules and powder form. It is also often combined with other body-building compounds such as creatine and whey protein. Dominant brands are EAS and Twinlab.

Cautions and Warnings

Since HMB is relatively new to the market, no information is available on its long-term safety.

Possible Side Effects

None known.

Drug Interactions

None known.

Food and Nutrient Interactions

Most often HMB supplementation is recommended in conjunction with a high protein intake (e.g., 120–175 g/day for athletes) to produce maximum results.

Usual Dosage

The typical dosage recommended for HMB is 3 g per day.

Overdosage

The effects of an overdosage of HMB are unknown. Do the following in case of accidental overdose: If the victim is unconscious or having convulsions, call for an ambulance immediately. If you take the victim to an emergency room, be sure to bring the bottle or container with you. If the victim is conscious, call your local poison control center or a health care professional. The poison control center may suggest inducing vomiting with ipecac syrup (available without a prescription at any pharmacy). *Do not* induce vomiting unless specifically instructed to do so.

Special Populations

Pregnant/breast-feeding women
As the effects of HMB during pregnancy and lactation have not been sufficiently evaluated, it should not be used during these times.

Children
There does not appear to be any appropriate use of HMB in children.

Seniors
No special precautions are known.

Hydroxytryptophan (5-HTP)

Used For

Depression
Effectiveness: A   Safety: D

Fibromyalgia
Effectiveness: A   Safety: D

Headaches
Effectiveness: A   Safety: D

Insomnia
Effectiveness: B+   Safety: D

Weight loss
Effectiveness: A   Safety: D

General Information

5-hydroxytryptophan (5-HTP) is an amino acid that is the middle step in the production of the important brain chemical serotonin from the amino acid tryptophan. Considerable scientific evidence indicates that low serotonin levels are linked to a number of common conditions, including depression, obesity, fibromyalgia, and headaches. 5-HTP boosts serotonin levels and may offer benefits in conditions linked to low serotonin levels. Commercially available 5-HTP is isolated from a seed from an African plant *(Griffonia simplicifolia)*.

Depression

There is excellent documentation that 5-HTP is an effective antidepressant agent. 5-HTP often produces very good results in patients who are unresponsive to standard antidepressant drugs. Several double-blind studies show that 5-HTP is equal to or better than standard antidepressant drugs. The study with the most significance was one that compared 5-HTP to fluvoxamine (Luvox), a selective serotonin reuptake inhibitor (SSRI) like fluoxetine (Prozac), paroxetine (Paxil), and sertraline (Zoloft). In the study, subjects received either 5-HTP (100 mg) or fluvoxamine (50 mg) three times daily for six weeks. The percentage decrease in overall depression scores was slightly better in the 5-HTP group (60.7

percent versus 56.1 percent). More patients responded to 5-HTP than fluvoxamine, and 5-HTP was quicker-acting than the fluvoxamine.

The real advantage of 5-HTP in this study was the low rate of side effects. The most frequent side effect with 5-HTP was mild nausea, but this occurred in less than one out of ten subjects. In contrast, antidepressant drugs usually produce moderate to severe side effects in 20 to 65 percent of subjects.

Fibromyalgia

Fibromyalgia is a recently recognized disorder. It causes chronic musculoskeletal pain and fatigue. Fibromyalgia is a relatively common condition, estimated to affect about 4 percent of the general population. 5-HTP can largely improve the painful picture of fibromyalgia, as demonstrated in several double-blind studies.

Headaches

Because chronic headache sufferers have low levels of serotonin in their tissues, some researchers refer to migraine and chronic headaches as "low serotonin syndrome." There have been several clinical studies demonstrating excellent results with 5-HTP in the treatment of headaches, both migraine and tension. In particular, 5-HTP is very effective in the prevention of migraine headache.

Insomnia

Several clinical studies have shown 5-HTP to produce good results in promoting and maintaining sleep in normal subjects as well as those experiencing insomnia. One of the key benefits with 5-HTP in the treatment of insomnia is its ability to increase sleep quality.

Weight loss

As far back as 1975, researchers demonstrated that administering 5-HTP to rats that were bred to overeat and be obese resulted in significant reduction in food intake. It turns out that these genetically obese rats have decreased activity of the enzyme that converts tryptophan to 5-HTP and subsequently to serotonin. As a result, these rats never get the message to stop eating until they have consumed far greater amounts of food than normal rats.

There is much circumstantial evidence that many humans are genetically predisposed to obesity. This predisposition may involve the same mechanism as that observed in rats genetically predisposed to obesity. In other words, many people may be predisposed to being overweight because they have a decreased ability to convert tryptophan to 5-HTP and, as a result, decreased serotonin levels. By providing preformed 5-HTP, this genetic defect is bypassed and more serotonin is manufactured. 5-HTP literally turns off hunger.

The early animal studies that used 5-HTP as a weight loss aid have been followed by a series of four human clinical studies of overweight women conducted at the University of Rome. These studies have shown that 5-HTP is able to reduce caloric intake and promote weight loss even if the women made no conscious effort to lose weight. 5-HTP appears to promote weight loss by promoting satiety (the feeling of satisfaction), leading to fewer calories being consumed at meals. In one study, the group that received the 5-HTP had lost an average of 4.39 pounds at six weeks and an average of 11.63 pounds at twelve weeks. In comparison, the placebo group had lost an average of only 0.62 pounds at six weeks and 1.87 pounds at twelve weeks.

Available Forms

5-HTP is available in capsules and tablets, including enteric-coated capsules or tablets (pills prepared in a manner so that they will dissolve in the intestine rather than the stomach). Using enteric-coated capsules or tablets significantly reduces the likelihood of nausea.

Cautions and Warnings

Do not use 5-HTP if you are taking an antidepressant drug unless under direct supervision of a physician.

Do not use 5-HTP if you are pregnant or lactating.

Do not use 5-HTP if you have Parkinson's disease and are not taking the drug Sinemet.

Do not use 5-HTP if you have scleroderma.

Possible Side Effects

5-HTP is generally very well tolerated at recommended dosages. At higher dosages (e.g., 300 mg or more as one dose) nausea is an extremely common side effect. At the recommended dosage of 50 to 100 mg three times daily, any nausea is usually quite mild, as are other possible side effects such as drowsiness, dry mouth, and stomach irritation. 5-HTP can worsen Parkinson's disease symptoms unless the person is also on the drug Sinemet.

The major concern with 5-HTP is a possible link to L-tryptophan and eosinophilia-myalgia syndrome (EMS). For more than thirty years, tryptophan was used safely and effectively by over thirty million people in the United States and around the world to treat insomnia and depression. But in October 1989 some people who were taking tryptophan started reporting strange symptoms to physicians: severe muscle and joint pain, high fever, weakness, swelling of the arms and legs, and shortness of breath. The syndrome was dubbed EMS (eosinophilia-myalgia syndrome), because the blood of those affected contained a very high level of eosinophils—white blood cells involved in allergic/inflammatory reactions.

Detailed analysis of all the evidence by the Centers for Disease Control (CDC) led to the conclusion that the cause of the EMS epidemic could be traced to one Japanese manufacturer. The tryptophan produced from October 1988 to June 1989 by this manufacturer became contaminated due to changes in the filtration process and in the bacteria being used to produce the tryptophan.

While L-tryptophan is produced via bacterial fermentation and filtration, 5-HTP is commercially available through an extraction process from the seed of *Griffonia simplicifolia*, an African plant. 5-HTP extracted from this natural source avoids the contamination problem associated with past L-tryptophan manufacturing problems. There was a single case report linking 5-HTP to a condition similar to EMS in 1980. However, this case involved the use of very high dosages of 5-HTP (1,400 mg) over a twenty-month period.

In 1998 researchers at the Mayo Clinic claimed that they identified trace levels of peak X, a substance linked to EMS-like illness, in commercially available 5-HTP. As a result, manufacturers of 5-HTP now screen for the presence of this compound to ensure that all of the 5-HTP on the marketplace is free from peak X. There have been no reports of a single person developing EMS from 5-HTP despite its popularity. Nonetheless, to be on the safe side, some experts recommend that long-term continual use of 5-HTP be monitored by regular (every six months) determination of eosinophil levels.

Drug Interactions

Because 5-HTP is the direct precursor to serotonin, it should not be used by individuals taking antidepressant drugs unless under the direct supervision of a physician. Although 5-HTP has been used safely in combination with prescription antidepressant drugs in clinical studies, taking this combination without medical supervision could result in too much serotonin in the body. The result is a condition known as serotonin syndrome, which is characterized by confusion, fever, shivering, sweating, diarrhea, and muscle spasms.

　5-HTP may antagonize the effects of drugs used in migraine headaches such as methysergide and cyproheptadine, which block serotonin's effects.

Food and Nutrient Interactions

Vitamin B_6 is required for the conversion of 5-HTP to serotonin.

Usual Dosage

For depression, weight loss, headaches, and fibromyalgia the dosage should be started at 50 mg three times per day. If the response is inadequate after two weeks, increase the dosage to 100 mg three times per day. Because 5-HTP does not rely on the same transport vehicle as L-tryptophan, it can be taken with food. However, if taking 5-HTP for weight loss, it is best to take it twenty minutes before meals.

For insomnia, the recommended dosage is 100 to 300 mg thirty to forty-five minutes before retiring. Start with the lower dose for at least three days before increasing the dosage.

Overdosage

Overdosage can produce severe nausea, vomiting, and diarrhea. Do the following in case of accidental overdose: If the victim is unconscious or having convulsions, call for an ambulance immediately. If you take the victim to an emergency room, be sure to bring the bottle or container with you. If the victim is conscious, call your local poison control center or a health care professional. The poison control center may suggest inducing vomiting with ipecac syrup (available without a prescription at any pharmacy). *Do not* induce vomiting unless specifically instructed to do so.

Special Populations

Pregnant/breast-feeding women
5-HTP is not recommended during pregnancy and lactation.

Children
5-HTP is suitable for children at a dosage of 5 mg per kg (2.2 pounds) of body weight.

Seniors
No special precautions are known.

7-keto DHEA

Used For

Weight loss
Effectiveness: B   Safety: B

General Information

7-keto DHEA (3-acetyl-7-oxo-dehydroepiandrosterone) is a naturally occurring metabolite (breakdown product) of the hormone DHEA (dehydroepiandrosterone). DHEA is the most abundant of the adrenal steroid hormones and serves as a precursor for sex hormones such as estrogen and testosterone. 7-keto was developed by researchers who were looking for biologically active metabolites of DHEA that could not be converted to estrogen and testosterone, which may be cancer-causing under certain circumstances. Tests in animals and test tubes were performed in the areas of immune modulation, memory enhancement, and thermogenesis (the process the body uses to convert stored calories into energy). In all cases, the effects of 7-keto were stronger than those produced by DHEA.

The capacity of 7-keto to promote weight loss in overweight adults has been investigated in a double-blind study. Participants in the study were advised to exercise three times per week for forty-five minutes and to eat a 1,800-calorie diet. Each individual was given either a placebo or 100 mg of 7-keto twice daily. After eight weeks, those receiving 7-keto had lost an average of 6.34 pounds, compared with 2.13 pounds in the placebo group. In addition, the percentage of body fat decreased by 1.8 percent in the 7-keto group, compared with only

0.57 percent in the placebo group. The increased weight loss in the 7-keto group was associated with a significant increase in levels of T_3 (a thyroid hormone that plays a major role in determining a person's metabolic rate), although the levels of T_3 did not exceed the normal range.

Available Forms

7-keto is currently available as a dietary supplement in capsules. Dominant brands are Twinlab and Enzymatic Therapy.

Cautions and Warnings

Because 7-keto has not been studied in individuals who are taking thyroid hormone medications and because of its noted effect on T_3 levels, individuals taking thyroid medications are encouraged to have their physician check blood levels of thyroid hormones (including T_3) after six weeks of 7-keto use.

Possible Side Effects

A safety study in humans has shown that 7-keto does not raise estrogen or testosterone levels or produce any other negative effects at levels up to 200 mg per day. Animal studies have also shown it to be extremely safe and nontoxic. In a toxicity study in monkeys, oral administration of 7-keto to monkeys at a dosage of up to 1,000 mg per kg (2.2 pounds) body weight demonstrated no adverse effect.

Drug Interactions

7-keto may increase the effect of thyroid hormone medications (see "Cautions and Warnings," above).

Food and Nutrient Interactions
None known.

Usual Dosage
The recommended level for weight loss is 100 mg twice daily.

Overdosage
None known.

Special Populations

Pregnant/breast-feeding women
As the effects of 7-keto during pregnancy and lactation have not been sufficiently evaluated, it should not be used during these times.

Children
There is no known application for 7-keto in children.

Seniors
No special precautions are known.

Indole-3-carbinol

Used For

Cancer prevention and treatment
Effectiveness: B+   Safety: B

General Information

Indole-3-carbinol is one of the major anticancer substances found in cruciferous vegetables (members of the cabbage family). It is a member of the class of sulfur-containing chemicals called glucosinolates. It is formed from parent compounds whenever cruciferous vegetables are crushed or cooked. Indole-3-carbinol and other glucosinolates (e.g., other indoles and isothiocyanates such as sulforaphane) are antioxidants and potent stimulators of natural detoxifying enzymes in the body and are believed to be responsible for the lowered risk of cancer in humans that is associated with the consumption of broccoli and other cruciferous vegetables such as cauliflower, cabbage, and kale.

Feeding indole-3-carbinol or broccoli extracts rich in indole-3-carbinol has dramatically reduced the frequency, size, and number of tumors in laboratory rats exposed to a carcinogen. It appears to be especially protective against breast and cervical cancer because of a number of actions, including an ability to increase the breakdown of estrogen. In preliminary clinical studies, indole-3-carbinol has shown promising results in the treatment of precancerous lesions.

Available Forms

Indole-3-carbinol is available most often in capsules or tablets.

Cautions and Warnings

None known.

Possible Side Effects

None known.

Drug Interactions

Since indole-3-carbinol and dietary consumption of cruciferous vegetables interact with drug-detoxifying enzymes in a manner that may increase or decrease the breakdown of certain medications, anyone taking medication should consult a nutritionally oriented practitioner before supplementing with indole-3-carbinol or before greatly increasing their intake of cruciferous vegetables.

Since stomach acid is required in the conversion of indole-3-carbinol to active metabolites, drugs that inhibit stomach acid such as antacids, ranitidine (Zantac), famotidine (Pepcid), and omeprazole (Prilosec) may decrease the effectiveness of indole-3-carbinol.

Food and Nutrient Interactions

Indole-3-carbinol is found in highest concentrations in broccoli, but is also found in other cruciferous vegetables, such as cauliflower, cabbage, and kale.

Usual Dosage

The typical dosage recommendation is 100 to 400 mg daily.

Overdosage

None known.

Special Populations

Pregnant/breast-feeding women
As the effects of indole-3-carbinol during pregnancy and lactation have not been sufficiently evaluated, it should not be used during these times.

Children
It appears that indole-3-carbinol can be used by children over the age of two years even at the adult dosage.

Seniors
No special precautions are known.

Inositol

Used For

Depression
Effectiveness: A   Safety: A

Diabetes
Effectiveness: B   Safety: A

Panic attacks
Effectiveness: B+   Safety: A

General Information

Inositol is an unofficial member of the B vitamin group that functions as a primary component of cell membranes. With phosphate groups attached, it acts as an important regulator of cell division (see

Ip6 [inositol hexaphosphate]). Although inositol has not been shown to be essential in the human diet, supplementation has been shown to exert some beneficial effects in cases of depression, panic attacks, and diabetes.

Depression and panic attacks

Inositol is required for the proper action of several brain neurotransmitters, including serotonin and acetylcholine. It is currently thought that a reduction of brain inositol levels may induce depression, as inositol levels in the cerebrospinal fluid have been shown to be low in patients with depression. In double-blind studies, inositol at a dosage of 12 g per day has demonstrated therapeutic results (e.g., reduction in score on the Hamilton Depression Scale) similar to those of tricyclic antidepressant drugs but without the side effects.

Because of the effect of inositol on depression, a double-blind study was designed to test inositol's effectiveness in panic disorder. The frequency and severity of panic attacks declined significantly more after inositol (12 g per day) than after placebo administration. Further studies are needed to document this effect.

Diabetes

Inositol is showing some promise in diabetic neuropathy, a nerve disease caused by diabetes. Diabetic neuropathy is the most frequent complication of long-term diabetes. Much of the decreased nerve function is due to loss of inositol from the nerve cell. Inositol supplementation may improve nerve conduction velocities in diabetics, but it should not be relied upon as the sole therapy.

Available Forms

Inostil is available commercially as inositol mono-phosphate, **inositol hexaphosphate,** and inositol hexaniacinate (see **niacin**).

Cautions and Warnings

None known.

Possible Side Effects

None known.

Drug Interactions

None known.

Food and Nutrient Interactions

None known.

Usual Dosage

The dosage for general support is 100 to 500 mg daily. The dosage for depression or panic disorder is 12 g daily; the dosage in the treatment of diabetic neuropathy is 1,000 to 2,000 mg daily.

Overdosage

None known.

Special Populations

Pregnant/breast-feeding women
Considered safe during pregnancy and lactation.

Children
Suitable for children at one-half the adult dosage.

Seniors
No special precautions are known.

Ip6 (Inositol Hexaphosphate)

Used For

Cancer prevention and treatment adjunct
Effectiveness: C   Safety: A

General Information

Ip6—short for inositol hexaphosphate—is a component of fiber that is found primarily in whole grains
and legumes. It appears that some of the cancer-
protective effects of a high-fiber diet are due to the
presence of higher levels of Ip6. Although Ip6 is
found in substantial amounts in these whole foods,
supplementation with purified Ip6 offers several advantages. First of all, in grains and beans the Ip6-
exists primarily as a complex with protein and
minerals such as calcium, magnesium, or potassium,
and as such it is poorly absorbed. Studies have
shown that pure Ip6 is significantly more bioavail-

able than the Ip6 found in whole grains and beans. In animal studies, the degree of protection against cancer offered by supplementing the diet with Ip6 is substantially greater than that provided by a high-fiber diet containing an identical amount of Ip6.

It is very important to note that while Ip6 has shown good results in test tube and animal studies, there are no human studies in cancer patients. In these extensive experimental studies in animals and cell cultures, Ip6 has been shown to exert anticancer effects against virtually all types of cancers, including cancers of the breast, prostate, lung, skin, and brain as well as lymphomas and leukemias. The positive effects noted in these preliminary studies need to be followed up with clinical studies in humans.

Although Ip6 is gaining all of the attention, it is really a derivative compound, Ip3, that is doing all the work. Inositol, the backbone structure of Ip6, has six carbon atoms that are capable of binding phosphate molecules; when all of the six carbons are occupied by six phosphate groups, it forms Ip6. When only three of the carbons are bound by phosphate, it is called Ip3. When taken with plain inositol in the proper proportions, Ip6 forms two molecules of Ip3 in the body. Ip3 basically functions as an on/off switch for human cancer cells, according to experimental studies in cell cultures (test tube studies). When Ip3 levels are low (as in cancer cells), the cells replicate out of control. When cancer cells are bathed in a broth with Ip3, they literally turn themselves off. This action reflects the central role that Ip3 plays in controlling key cell functions, including replication and communication between cells.

In animal studies, Ip6 has also been shown to be an effective antioxidant and booster of immune function. It is especially helpful in boosting the activity of a type of white blood cell known as a natural killer cell. These white blood cells get their name because they literally kill cancer cells, viruses, and other infecting organisms. They play a major role in protecting the body against cancer and infection.

Available Forms

Ip6 is derived from rice bran. It is available in tablets, in capsules, and as a bulk powder. For maximum benefit Ip6 should be combined with inositol at a 4:1 ratio of Ip6 to inositol. This combination is available as Cell Forté and Cellular Forté.

Cautions and Warnings

Due to the lack of human data in cancer treatment with Ip6, it should not be used as a primary therapy in cancer. Cancer is a potentially life-threatening disease that requires proper medical treatment.

Possible Side Effects

None known.

Drug Interactions

Animal studies have also shown that Ip6 can be used in combination with conventional cancer treatments such as radiation and chemotherapy. In fact, Ip6 has been shown to increase the effectiveness of these therapies.

Food and Nutrient Interactions

Since Ip6 can form complexes with various food components, especially minerals, it is recommended that it be taken on an empty stomach.

Usual Dosage

For prevention: 800–1,200 mg Ip6 plus 200–300 mg inositol. As an adjunct to therapy in cancer patients: 4,800–7,200 mg Ip6 plus 1,200–1,800 mg inositol.

Overdosage

None known. Ip6 is extremely safe even at high dosages (e.g., 8 g per day) based upon extensive animal testing and human studies.

Special Populations

Pregnant/breast-feeding women
Considered safe during pregnancy and lactation.

Children
Suitable for children at one-half the adult dosage.

Seniors
No special precautions are known.

Ipriflavone

Used For

Osteoporosis
Effectiveness: A   Safety: A

General Information

Ipriflavone is a naturally occurring bioflavonoid (plant pigment) that is utilized as a nutritional supplement to promote bone health. Ipriflavone has exceptional documentation of effectiveness and safety. Over sixty clinical studies that involved a total of more than three thousand patients treated with ipriflavone show that long-term treatment with ipriflavone along with 1,000 mg supplemental calcium is safe and effective in halting bone loss. In addition, ipriflavone has been shown to actually increase bone density even in women with confirmed osteoporosis.

It appears that ipriflavone promotes the utilization of calcium in bone and reduces the bone turnover rate (bone is constantly remodeling, or breaking down and re-forming, and ipriflavone slows bone breakdown). Results from the clinical studies indicate that while calcium alone can slow down the loss of bone density, ipriflavone can actually stop bone loss, and in women with osteoporosis it can lead to an increase in bone density, substantially lessen the risk of fractures, and reduce bone pain.

The results from these studies suggest that ipriflavone can provide the same sort of bone-protecting effects of estrogen without the risk of breast cancer (ipriflavone exerts no estrogenic effect).

Available Forms

Ipriflavone is available in tablets and capsules. It is often an ingredient in nutritional formulas designed to build bone. The dominant brand is Ostivone.

Cautions and Warnings

Ipriflavone may increase the blood-thinning activity of the drug warfarin (Coumadin). Patients taking warfarin are encouraged to have their dosages of this drug closely monitored by their physician if they elect to use ipriflavone.

Lower dosages are recommended to individuals with impaired kidney function. For mild to moderate kidney impairment the dosage recommendation is 400 mg per day. For more severe kidney impairment the dosage recommendation is 200 mg per day.

Possible Side Effects

The frequency of adverse reactions in ipriflavone-treated patients (14.5 percent in the double-blind studies) is actually less than that observed in subjects receiving the placebo (16.1 percent). Side effects were mainly stomach upset.

Drug Interactions

No adverse drug interactions have been reported. Ipriflavone may increase the blood-thinning activity of the drug warfarin (Coumadin). Patients taking warfarin are encouraged to have their dosages of this drug closely monitored by their physician if they elect to use ipriflavone. Ipriflavone may also potentiate the effects of theophylline (a drug used in asthma) as well as caffeine by inhibiting the breakdown of these drugs. Ipriflavone can reduce the dosage or need for estrogen therapy in the treatment of osteoporosis.

Food and Nutrient Interactions

Ipriflavone exerts positive interactions with calcium and vitamin D in promoting bone health. No other interactions with food are known.

Usual Dosage

The typical dosage of ipriflavone is 200 mg three times daily.

Overdosage

None known.

Special Populations

Pregnant/breast-feeding women

The safety of ipriflavone has not been established during pregnancy and lactation.

Children

The appropriate use of ipriflavone in children has not been established.

Seniors

No special precautions are known.

Kombucha

Used For

Boosting energy levels
Effectiveness: C   Safety: C

Low immunity and immune support
Effectiveness: C   Safety: C

General Information

Kombucha is a tea made from a Manchurian mushroom. Traditionally kombucha is prepared by fermenting the mushroom in sugared tea for seven days. There has been a tremendous amount of anecdotal reports and marketing materials claiming it as a panacea, but there is little scientific information on the benefits of the tea. In its traditionally prepared form there are significant safety concerns about contamination. Most experts agree that the danger of kombucha in its traditional form is greater than any potential benefit. Commercially available forms must be prepared with the utmost attention to sanitation and purity of the culture to remove these safety concerns.

Available Forms

Kombucha is available in liquid form as well as in dehydrated form for use in capsules and tablets.

Cautions and Warnings

Do not use traditionally prepared kombucha if you suffer from HIV infection or AIDS because of increased susceptibility to any infectious contaminant.
   Do not culture kombucha at home.

Possible Side Effects

Using uncontaminated commercial products is thought to be safe. However, culturing kombucha at home creates a significant safety issue because it is easy for the culture to become contaminated with other microorganisms, including some associated with serious infections. Although kombucha appears to be well tolerated, there has been one case report in the medical literature citing liver damage.

Drug Interactions

None known.

Food and Nutrient Interactions

None known.

Usual Dosage

The equivalent of 3 to 4 fluid ounces up to three times daily is the usual dosage recommendation. Pill or liquid extracts usually give equivalences to the tea.

Overdosage

None known.

Special Populations

Pregnant/breast-feeding women
As the effects of kombucha during pregnancy and lactation have not been sufficiently evaluated, it should not be used during these times.

Children
Suitable for children at one-half the adult dosage.

Seniors
No special precautions are known.

Lactaid

Used For

Lactose intolerance
Effectiveness: B   Safety: A

General Information

Lactaid contains the enzyme lactase, which is necessary for digesting the sugar lactose from dairy products. The enzyme is derived from a yeast. Deficiency in the enzyme lactase is common worldwide. It has been estimated that 70 to 90 percent of Asian, black, American Indian, and Mediterranean adults lack this enzyme. The frequency of the deficiency is believed to be approximately 10 to 15 percent in northern and western Europeans. While almost all infants are able to digest milk and other dairy products, many children lose their ability to produce lactase by three to seven years of age. Symptoms of lactose intolerance range from minor abdominal discomfort and bloating to severe diarrhea in response to even small amounts of lactose. Lactaid allows people with lactase deficiency to eat or drink dairy foods without experiencing the symptoms of lactose intolerance.

Available Forms

Lactaid is available in caplets and liquid form.

Cautions and Warnings

None known.

Possible Side Effects

None known.

Drug Interactions

None known.

Food and Nutrient Interactions

Lactaid aids in the digestion of dairy foods containing lactose.

Usual Dosage

Here are the recommendations for the various forms of Lactaid. Because the degree of enzyme deficiency may vary from person to person, the dosage may have to be adjusted for individual needs.

Lactaid Original: Swallow or chew 3 caplets with the first bite of dairy food.

Lactaid Extra: Swallow or chew 2 caplets with the first bite of dairy food.

Lactaid Ultra: Swallow 1 caplet with the first bite of dairy food.

Lactaid drops: Add 5 to 7 drops to a quart of milk and refrigerate for twenty-four hours before use.

Overdosage

None known.

Special Populations

Pregnant/breast-feeding women
Lactaid is considered safe during pregnancy and lactation.

Children
Suitable for children at the adult dosage.

Seniors
No special precautions are known.

Lactobacillus acidophilus and Lactobacillus rhamnosus

Used For

Antibiotic-induced diarrhea and infectious diarrhea
Effectiveness: A   Safety: A

Cancer prevention
Effectiveness: B   Safety: A

Promotion of proper intestinal environment
Effectiveness: B   Safety: A

Traveler's diarrhea
Effectiveness: B+   Safety: A

Urinary tract (bladder) infections
Effectiveness: B   Safety: A

Vaginal yeast infections
Effectiveness: B+   Safety: A

General Information

Lactobacillus acidophilus and *L. rhamnosus* are "friendly" bacteria valued for their health-promoting properties. Lactobacilli are key components of proper intestinal flora. Lactobacilli have long been noted for the role they play in the defense against disease, particularly gastrointestinal tract infections. Lactobacilli produce a variety of factors that inhibit or antagonize other bacteria. These include metabolic end products such as organic acids (lactic and acetic acid), hydrogen peroxide, and compounds known as bacteriocins—proteins produced by certain bacteria that exert a lethal effect on closely related bacteria. In general, bacteriocins have a narrower range of activity than antibiotics but are often more lethal.

Antibiotic-induced diarrhea and infectious diarrhea

Lactobacillus supplementation has shown good results in preventing and treating antibiotic-induced diarrhea and infectious diarrheas. Antibiotics often cause diarrhea by altering the type of bacteria in the colon or by promoting the overgrowth of *Candida albicans.* Antibiotic use can result in a severe form of diarrhea known as pseudomembranous enterocolitis. This condition is attributed to overgrowth of a bacterium *(Clostridium difficile),* resulting from the death of the bacteria that normally keep *C. difficile* under control.

It appears that when antibiotics are necessary, it is important to supplement with lactobacilli. Although it is commonly believed that acidophilus supplements are not effective if taken during antibiotic therapy, research actually supports the use of *L. acidophilus* during antibiotic administration. Reductions of friendly bacteria and/or infection with antibiotic-resistant bacteria may be prevented by administering lactobacillus products during antibiotic therapy. A dosage of at least 15 billion to 20 billion organisms is required. It is recommended that the lactobacillus supplement be taken several hours before or after the antibiotic.

The effectiveness of lactobacillus supplementation in infectious diarrhea may be dependent upon strain and dosage. For example, in traveler's diarrhea—a diarrhea caused by *E. coli*—two double-blind studies failed to demonstrate benefit of one commercial preparation (Lactinex), but two other double-blind studies did demonstrate small protective effects with another product (Culturelle) at a daily dosage of 10 billion live bacteria. The same is true with other infectious diarrhea, as several double-blind studies have demonstrated positive results with the particular strain found in Culturelle, Lactobacillus GG, in cases where other strains/products failed to produce benefit. Lactobacillus GG also appears quite useful in helping the recovery from rotavirus-caused diarrhea in children.

Cancer prevention

A series of population studies has suggested that the consumption of high levels of cultured milk products containing lactobacilli may reduce the risk of colon cancer. Various species of lactobacilli have demonstrated antitumor activity. In human studies, ingestion of *L. acidophilus* resulted in reduced activity of bacterial enzymes associated with the formation of cancer-causing compounds in the gut. In one double-blind trial in patients surgically treated for bladder cancer, lactobacillus supplementation was shown to prevent recurrences in those patients with bladder cancer as long as the patient was not suffering from recurring multiple tumors.

L. acidophilus preparations are also of value in cancer patients receiving chemotherapy drugs or radiation therapy involving the gastrointestinal tract. Double-blind studies indicate that lactobacillus supplementation can help prevent diarrhea caused by chemotherapy or radiation.

Urinary tract (bladder) infections

One of the problems with antibiotic therapy for urinary tract infections is that it results in disturbance in the bacterial flora that protect against those same infections, which may lead to recurrent infections. The insertion of lactobacilli suppositories into the vagina of women after they had been treated with antibiotics has been shown to significantly reduce the recurrence rate. Women given antibiotics should routinely reestablish proper vaginal flora by following the guidelines for vaginal infections (see "Usual Dosage"). Oral therapy is also often recommended.

Vaginal yeast infections

L. acidophilus has been shown to retard the growth of *Candida albicans,* the major yeast involved in vaginal yeast infections. Clinical studies have suggested that the introduction of lactobacilli to the vagina can assist in clearing up yeast infections and preventing recurrent infections as well as preventing bacterial vaginosis.

Available Forms

Lactobacillus preparations are available in powder, liquid, capsule, and tablet form. Proper manufacturing, packaging, and storing of the product is necessary to ensure viability, the right amount of moisture, and freedom from contamination. Lactobacilli do not respond well to freeze-drying (lyophilization), spray drying, or conventional frozen storage. Excessive temperature during packaging or storage can dramatically reduce viability. Also, unless the product has been shown to be stable, refrigeration is necessary, though some products do not have to be refrigerated until after the bottle has been opened. Brands available include Culturelle.

Cautions and Warnings

None known.

Possible Side Effects

Generally lactobacillus products are well tolerated. At higher dosages (e.g., more than 20 billion live bacteria) they may produce excessive flatulence and possibly diarrhea.

Drug Interactions

Studies in humans indicate that lactobacillus preparations do not appear to interfere with the effectiveness of antibiotics, but they may prevent antibiotic-induced diarrhea.

Food and Nutrient Interactions

None known.

Usual Dosage

The dosage is based upon the number of live organisms. The ingestion of 1 billion to 10 billion viable lactobacillus cells daily is sufficient for most people. Amounts exceeding this may induce mild gastrointestinal disturbances, while smaller amounts may not be able to colonize the gastrointestinal tract.

As a douche in the reestablishment of normal vaginal flora, it is generally recommended that 10 billion live organisms be dissolved in 10 ml of warm water. Use a syringe to douche the material into the vagina and retain for at least five minutes or as long as desired.

Overdosage

Overdosage generally results in excessive flatulence and possibly diarrhea.

Special Populations

Pregnant/breast-feeding women
   Generally regarded as safe for use during pregnancy and lactation.

Children
   Suitable for children at one-half the adult dosage.

Seniors
   No special precautions are known.

Lactobacillus GG *(see Lactobacillus acidophilus, Lactobacillus rhamnosus)*

General Information

Lactobacillus GG (LGG) is a patented strain of *Lactobacillus rhamnosus* bacteria that is the most extensively researched and clinically proven strain available. LGG takes its name from its discoverers, Drs. Sherwood Gorbach and Barry Goldin of Tufts University. Several studies have shown that LGG is better able to withstand stomach acid and colonize the large intestine than other lactobacillus varieties.

LGG is found in the commercial product Culturelle; each capsule contains a minimum of 10 billion live bacteria.

Lactoferrin

Used For

Antiviral and immune-enhancing effects
Effectiveness: B–   Safety: C

General Information

Lactoferrin is an iron-binding protein that is one of the key components of **bovine colostrum,** often cited for its immune-enhancing and antiviral effects. However, while it is true that lactoferrin has demonstrated activity against bacteria and viruses, including human immunodeficiency virus (HIV) and the hepatitis C virus (HCV), in test tube studies, the clinical effectiveness of even purified bovine lactoferrin is questionable. For example, in one open clinical trial eleven patients with chronic hepatitis C who received an eight-week course of bovine lactoferrin (1.8 or 3.6 g/day) the results did not demonstrate any significant benefit.

Available Forms

Lactoferrin is available in capsules and tablets.

Cautions and Warnings

None known.

Possible Side Effects

None known.

Drug Interactions

None known.

Food and Nutrient Interactions

None known.

Usual Dosage

The typical recommendation is 250 to 500 mg daily, but the effective dosage is not known at this time.

Special Populations

Pregnant/breast-feeding women
As the effects of lactoferrin during pregnancy and lactation have not been sufficiently evaluated, it should not be used during these times.

Children
Suitable for children at one-half the adult dosage.

Seniors
No special precautions are known.

Lecithin (see Phosphatidylcholine)

General Information

Lecithin is a mixture of fatty substances derived from soy. It is a rich source of phospholipids. A phospholipid is a molecule that has a glycerol backbone with two fatty acids and either choline or serine attached. Although we can ingest preformed phospholipids such as phosphatidylserine or phosphatidylcholine, most of these phospholipids are broken down into glycerol, free fatty acids, and the phosphate group rather than being absorbed intact. Most commercial lecithin contains only 10–20 percent phosphatidylcholine and trace amounts of phosphatidylserine; however, some newer preparations are available that contain up to 55 percent phosphatidylcholine and 90 percent phosphatidylserine. Ideally these higher-concentration preparations are the ones that should be used, since they are associated with fewer of the side effects (loss of appetite, nausea, abdominal bloating, gastrointestinal pain, and diarrhea) found with higher doses of lecithin.

Lipoic Acid

Used For

Diabetic neuropathy
Effectiveness: A   Safety: A

HIV infection and AIDS
Effectiveness: B   Safety: A

Liver disorders
Effectiveness: B   Safety: A

General Information

Lipoic acid (also known as alpha-lipoic acid and thioctic acid) is a sulfur-containing vitaminlike substance that plays an important role as the necessary cofactor in two vital energy-producing reactions involved in the production of cellular energy (ATP). Lipoic acid is not considered a vitamin, but because it is an accessory nutrient, a relative deficiency can occur in certain situations. Lipoic acid is an effective antioxidant. It is unique in that it is effective against both water- and fat-soluble free radicals.

Diabetic neuropathy
Lipoic acid is an approved drug in Germany for the treatment of diabetic neuropathy (nerve disease). Several double-blind studies have shown that lipoic acid supplementation (300 to 600 mg daily) does improve diabetic neuropathy. Lipoic acid's primary effect in improving diabetic neuropathy is thought to be the result of its antioxidant effects. However, it has also been shown to lead to an improvement in blood sugar metabolism, improve blood flow to peripheral nerves, and actually stimulate the regeneration of nerve fibers. Its ability to improve blood sugar metabolism is a result of its effects on glucose metabolism and an ability to increase insulin sensitivity.

HIV infection and AIDS

Several studies have shown that individuals infected with HIV and suffering from AIDS have low lipoic acid levels and a compromised antioxidant defense system. Preliminary studies have shown that lipoic acid supplementation exerts a significant beneficial effect in the blood of HIV-infected patients. Specifically, supplementation increased plasma vitamin C in nine of ten patients, total glutathione in seven of seven patients, and helper T lymphocytes and the helper/suppressor T cell ratio in six of ten patients, while an indicator of lipid peroxidation (malondialdehyde) decreased in eight of nine patients. Larger, double-blind studies are needed to support these encouraging results. In addition, in test tube studies lipoic acid has been shown to significantly inhibit the replication of HIV by reducing the activity of reverse transcriptase, the enzyme responsible for manufacturing the virus from the DNA of lymphocytes.

Liver disorders

Lipoic acid protects the liver from free-radical damage and also helps promote detoxification reactions. Preliminary studies suggest a possible role in the treatment of hepatitis and cirrhosis of the liver, but more clinical research is needed to confirm these effects.

Available Forms

Lipoic acid is available in tablets and capsules.

Cautions and Warnings

Individuals with diabetes need to be aware that taking lipoic acid may alter insulin or drug require-

ments. Consult a physician to discuss proper monitoring of blood sugar levels before taking lipoic acid.

Possible Side Effects

None known.

Drug Interactions

Lipoic acid may affect insulin in insulin-dependent
diabetics or drugs that lower blood sugar levels in
non-insulin-dependent diabetics, such as glyburide
(Diabeta, Micronase) and metformin (Glucophage).
Consult a physician to discuss proper monitoring of
blood sugar levels before taking lipoic acid.

Food and Nutrient Interactions

None known.

Usual Dosage

For general antioxidant support, the recommended
dosage is 20 to 50 mg. In the treatment of diabetic
neuropathy and liver disorders, the recommended
dosage is 300 to 600 mg daily. In the treatment of
HIV infection and AIDS, the recommended dosage is
150 to 200 mg three times daily.

Overdosage

None known.

Special Populations

Pregnant/breast-feeding women
As the effects of lipoic acid during pregnancy and lactation have not been sufficiently evaluated, it should not be used during these times unless directed to do so by a physician.

Children
Suitable for children at one-half the adult dosage.

Seniors
No special precautions are known.

Liver Extracts

Used For

Iron deficiency anemia
Effectiveness: A   Safety: C

Hepatitis
Effectiveness: B   Safety: C

General Information

Extracts of beef (bovine) liver are a rich natural source of many vitamins and minerals including iron. Liver extracts provide the most absorbable form of iron—heme iron—and other nutrients critical in building blood, including vitamin B_{12} and folic acid. Liver extracts can contain as much as 3–4 mg of heme iron per gram. In addition to its use as a source of iron, liver extracts are also used to support liver function and boost energy levels.

Most clinical studies have utilized hydrolyzed liver extracts, produced by exposing the liver material to enzymes that hydrolyze (add water to) the protein bonds. This process basically liquefies the liver and is the reason why hydrolyzed extracts are often referred to as "liquid liver extracts."

Hydrolyzed liver extracts have been shown to improve fat utilization, promote tissue regeneration, and prevent damage to the liver in animal studies. Double-blind studies in humans have shown that hydrolyzed liver extracts are effective orally in the treatment of chronic liver disease. For example, in one double-blind study involving 556 patients with chronic hepatitis, subjects were given either 70 mg of hydrolyzed liver extract or a placebo three times daily. At the end of three months of treatment, the group receiving the liver extract was shown to have far lower liver enzyme levels. Since the level of liver enzymes in the blood reflects damage to the liver, it was concluded that the liver extract improved the function of damaged liver cells as well as prevented further damage to the liver.

Available Forms

Liver extracts are available as nutritional supplements in capsules and tablets. The highest-quality liver extracts are aqueous (hydrolyzed) extracts, which have had the fat-soluble components removed, and typically contain more than twenty times the nutritional content of raw liver, including 3–4 mg of heme iron per gram.

Cautions and Warnings

Liver extracts should not be used in patients suffering from an iron storage disorder such as hemochromatosis.

Possible Side Effects

None known.

Drug Interactions

None known.

Food and Nutrient Interactions

None known.

Usual Dosage

The recommended dosage is entirely dependent upon the concentration, method of preparation, and quality of the liver extract. Follow the manufacturer's recommendation on the label.

Overdosage

None known.

Special Populations

Pregnant/breast-feeding women
Considered safe during pregacy and lactation.

Children
Suitable for children at one-half the adult dosage.

Seniors
No special precautions are known.

Lutein

Used For

Prevention of macular degeneration
Effectiveness: B   Safety: B

General Information

Lutein is a yellow-orange carotene that appears to
offer significant protection against macular degeneration. The macula is the area of the retina where
images are focused. It is the portion of the eye responsible for fine vision. Degeneration of the macula is the leading cause of severe vision loss in the
United States. The macula, especially the central
portion of the macula (the fovea), owes its yellow
color to its high concentration of lutein.

A low level of lutein in the macula is thought to be
a major risk factor for age-related macular degeneration. Therefore, the possibility of increasing the
concentration of lutein within the macula may offer
significant protective effects against the development of macular degeneration. Lutein supplementation has been able to increase blood and macular
lutein concentrations. However, whether or not
lutein supplementation can actually prevent or treat
macular degeneration has not been sufficiently determined.

There is also evidence that lutein intake may

protect against cataract formation and coronary artery disease because of its antioxidant effects.

Available Forms

Lutein supplements are either derived from the
marigold flower or manufactured synthetically.
Lutein is most often available in soft gelatin capsules
but may also be found in hard gelatin capsules and
tablets. Brand names available include FloraGLO.

Cautions and Warnings

None known.

Possible Side Effects

None known.

Drug Interactions

None known.

Food and Nutrient Interactions

Lutein is most often recommended to be taken with
food to possibly improve absorption. High dosages
of beta-carotene may reduce the absorption of
lutein.

Usual Dosage

In population studies, the people showing protection from macular degeneration were estimated to
have eaten about 6 mg of lutein per day from food.
This amount appears to be a reasonable level for
supplementation.

Overdosage

None known.

Special Populations

Pregnant/breast-feeding women
As the effects of lutein supplementation during pregnancy and lactation have not been sufficiently evaluated, it should not be used during these times.

Children
Suitable for children at one-half the adult dosage.

Seniors
No special precautions are known.

Lycopene

Used For

Cancer prevention
Effectiveness: B+   Safety: A

Heart disease (atherosclerosis) prevention
Effectiveness: B   Safety: A

General Information

Lycopene is a red-colored carotene found primarily in tomatoes that has potent antioxidant and anticancer properties. In one study conducted by Harvard researchers of all of the carotenoids, only lycopene was clearly linked to protection against prostate cancer. The men who had the greatest amounts of lycopene (6.5 mg per day) in their diet showed a 21 percent lower risk of prostate cancer compared with those eating the least. When the researchers looked at only advanced prostate cancer, those with a high lycopene intake had an 86 percent lower risk (although this result was not statistically significant due to the small number of cases). Similar results were seen with cancers of the gastrointestinal tract, cervical cancer, and breast cancer. Researchers have also found a statistically significant association between high dietary lycopene and a lower risk of heart disease.

Lycopene supplementation may actually decrease the size of prostate tumors and lower the blood levels of prostate-specific antigen (PSA, an indicator of cancer activity) in men with prostate cancer. In a small pilot study of 26 men with newly diagnosed prostate cancer, the men were randomly assigned to receive 15 mg of lycopene twice daily or no supplementation for three weeks before surgery to remove their prostate. PSA levels decreased by 18 percent in the intervention group, whereas they increased by 14 percent in the control group.

Available Forms

Supplemental lycopene is either derived from natural sources (tomato extracts) or manufactured synthetically. Most often lycopene supplements are available in soft gelatin capsules, but hard gelatin capsules and tablets are also available. Brands on the market include Lyc-O-Mato.

Cautions and Warnings

None known.

Possible Side Effects

None known.

Drug Interactions

None known.

Food and Nutrient Interactions

Lycopene is most often recommended to be taken with food, which may improve absorption.

Usual Dosage

In population studies, groups with a lower incidence of various cancers and heart disease were estimated to have eaten about 6 mg of lycopene per day from food. This amount appears to be a reasonable level for supplementation.

Overdosage

None known.

Special Populations

Pregnant/breast-feeding women

As the effects of lycopene supplementation during pregnancy and lactation have not been sufficiently evaluated, it should not be used during these times unless directed by your physician.

Children

Suitable for children at one-half the adult dosage.

Seniors

No special precautions are known.

Lysine

Used For

Herpes
Effectiveness: B+   Safety: B

General Information

Lysine supplementation has become a popular treatment for herpes simplex virus (HSV) infections including cold sores (HSV-1) and genital herpes (HSV-2). This popularity arose from research showing that lysine has antiviral activity in test tube studies. Lysine blocks arginine, another amino acid.

In order for lysine to be effective, it appears that the dietary intake of arginine must be restricted, as double-blind studies on the effectiveness of lysine supplementation without avoiding arginine-rich foods have shown inconsistent results. When lysine has been given at a dosage of 1 g three times daily along with dietary restriction of nuts, chocolate, and gelatin, very good results have been seen. In one double-blind study, after six months of use lysine was rated as effective or very effective in 74 percent of subjects, compared to only 28 percent for those who received the placebo. The mean number of herpes outbreaks was 3.1 in the lysine group, compared to 4.2 in the placebo group.

Available Forms

Lysine supplements are available in capsules and tablets.

Cautions and Warnings

Do not take lysine if you have severe liver or kidney disease without consulting your doctor first.

Possible Side Effects

At recommended dosage levels no side effects have been reported even with chronic use.

Drug Interactions

None known.

Food and Nutrient Interactions

For maximum benefit, it is often recommended that a diet low in arginine and high in lysine be consumed. Foods high in arginine are chocolate, peanuts, seeds, and almonds and other nuts. Foods high in lysine include most vegetables, legumes, fish, turkey, and chicken.

Usual Dosage

The recommended dosage is 1,000 mg (1 g) three times daily with meals.

Overdosage

Accidental overdosage of lysine may produce kidney damage. Do the following in case of accidental overdose: If the victim is unconscious or having convulsions, call for an ambulance immediately. If you take the victim to an emergency room, be sure to bring the bottle or container with you. If the victim is

conscious, call your local poison control center or a
health care professional. The poison control center
may suggest inducing vomiting with ipecac syrup
(available without a prescription at any pharmacy).
Do not induce vomiting unless specifically instructed to do so.

Special Populations

Pregnant/breast-feeding women
As the effects of lysine supplementation during
pregancy and lactation have not been sufficiently
evaluated, it should not be used during these times.

Children
Suitable for children at one-half the adult dosage.

Seniors
No special precautions are known.

Maitake *(Grifola frondosa)*

Used For

Cancer and immune system enhancement
Effectiveness: B   Safety: C

General Information

The maitake mushroom can grow to the size of a
basketball. Historically, maitake has been used as a
food to help promote wellness and vitality. Recent

scientific research has focused on its immune-enhancing and anticancer properties. The primary compounds responsible for its effects in test tube and animal studies are beta-glucans (see **beta 1,3-glucan**). The D-fraction of maitake refers to the portion of the hot-water extract that contains beta-1,3-glucan and beta-1,6-glucan. The M,D-fraction is a purer concentrate of the D-fraction. The beta-glucans of maitake have a unique structure, and test tube studies suggest they are among the most powerful immune stimulants known to date. Human studies are currently under way. Until the results from these studies are published, the effectiveness of maitake preparations in enhancing human immune function is largely unknown.

Maitake researchers have identified four primary mechanisms by which maitake may fight cancer: by protecting healthy cells from becoming cancerous; by enhancing the immune system's ability to seek out and destroy cancer cells; by helping the cell regain control of cell division and programmed cell death (apoptosis); and by helping to prevent the spreading (metastasis) of cancer.

Preliminary studies in animal models have shown that maitake fractions inhibit the growth of tumors in the colon, lungs, stomach, liver, prostate, cervix, bladder, and brain as well as leukemia. The significance for humans of this inhibition in animals is not yet clear.

At this time it appears that maitake beta-glucan fractions are best used in conjunction with conventional cancer therapies. Several studies have shown maitake D- or M,D-fraction helps reduce the side effects of conventional chemotherapy and radiation while at the same time enhancing its effectiveness. In one preliminary study, 165 patients with advanced cancer were given maitake extract. In the patients who were also on chemotherapy, 90 percent of the patients experienced a reduction in the side effects common to chemotherapy, including hair loss, decreased white blood cell counts, nausea, vomiting, and loss of appetite. Maitake was shown to effectively reduce pain levels in 83 percent of the patients. The results were best in breast, lung, and liver cancers. Larger, better controlled studies may be on the horizon, as the U.S. Food and Drug Administration has approved an Investigational New Drug Application for researchers to conduct a more detailed pilot study on maitake D-fraction's effects on advanced breast and prostate cancers.

Available Forms

Maitake is available as a fresh food as well as dried in bulk form and in capsules and tablets. Brands available include Grifon D-Fraction (an alcohol-free liquid preparation in a dropper bottle) and Maitake Gold 404.

Cautions and Warnings

Due to the lack of human data on the role of maitake in cancer treatment, it should not be used as a primary therapy in cancer. Cancer is a potentially life-threatening disease that requires proper medical treatment.

Possible Side Effects

None known.

Drug Interactions

According to preliminary data, maitake beta-glucan fractions appear to help reduce the side effects of conventional chemotherapy and radiation while at the same time enhancing their effectiveness.

Food and Nutrient Interactions

Generally it is recommended that maitake products be taken on an empty stomach.

Usual Dosage

The dosage of maitake extracts is based upon the level of the D- or M,D-fraction. The therapeutic dosage range is based upon body weight, 0.5 mg to 1.0 mg for every kg (2.2 pounds) per day. That translates to a daily dosage of approximately 35–70 mg of the D- or M,D-fraction. The dosage recommendation for prevention is typically 5 to 15 mg of the D- or M,D-fraction.

Overdosage

None known.

Special Populations

Pregnant/breast-feeding women
As the effects of maitake preparations during pregnancy and lactation have not been sufficiently evaluated, it should not be used during these times unless directed to do so by a physician.

Children
Suitable for children at one-half the adult dosage.

Seniors
No special precautions are known.

Maltsupex

Used For

Constipation
Effectiveness: A   Safety: A

General Information

Maltsupex is an extract of barley malt that contains non-absorbable sugars. It is an effective laxative similar in action to bulk-forming fiber supplements (see **Fiber**).

Available Forms

Maltsupex is available in powder, liquid, and tablet form.

Cautions and Warnings

Do not take for more than one week unless under a doctor's supervision. May cause laxative dependence.

Do not use laxative products when abdominal pain, nausea, or vomiting are present unless directed by a physician. If constipation persists, consult a physician.

Do not use the liquid preparation if you are on a sodium-restricted diet as it contains 36 mg of sodium per tablespoon.

Possible Side Effects

None known.

Drug Interactions

None known.

Food Interactions

None known.

Usual Dosage

Drink a full 8 ounces of liquid (preferably water) with each dose.

Tablets: For adults and children over 12 years of age the dosage is four tablets (750 mg each, 3 g total) four times daily. Dosage can be increased up to 48 tablets (36 grams) per day.
Powder: For adults and children over 12 years of age the dosage is up to 4 scoops twice daily.
Liquid: For adults and children over 12 years of age the dosage is 2 tablespoons twice daily.

Overdosage

None known.

Special Populations

Pregnant/breast-feeding women
Generally regarded as safe. But, as the effects of Maltsupex during pregnancy and lactation have not been sufficiently evaluated, it should not be used during these times unless directed to do so by a physician.

Children
   Suitable for children at the following dosages:

Powder: For children 6–12 years of age the dosage is
   up to 2 scoops twice daily; for children 2–6 years
   of age 1 scoop twice daily; and for children under
   2 years of age 2 to 3 level measuring teaspoonfuls, 3 to 4 times per day in water, juice, or formula.
Liquid: For children 6–12 years of age the dosage is
   up to 1 tablespoon twice daily; for children 2–6
   years of age 1/2 tablespoon twice daily; and for
   children under 2 years of age 1 to 2 level measuring teaspoonfuls, 2 to 3 times per day in water,
   juice, or formula.

Seniors
No special precautions are known.

Medium-Chain Triglycerides

Used For

Malabsorption syndromes
Effectiveness: A   Safety: A

Weight loss
Effectiveness: B+   Safety: A

General Information

Medium-chain triglycerides (MCTs) are special types
of saturated fats prepared from coconut oil that
range in length from six to twelve carbon chains.

The two primary uses of MCTs are as an easily absorbed energy source in malabsorption syndromes and to help promote weight loss.

Malabsorption syndromes

For almost fifty years MCTs have been used in the treatment of malabsorption syndromes such as occur after surgical resection of any portion of the intestinal tract or in inflammatory bowel disease (Crohn's disease and ulcerative colitis). Unlike other fats, MCTs do not require pancreatic enzymes and bile acids to be absorbed. If you have a condition associated with malabsorption and are having trouble maintaining your weight, please ask your doctor about the appropriateness of MCTs as an energy source.

Weight loss

MCTs promote weight loss by increasing the burning of calories (thermogenesis). In one study the thermogenic effect of a high-calorie diet containing 40 percent fat as MCTs was compared to one containing 40 percent fat composed of long-chain triglycerides (LCTs) found in most other vegetable oils. The thermogenic effect (calories burned six hours after the meal) of the MCTs was almost twice as high as that of the LCTs, 120 calories versus 66 calories. A follow-up study demonstrated that MCT oil given over a six-day period can increase diet-induced thermogenesis by 50 percent.

Available Forms

MCTs are available in liquid form, usually with flavoring agents (e.g., orange, butter, olive oil, and garlic).

Cautions and Warnings

MCTs should not be used by diabetics or individuals with severe liver disease unless under a doctor's supervision, as a high intake of MCTs may lead to acidosis in these cases.

Possible Side Effects

MCTs are generally regarded as safe and have a good safety record in clinical studies, with no significant side effects noted.

Drug Interactions

None known.

Food and Nutrient Interactions

None known.

Usual Dosage

The usual dosage when being used as a weight-loss aid is 1 to 2 tbsp. per day (roughly 14 to 28 g). MCTs can be used as an oil for salad dressing or as a bread spread, or simply taken as a supplement. MCTs can be used in cooking as long as the temperature is not greater than 160 degrees. At higher temperatures the MCTs give off an unpleasant odor and can give food a soapy flavor.

Overdosage

Overdosage is unlikely, except in diabetics and individuals with liver disease. In these individuals, a high intake of MCTs may lead to acidosis. Do the following in case of accidental overdose: If the victim is unconscious or having convulsions, call for an ambulance immediately. If you take the victim to an emergency room, be sure to bring the bottle or container with you. If the victim is conscious, call your local poison control center or a health care professional. The poison control center may suggest inducing vomiting with ipecac syrup (available without a prescription at any pharmacy). *Do not* induce vomiting unless specifically instructed to do so.

Special Populations

Pregnant/breast-feeding women
As the effects of MCTs during pregnancy and lactation have not been sufficiently evaluated, they should not be used during these times unless recommended by a physician.

Children
As the effects of MCTs in children have not been sufficiently evaluated, they should not be used in children unless recommended by a physician.

Seniors
No special precautions are known.

Melatonin

Used For

Adjunct to chemotherapy
Effectiveness: B+   Safety: A

Insomnia
Effectiveness: B+   Safety: A

Jet lag
Effectiveness: B+   Safety: A

General Information

Melatonin is a hormone secreted by the pineal gland, a pea-sized gland at the base of the brain. The exact function of melatonin is still poorly understood, but it is critically involved in regulating the body's circadian rhythms—the natural biorhythm of hormone secretion—as well as the sleep/wake cycle. Release of melatonin is stimulated by darkness and suppressed by light. The primary uses of melatonin are in the treatment of jet lag and insomnia and as an adjunct in cancer therapy. There are other possible indications for melatonin, but these other uses are based on very preliminary studies.

Adjunct to chemotherapy

Melatonin has been shown to inhibit several types of cancers in test tube and animal studies. In human studies, melatonin has also been shown to enhance the anticancer effects of chemotherapy drugs such as interleukin-2, interferon, and tamoxifen. More research is required on the use of melatonin in cancer patients.

Insomnia

Melatonin plays an important role in the induction of sleep. Low melatonin secretion at night can be a cause of insomnia, particularly in the elderly. Several double-blind trials have shown melatonin supplementation to be very effective in promoting sleep, but it appears the sleep-promoting effects of melatonin are most apparent when melatonin levels are low. Low melatonin levels are thought to be an extremely common cause of insomnia in the elderly, while in younger individuals this is less of a factor.

Jet lag

Several double-blind studies have shown melatonin to be very effective in relieving jet lag. Different dosage recommendations have been given. It appears the best results are achieved when melatonin is taken at a dosage of 5 mg in the evening at the new destination for up to five days.

Available Forms

Melatonin is most often available as a sublingual tablet. Timed-release preparations designed to replicate the body's own melatonin secretion may provide the best results in treating insomnia. Brands available include Melatonex.

Cautions and Warnings

Must not be used in children. Must not be used during pregnancy or lactation.

Cancer is a potentially life-threatening disease that requires proper medical treatment. If you are interested in using melatonin as an adjunct to cancer treatment, talk it over with your medical doctor.

Possible Side Effects

Although there appear to be no serious side effects at recommended dosages, conceivably melatonin supplementation above 8 mg daily could disrupt the normal circadian rhythm and lead to changes in the levels of key hormones.

Drug Interactions

Melatonin may enhance the anticancer effects of certain chemotherapy agents, including interleukin-2, interferon, and tamoxifen. Melatonin has been used to treat withdrawal reactions from people addicted to benzodiazepines, such as diazepam (Valium) and triazolam (Halcion). Melatonin levels are typically lowered by beta-blocker drugs such as propanolol (Inderal) and atenolol (Tenormin) as well as by other drugs used in treating high blood pressure or angina (e.g., verapamil), aspirin, and other nonsteroidal anti-inflammatory drugs. Melatonin levels may be increased by fluoxetine (Prozac).

Food and Nutrient Interactions

None known.

Usual Dosage

In the treatment of insomnia, a dosage of 3 mg at bedtime is the most common recommendation. This dosage appears to be more than enough, as dosages as low as 0.1 mg and 0.3 mg have been shown to produce a sedative effect in individuals with low melatonin levels.

Overdosage

None known.

Special Populations

Pregnant/breast-feeding women
As the effects of melatonin during pregnancy and lactation have not been sufficiently evaluated, it should not be used during these times.

Children
Melatonin is not suitable for use in children unless specifically recommended and monitored by a physician.

Seniors
No special precautions are known.

Methionine

Used For

Liver aid
Effectiveness: C   Safety: C

General Information

Methionine is a sulfur-containing essential amino acid (one of the required building blocks for many body proteins). Methionine is most often included in lipotropic formulas designed to promote the flow of bile and fat to and from the liver. Other compounds typically found in these formulas are cysteine, choline, inositol, and betaine. The effectiveness of methionine as a lipotropic agent has not been confirmed. Its use as a supplement is based upon its physiologic roles in the liver, primarily as **S-adeno-sylmethionine** (SAMe).

Available Forms

Methionine is available as L-methionine in tablets and capsules.

Cautions and Warnings

None known.

Possible Side Effects

None known. Supplementation of up to 2 g of methionine daily for long periods of time has not produced any serious side effects in humans.

Drug Interactions

None known.

Food and Nutrient Interactions

Excessive methionine intake combined with inadequate intake of folic acid, vitamin B_6, and vitamin B_{12} can increase the conversion of methionine to homocysteine—a substance linked to heart disease and stroke.

Usual Dosage

The typical recommendation is 250 to 1,000 mg daily.

Overdosage

None known.

Special Populations

Pregnant/breast-feeding women
As the effects of methionine supplementation during pregnancy and lactation have not been sufficiently evaluated, it should not be used during these times unless directed to do so by a physician.

Children
As the effects of methionine supplementation in children have not been sufficiently evaluated, it should not be used in children unless directed to do so by a physician.

Seniors
No special precautions are known.

MSM (methylsulfonylmethane)

Used for

Source of sulfur
Effectiveness: B   Safety: C

General Information

MSM (methylsulfonylmethane) is the major form of sulfur in the human body. Sulfur is an important element for all cells and body tissues and an especially important nutrient for joint tissue, where it functions in the stabilization of the connective tissue matrix of cartilage, tendons, and ligaments. As far back as the 1930s, researchers demonstrated that in-dividuals with arthritis are commonly deficient in this essential nutrient. Restoring sulfur levels brought about significant benefit to these patients. Many claims are being made regarding the use of a sulfur-containing supplement called methylsulfonyl-methane (MSM) in the treatment of a wide variety of disorders. These claims are based on anecdotal evidence involving individual cases of arthritis (both osteoarthritis and rheumatoid arthritis), lupus, muscle pain, and promotion of wound healing. To date, none of these claims have been substantiated in clinical research published in medical journals.

Available Forms

MSM is available in powder form, capsules, and tablets.

Cautions and Warnings

None known.

Possible Side Effects

MSM provides significant advantages over other forms of sulfur in that it is completely safe and at recommended levels (up to 8,000 mg daily) appears to be without side effects. Note: when people say they are allergic to sulfur, what they really mean is that they are allergic to the so-called sulfa drugs or sulfite-containing food additives. No allergies to MSM have been reported.

Drug Interactions

None known.

Food Interactions

None known.

Usual Dosage

The typical dosage of MSM is 1,500 to 8,000 mg per day.

Overdosage

Overdosage can result in headache, nausea, and diarrhea.

Special Populations

Pregnant/breast-feeding women

As the effects of MSM during pregnancy and lactation have not been sufficiently evaluated, it should not be used during these times.

Children

As the effects of MSM have not been sufficiently evaluated in children, it should be used only under direct medical supervision.

Seniors

No special precautions are known.

N-acetylcysteine (NAC)

Used For

Acetaminophen toxicity
Effectiveness: A   Safety: A

Antioxidant effects
Effectiveness: B–   Safety: D

Bronchial and lung disorders
Effectiveness: B   Safety: A

HIV and AIDS
Effectiveness: D   Safety: C

General Information

N-acetylcysteine (NAC) is a derivative of the naturally occurring amino acid cysteine. It is used as a nutritional supplement primarily for its potential role in boosting tissue levels of **glutathione,** an important antioxidant that is composed of the amino acids cysteine, glutamic acid, and glycine.

Acetaminophen toxicity

Acetaminophen (Tylenol, paracetamol) overdose is capable of injuring the liver, kidneys, heart, and central nervous system. Overdose can also produce fatal results, typically in individuals who intentionally consume more than 10 g. Liver damage usually develops within several hours of ingestion as a result of oxidation of acetaminophen, which produces toxic compounds that deplete liver glutathione stores and subsequently damage the liver. NAC is the treatment of choice in conventional medicine for acetaminophen overdose. This treatment, however, requires strict medical supervision, as extremely high dosages of NAC are required.

Antioxidant effects

Although NAC has shown some antioxidant activity in preliminary human studies, it may not be as useful as less expensive antioxidants such as vitamin C. Individuals with a hereditary deficiency of glutathione due to a defect in synthesis respond better to vitamin C (3 g per day) than to NAC (800 mg per day). The same may be true in normal individuals. There is evidence that NAC supplementation at higher dosages (greater than 600 mg) may act as a pro-oxidant—a substance that causes oxidative damage. One study found that when NAC was given orally to six volunteers at a dosage of 1.2 g per day for four weeks, followed by 2.4 grams per day for an additional two weeks, it actually increased oxidative stress by 83 percent and reduced glutathione concentrations by 48 percent. Until this issue is resolved, NAC supplementation at dosages greater than 600 mg should be avoided in healthy individuals.

Bronchial and lung disorders

NAC has an extensive history of use as a mucolytic in the treatment of acute and chronic lung conditions such as emphysema, bronchitis, chronic asthma, and cystic fibrosis. It directly splits the sulfur linkages of mucoproteins, thereby reducing the viscosity of bronchial and lung secretions. As a result, it helps improve bronchial and lung function, reduce cough, and improve oxygen saturation in the blood. Most but not all of the studies with oral NAC in respiratory tract diseases have shown these positive effects. Better results have been achieved administering NAC via a ventilator.

HIV and AIDS

Numerous studies have shown that individuals infected with HIV have a compromised antioxidant defense system. Since glutathione has been shown to inhibit the virus, it was originally proposed that NAC may act as an effective antioxidant and raise tissue glutathione levels in AIDS. However, supplementation with NAC at a dosage of 1.8 g per day failed to increase glutathione in white blood cells in patients with AIDS.

Available Forms

NAC is available as a nutritional supplement in capsules and tablets.

Cautions and Warnings

NAC may reduce the effectiveness of carbamazepine (Tegretol). Do not use NAC while taking this drug. It also should not be used while taking nitroglycerine, as severe headaches may result.

Possible Side Effects

At recommended levels, NAC is generally well tolerated. At higher dosages, such as those required to treat acetaminophen toxicity, NAC may cause headache, nausea, vomiting, and other gastrointestinal symptoms.

Drug Interactions

Do not use NAC while taking carbamazepine (Tegretol), as NAC may reduce the drug's effectiveness.

Use of NAC with nitroglycerine can cause severe

headache. Do not use NAC while taking nitroglycerine.

NAC may interfere with several classes of chemotherapy drugs and should not be used with any active chemotherapy treatment program.

Food and Nutrient Interactions

None known.

Usual Dosage

The recommended dosage for bronchial and lung disorders is usually 200 mg three times daily.

Overdosage

Accidental overdosage with NAC may cause headache, nausea, vomiting, and other gastrointestinal symptoms.

Special Populations

Pregnant/breast-feeding women

As the effects of NAC during pregnancy and lactation have not been sufficiently evaluated, it should not be used during these times unless recommended by a physician.

Children

As the effects of NAC in children have not been sufficiently evaluated, it should not be used in children unless recommended by a physician.

Seniors

No special precautions are known.

N-acetyl-glucosamine (NAG)

General Information

N-acetyl-glucosamine (NAG) is a form of glucosamine that lacks the scientific documentation of **glucosamine sulfate**. NAG differs from glucosamine sulfate in that instead of a sulfur molecule, NAG has a portion of an acetic acid molecule attached to it. Glucosamine sulfate and NAG are entirely different molecules and appear to be handled by the body differently. The absorption of NAG is questionable in humans for several reasons: (1) NAG is quickly digested by intestinal bacteria; (2) NAG is known to bind to dietary compounds (lectins) in the gut, with the resultant complex being excreted in the feces; and (3) a large percentage of NAG is broken down by intestinal cells.

Octacosanol

Used For

Amyotrophic lateral sclerosis
Effectiveness: D   Safety: C

Enhancing physical performance
Effectiveness: B   Safety: C

General Information

Octacosanol is a waxy substance naturally present in wheat germ oil, rice bran, and the wax layer of many plants. Animal research indicates that it shares many common features with vitamin E and plays a role in enhancing energy production within cells. Early research suggested that octacosanol might help in improving amyotrophic lateral sclerosis (Lou Gehrig's disease), but this possible treatment was subsequently disproved. More recent research has focused on octacosanol as an ergogenic (performance-enhancing) agent. Preliminary studies found that octacosanol had promising effects on endurance, reaction time, and other measures of exercise capacity. In one study, 1,000 mcg per day of octacosanol for eight weeks was found to improve grip strength and visual reaction time but had no effect on chest strength, auditory reaction time, or endurance. More research is required to verify these effects.

Available Forms

Octacosanol is available from wheat germ oil, rice bran oil, and spinach extract, usually in soft gelatin capsules. **Policosanol** is a mixture of octacosanol and related compounds derived from sugar cane wax.

Cautions and Warnings

None known.

Possible Side Effects

None known.

Drug Interactions

None known.

Food and Nutrient Interactions

None known.

Usual Dosage

The usual dosage is 1 to 8 mg daily.

Overdosage

None known.

Special Populations

Pregnant/breast-feeding women

As the effects of octacosanol during pregnancy and lactation have not been sufficiently evaluated, it should not be used during these times.

Children

Suitable for children at one-half the adult dosage.

Seniors

No special precautions are known.

Ostivone (*see* Ipriflavone)

General Information

Ostivone is a popular brand of the generic compound ipriflavone, a naturally occurring flavonoid (plant pigment) that is utilized as a nutritional supplement to promote bone health.

Pancreatin

Used For

Cancer
Effectiveness: B   Safety: A

Digestive aid
Effectiveness: B   Safety: A

Food allergies
Effectiveness: B   Safety: A

Herpes zoster (shingles)
Effectiveness: B   Safety: A

Inflammation, sports injuries, and trauma
Effectiveness: B   Safety: A

Multiple sclerosis and autoimmune disorders
Effectiveness: B   Safety: A

Pancreatic insufficiency
Effectiveness: B+   Safety: A

General Information

Pancreatin is a name for pancreatic enzymes prepared from fresh hog pancreas. The pancreas is a digestive tract gland that produces enzymatic secretions required for the digestion and absorption of food. There are three major classes of pancreatic enzymes:

Lipases: The pancreatic lipases, along with bile, function in the digestion of fats. Deficiency of lipase results in malabsorption of fats and fat-soluble vitamins.

Amylases: Amylases are enzymes that break down
  starch molecules into smaller sugars. Amylases
  are secreted by the salivary glands as well as the
  pancreas.
Proteases: The proteases secreted by the pancreas
  (trypsin, chymotrypsin, and carboxypeptidase)
  function in digestion by breaking down protein
  molecules into single amino acids.

The most obvious use of pancreatic extracts is in
cases of pancreatic insufficiency, characterized by
impaired digestion, malabsorption, nutrient deficiencies, and abdominal discomfort. Pancreatin is a
well-accepted medical treatment for cystic fibrosis, a
genetic disorder characterized by severe pancreatic
insufficiency. While cystic fibrosis is relatively rare,
pancreatic insufficiency is thought to be relatively
common in the elderly. Given its ability to improve
digestive function in more severe pancreatic enzyme insufficiency, it is reasonable to assume that
pancreatin may help improve digestion in milder
cases as well.

Cancer

Pancreatin and other proteases (papain and
bromelian) have a long history of use in cancer
treatment. Current clinical research suggests significant benefits from their use in the treatment of
many forms of cancer. Specifically, these studies
have shown improvements in the general condition
of patients, quality of life, and modest to significant
improvements in life expectancy. Studies have consisted of patients with cancers of the breast, lung,
stomach, head and neck, ovaries, cervix, and colon;
and lymphomas and multiple myeloma. The proteases were used in conjunction with surgery,

chemotherapy, and/or radiation indicating that pancreatin and proteases can be used safely and effectively with conventional treatments.

Food allergies

In studies performed in the 1930s and 1940s, pancreatin was shown to be effective in preventing food allergies. Unfortunately, there are no more-recent studies in this area.

Herpes zoster (shingles)

Orally administered pancreatic enzyme preparations have been used in Germany in the treatment of herpes zoster (shingles) for over thirty years. The positive results obtained in earlier studies with proteolytic enzymes led to a double-blind study comparing enzyme therapy versus acyclovir (Zovirax). Ninety patients were randomly assigned to receive either acyclovir (800 mg) or an enzyme preparation (120 mg trypsin, 40 mg chymotrypsin, and 320 mg papain) five times per day for a treatment period of seven days. The parameters of pain and skin lesions were measured over fourteen to twenty-one days. Results indicated no statistically significant differences between the two groups, indicating that the enzyme preparation is as effective as acyclovir. The proposed mechanism of action for the enzyme preparation is stimulation of the breakdown of immune complexes as well as enhancement of immune function.

Inflammation, sports injuries, and trauma

Pancreatin and protease enzyme preparations have been shown to be useful in the treatment of many acute and chronic inflammatory conditions, including sports injuries, tendinitis, and rheumatoid arthritis.

Multiple sclerosis and other autoimmune diseases

The proteases are also essential in preventing the deposit of immune complexes in body tissues. Diseases associated with high levels of circulating immune complexes include rheumatoid arthritis, systemic lupus erythematosus, periarteritis nodosa, scleroderma, ulcerative colitis, Crohn's disease, multiple sclerosis, and AIDS. The presence of immune complexes is thought to contribute greatly to the disease process, even in AIDS. Experimental and clinical studies have shown that protease enzyme preparations are extremely effective in reducing circulating immune complex levels in several of these diseases. Furthermore, clinical improvements correspond with decreases in immune complex levels.

For example, in the treatment of multiple sclerosis, pancreatic enzyme preparations have been shown to produce good effects in reducing the severity and frequency of symptom flare-ups. Especially good results were noted in cases of visual disturbance, urinary and intestinal malfunction, and sensory disturbances. However, it should be pointed out that there was little effect on spasticity, dizziness, or tremor.

Available Forms

The United States Pharmacopoeia (USP) has set strict definitions for level of activity. A 1X pancreatic enzyme (pancreatin) product has in each milligram not less than 25 USP units of amylase activity, not less than 2 USP units of lipase activity, and not less than 25 USP units of protease activity. Pancreatin of higher potency is given a whole-number multiple indicating its strength. For example, a full-strength undiluted pancreatic extract that is ten times stronger than the USP standard would be referred to as 10X USP. Full-strength products are preferred to lower-potency pancreatin products because lower-potency products are often diluted with salt, lactose, or galactose to achieve the desired strength.

Pancreatin products are often enteric-coated—that is, coated to prevent digestion in the stomach, so that the enzymes will be liberated in the small intestine. However, non-enteric-coated enzyme preparations actually outperform enteric-coated products if they are given prior to a meal (for digestive purposes) or on an empty stomach (for anti-inflammatory effects).

Brands available include Wobenzyme N.

Cautions and Warnings

If you are allergic to pork, do not use pancreatin or any other enzyme derived from pork sources.

Possible Side Effects

Pancreatin is generally well tolerated at recommended dosage levels and is not associated with any significant side effects.

Drug Interactions

Pancreatin may interfere with the blood-sugar-lowering effect of acarbose (Precose) and miglitol (Glyset).

Food and Nutrient Interactions

Generally pancreatin is recommended to be taken on an empty stomach when being used for effects other than as a digestive aid.

Usual Dosage

The dosage recommendation for full-strength 8–10X USP pancreatic enzyme is typically 300–500 mg three times a day immediately before meals when used as a digestive aid and ten to twenty minutes before meals or on an empty stomach when other effects are desired.

Overdosage

Excessive dosages are associated with nausea, vomiting, and diarrhea.

Special Populations

Pregnant/breast-feeding women

As the effects of pancreatin during pregnancy and lactation have not been sufficiently evaluated, it should not be used during these times unless directed to do so by a physician.

Children

Suitable for children at one-half the adult dosage.

Seniors

No special precautions are known.

PABA
(Para-aminobenzoic Acid)

Used For

Scleroderma and other connective tissue diseases
Effectiveness: B–   Safety: D

General Information

PABA is an essential nutrient for many microorganisms and some animals, but its role in human nutrition has not yet been demonstrated. PABA is often used to help prevent or even reverse accumulation of abnormal fibrous tissue, as occurs in various connective tissue diseases. Although uncontrolled studies have reported that high dosages of PABA (8 to 12 g per day) were helpful to people with scleroderma and Peyronie's disease (accumulation of abnormal fibrous tissue in the penis), a double-blind study of scleroderma failed to show any improvement from supplementation with PABA. Until additional research is conducted, PABA cannot be considered effective.

Available Forms

PABA is available in tablets and capsules. PABA is often an ingredient used in topical sunscreen products. (Taking PABA internally offers no protection from the sun.)

Cautions and Warnings

Do not take dosages greater than 400 mg withou
consulting a physician.

Possible Side Effects

No significant side effects have been reported with
dosages in the range of 300 to 400 mg per day
However, at higher dosages (such as 8 g per day or
more) PABA may cause low blood sugar, rash, fever
and (on rare occasions) liver damage. Use o'
amounts over 20 g per day in small children has re
sulted in death.

Drug Interactions

Theoretically, PABA may interfere with the following
drugs (primarily antibiotics): sulfasalazine (Azulfidine),
sulfamethoxazole/trimethoprim (Septra, Bactrim),
dapsone, and methotrexate.

Food and Nutrient Interactions

None known.

Usual Dosage

PABA is often included at low dosages (i.e., 10 to 100
mg) in B vitamin complexes and multiple vitamin
formulas. Higher dosages should only be used
under the direction of a physician.

Overdosage

Overdosage is most likely to occur in children. Do
the following in case of accidental overdose: If the

victim is unconscious or having convulsions, call for an ambulance immediately. If you take the victim to an emergency room, be sure to bring the bottle or container with you. If the victim is conscious, call your local poison control center or a health care professional. The poison control center may suggest inducing vomiting with ipecac syrup (available without a prescription at any pharmacy). *Do not* induce vomiting unless specifically instructed to do so.

Special Populations

Pregnant/breast-feeding women

As the effects of PABA during pregnancy and lactation have not been sufficiently evaluated, it should not be used at dosages greater than 100 mg (if at all) during these times.

Children

PABA is not suitable for use in children unless specifically directed by a physician.

Seniors

No special precautions are known.

Pectin (*see* Fiber)

General Information

Pectin is found in all plant cell walls as well as in the outer skin and rind of fruits and vegetables. For example, the rind of an orange contains 30 percent pectin, an apple peel is 15 percent pectin, and onion skin is 12 percent pectin. The gel-forming properties of pectin are well known to anyone who has made a jelly or jam. These same gel-forming qualities are responsible for the laxative and cholesterol-lowering effects of pectin. Most pectin used for supplementation is derived from citrus sources.

Phosphatidylcholine

Used For

Alzheimer's disease
Effectiveness: B–   Safety: A

Bipolar disorder
Effectiveness: B   Safety: A

Elevated cholesterol levels
Effectiveness: B   Safety: A

Liver disease
Effectiveness: B   Safety: A

General Information

All cells throughout the human body are enveloped by a membrane composed chiefly of essential fatty acids in the form of compounds known as phospholipids. The major phospholipid of the human body is phosphatidylcholine. Commercially available phosphatidylcholine preparations are derived from soy lecithin. These preparations are used in the treatment of Alzheimer's disease, bipolar disorder, elevated cholesterol levels, and liver disorders. The beneficial effects are likely due primarily to the essential fatty acid components of phosphatidylcholine and lecithin preparations.

Alzheimer's disease

Alzheimer's disease is characterized by the general destruction of nerve cells in several key areas of the brain. This destruction results in the formation of neurofibrillary tangles and plaques. The disease's clinical features are believed to be related to a decrease in brain acetylcholine levels. Since phosphatidylcholine can increase acetylcholine levels in the brain in normal patients, it seemed reasonable to assume phosphatidylcholine supplementation would be of benefit to Alzheimer's patients. However, the basic defect in cholinergic transmission in Alzheimer's disease relates to impaired activity of the enzyme acetylcholine transferase. This enzyme combines choline (as provided by phosphatidylcholine) with an acetyl molecule to form acetylcholine, the neurotransmitter. Since providing more choline will not necessarily increase the activity of this key enzyme, phosphatidylcholine supplementation will not be beneficial in the majority of patients with Alzheimer's disease. Not surprisingly, clinical trials using phosphatidylcholine for the treatment of this disorder have largely been disappointing. Studies have shown inconsistent improvements in memory from phosphatidylcholine supplementation in both normal and Alzheimer's patients. Inconsistent positive effects have been noticed only when using very high dosages (25–30 g). If phosphatidylcholine supplementation is going to be of value, it will produce noticeable improvement within the first two weeks of use.

Bipolar disorder

Bipolar disorder, also referred to as manic-depression, is a disorder characterized by periods of major depression alternating with periods of abnormally elevated mood. Phosphatidylcholine supplementation (15 to 30 g a day) has shown good results in the treatment of bipolar disorder. The use of phosphatidylcholine to increase brain choline levels may result in significant improvement or amelioration of symptoms in some patients but should be used only under the direct supervision of a physician.

Elevated cholesterol levels

Phosphatidylcholine has many important functions in the body, including increasing the solubility of cholesterol, thereby decreasing its ability to induce atherosclerosis. Phosphatidylcholine also aids in lowering cholesterol levels and removal of cholesterol from tissue deposits. In a total of fifteen clinical trials with a duration ranging from one to twelve months, phosphatidylcholine lowered total serum cholesterol by 8.8 to 28.2 percent, decreased triglyceride levels by 25 percent, and increased HDL cholesterol levels by 13.4 to 20 percent. The typical dosage was 1.5 to 2.7 g daily.

Liver disease

In Germany, phosphatidylcholine is marketed for the treatment of the following liver disorders: acute viral hepatitis; alcohol-induced fatty liver; chronic hepatitis; cirrhosis of the liver; decreased bile solubility; diabetic fatty liver; drug-induced liver damage; and toxic liver damage.

Good clinical data has been generated to support these clinical applications, and this use has received proper authorization from the BGA, the German equivalent of the FDA. The phosphatidylcholine preparations approved for use in these liver diseases are of high quality (90 percent phosphatidylcholine, with 50 percent of the molecule having the essential fatty acid linoleic acid bound at the first and second positions).

Available Forms

Phosphatidylcholine is available as soy lecithin granules and soft gelatin capsules. The phosphatidylcholine content in cruder products is approximately 10–20 percent. There are some products on the market that contain up to 90 percent phosphatidylcholine. These higher-content preparations should be used for most therapeutic applications, since they are associated with fewer side effects compared to lecithin.

Cautions and Warnings

Phosphatidylcholine is not indicated in patients with unipolar or clinical depression unless under the supervision of a physician, as high-dosage phosphatidylcholine supplementation has been shown to worsen depression in some cases.

Possible Side Effects

Phosphatidylcholine is generally well tolerated. At higher dosages (greater than 10 g) lecithin preparations may cause reduced appetite, nausea, abdominal bloating, gastrointestinal pain, and diarrhea.

Drug Interactions

None known.

Food and Nutrient Interactions

Generally it is recommended that phosphatidyl-choline be taken with food to enhance absorption.

Usual Dosage

Dosage is based upon the phosphatidylcholine content of the preparation used. Since large doses of phosphatidylcholine are often required in some clinical conditions, higher-phosphatidylcholine-content preparations are recommended over lecithin. For the treatment of Alzheimer's disease and bipolar disorder, the dosage would be 4,500 to 9,000 mg three times daily with meals. That would mean a dosage of 9 to 18 g for a product containing 50 percent phosphatidylcholine. For lowering cholesterol, the dosage would be 500 to 900 mg three times daily with meals. In the treatment of liver disorders, the dosage would be 350 to 500 mg three times daily with meals.

Overdosage

None known.

Special Populations

Pregnant/breast-feeding women
Considered safe during pregnancy and lactation.

Children
Suitable for children at one-half the adult dosage.

Seniors
No special precautions are known.

Phosphatidylserine

Used For

Aging-related memory impairment and Alzheimer's disease
Effectiveness: B+   Safety: A

Depression
Effectiveness: B+   Safety: A

General Information

Phosphatidylserine is the major phospholipid in the brain, where it plays a major role in determining the integrity and fluidity of cell membranes. Normally the brain can manufacture sufficient levels of phosphatidylserine, but there is evidence that insufficient production in the elderly may be linked to depression and/or impaired mental function. Good results have been obtained in numerous double-blind studies, where phosphatidylserine supplementation has been shown to improve mental function, mood, and behavior in elderly subjects, including those with early stages of Alzheimer's disease and Parkinson's disease. Unlike typical antidepressant drugs, phosphatidylserine does not influence serotonin and other neurotransmitters, suggesting another mechanism of action, such as a reduction in the secretion of the stress hormone cortisol.

Available Forms

Commercially available phosphatidylserine is manufactured from soy lecithin and contains the following:

Phosphatidylserine	100 mg
Phosphatidylcholine	45 mg
Phosphatidylethanomine	25 mg
Phosphatidylinositol	5 mg

Brand names available include Leci-PS.

Cautions and Warnings

None known.

Possible Side Effects

None known.

Drug Interactions

None known.

Food and Nutrient Interactions

None known.

Usual Dosage

The typical recommendation is 100 mg of phosphatidylserine three times daily.

Overdosage

None known.

Special Populations

Pregnant/breast-feeding women
As the effects of phosphatidylserine during pregnancy and lactation have not been sufficiently evaluated, it should be used during these times only if specifically recommended by a physician.

Children
Suitable for children at one-half the adult dosage.

Seniors
No special precautions are known.

Propolis

Used For

Low immunity and immune support
Effectiveness: C   Safety: D

Wound healing
Effectiveness: B   Safety: D

General Information

Propolis is the resinous substance collected by bees from the leaf buds and bark of trees, especially poplar and conifer trees. The bees utilize the propolis along with beeswax to construct the hive. Propolis has antibiotic activities that help the hive block out viruses, bacteria, and other organisms.

Like **bee pollen,** propolis is also used as a general

nutritional supplement. The composition of propolis products is typically 60 percent resins, 20 percent beeswax, 10 percent essential oils, 5 percent pollen, and 5 percent various organic and mineral matter. Propolis is also used orally to help stimulate the body's immune system and wound-healing ability. However, there is little clinical evidence to support either use. One clinical study did find propolis to be quite effective in healing surgical wounds in the mouth when used as a mouth rinse.

Available Forms

Propolis is available in liquid extract form as well as in capsules and tablets.

Cautions and Warnings

If you are allergic to bee pollen, honey, or conifer or poplar trees, do not use propolis. Severe allergic reactions have been reported.

Possible Side Effects

Allergic reactions are the most common side effects (see "Cautions and Warnings"). Allergic reactions can range from very mild (e.g., mild gastrointestinal upset) to more severe reactions including asthma, anaphylaxis (shock), and even death in people who are extremely allergic to bee products. Use with caution.

Drug Interactions

None known.

Food and Nutrient Interactions

None known.

Usual Dosage

The typical recommended dosage is 500 mg once or twice daily.

Overdosage

None known.

Special Populations

Pregnant/breast-feeding women
As the effects of propolis during pregnancy and lactation have not been sufficiently evaluated, it should not be used during these times unless directed to do so by a physician.

Children
Suitable for use in children at one-half the adult dosage.

Seniors
No special precautions are known.

Prostex

Used For

***Benign prostatic hyperplasia (prostate
enlargement)***
Effectiveness: B+   Safety: A

General Information

Prostex, a combination of the amino acids glycine, alanine, and glutamic acid, has been shown in several
studies to relieve many of the symptoms of BPH. For
example, in one study of forty-five men, nighttime urinary frequency (nocturia) was relieved or reduced in
95 percent of subjects, urgency was reduced in 81 percent, frequency was reduced in 73 percent, and de-
layed urination was alleviated in 70 percent. The
mechanism of action is unknown but is likely related to
the amino acids acting as inhibitory neurotransmitters
and reducing the feelings of a full bladder. This therapy, therefore, appears to only address the symptoms.

Available Forms

Prostex is available in capsule form, with each capsule containing 405 mg of the mixture of glycine,
alanine, and glutamic acid.

Cautions and Warnings

Prostate disorders can only be diagnosed by a physician; do not self-diagnose. If you are experiencing
any symptom such as increased urinary frequency,
feelings of bladder fullness or incomplete emptying,

or pain on urination, consult a physician immediately for proper diagnosis.

Possible Side Effects

None known.

Drug Interactions

None known.

Food and Nutrient Interactions

None known. Generally, amino acid supplements such as Prostex are recommended to be taken on an empty stomach to enhance utilization.

Usual Dosage

The recommended dosage is two capsules three times daily.

Overdosage

None known.

Special Populations

Pregnant/breast-feeding women
Prostex is not indicated for use by women.

Children
Prostex is not recommended for use in children.

Seniors
No special precautions are known.

Psyllium (*see* Fiber)

General Information

Psyllium is derived from the seed of the plant *Plantago ovata,* native to Iran and India. Psyllium is a bulk-forming laxative and is high in both fiber and mucilage. The laxative properties of psyllium are due to the swelling of the husk when it comes in contact with water. This forms a gelatinous mass and keeps the feces hydrated and soft. The resulting bulk stimulates a reflex contraction of the walls of the bowel, followed by emptying. In addition to relieving constipation, numerous double-blind studies have shown psyllium can lower total cholesterol.

Brands available include Metamucil, Konsyl, and Perdiem.

Pyruvate

Used For

Weight loss
Effectiveness: B   Safety: B

General Information

Pyruvate is an intermediate energy source generated in the conversion of sugars to energy. It has recently been touted as a natural dietary agent that can enhance weight loss while increasing lean body mass. The majority of the human trials that have been done have used very high dosages (19–44 g) of pyruvate. Although these studies were positive, the feasibility of giving such large doses was questionable. According to the results of one double-blind study, lower dosages (6 g) may be equally effective, but these results are controversial because pyruvate was not the sole compound in the test formula—in addition to providing 6,000 mg of pyruvate, the formula also provided zinc (50 mg), vitamin B_6 (15 mg), chromium (500 mcg), corn silk (300 mg), cranberry powder (50 mg), and DHA (50 mg). The problem is that chromium supplementation has also been shown to promote weight loss while increasing lean body mass. The pyruvate group experienced a 2.4 percent increase in lean body mass and a loss of roughly 4 pounds of body fat. Although these results are positive, there remains many questions to answer.

Available Forms

Pyruvate is available in powder, capsule, and tablet form.

Cautions and Warnings

None known.

Possible Side Effects

None known.

Drug Interactions

None known.

Food and Nutrient Interactions

None known.

Usual Dosage

Most studies have used dosages from 22 to 44 g daily.

Overdosage

None known.

Special Populations

Pregnant/breast-feeding women
As the effects of pyruvate during pregnancy and lactation have not been sufficiently evaluated, it should not be used during these times.

Children
As the effects of pyruvate during childhood have not been sufficiently evaluated, it should not be used in children unless directed by a physician.

Seniors
No special precautions are known.

Quercetin

Used For

Allergy and inflammation
Effectiveness: C   Safety: B

Cancer
Effectiveness: B   Safety: B

Prostatitis
Effectiveness: B   Safety: B

General Information

Quercetin is a bioflavonoid that serves as the backbone for many other flavonoids, including the citrus flavonoids rutin, quercitrin, and hesperidin (see **bioflavonoids**). These derivatives differ from quercetin in that they have sugar molecules attached to the quercetin backbone. Quercetin is consistently the most active of the flavonoids in experimental studies, and many medicinal plants owe much of their activity to their high levels of quercetin.

Allergy and inflammation

Quercetin has demonstrated significant anti-inflammatory and antiallergy activity in test tube studies. It directly inhibits several of the initial steps of inflammation and allergy. For example, it inhibits both the manufacture and release of histamine and other allergic/inflammatory mediators. In addition, it exerts potent antioxidant activity and vitamin-C-sparing action. Based on these test tube studies, quercetin is often recommended for use in virtually all inflammatory and allergic conditions, including asthma, hay fever, rheumatoid arthritis, and lupus, as well as in diabetes and cancer. However, the main shortcoming with quercetin is the lack of clinical studies in these and other applications.

Cancer

Many flavonoids have been shown to inhibit tumor formation, but quercetin has consistently been shown to be the most effective. In experimental models quercetin has demonstrated significant antitumor activity against a wide range of cancers, including cancers of the breast, lung, skin, ovaries, colon, rectum, and brain. Unfortunately, there are few human studies to support the impressive results noted in animal and in vitro studies. The preliminary studies that do exist are encouraging, but much more research is needed.

Prostatitis

Quercetin has been shown to be effective in non-bacterial chronic prostatitis (inflammation of the prostate gland) in a double-blind study. This condition is characterized by chronic pelvic pain that is worse upon urination. In patients taking quercetin, more than 67 percent of subjects had an improvement of symptoms of at least 25 percent. Combining quercetin with bromelain (see "Available Forms," below) produced slightly better results (82 percent had at least a 25 percent improvement in symptoms).

Available Forms

Quercetin is available alone in powder, tablet, and capsule form. Many products contain quercetin in combination with the enzyme **bromelain**. This combination is thought to provide additional benefit, as bromelain exerts antiallergy and anti-inflammatory activity on its own and may also enhance the absorption of quercetin. The amount of bromelain (1,800 MCU) is usually equal to the amount of quercetin.

Cautions and Warnings

None known.

Possible Side Effects

None known.

Drug Interactions

None known.

Food and Nutrient Interactions

None known.

Usual Dosage

The typical dosage recommendation for quercetin is 200 to 400 mg three times per day, twenty minutes before meals.

Overdosage

None known.

Special Populations

Pregnant/breast-feeding women

As the effects of quercetin during pregnancy and lactation have not been sufficiently evaluated, it should not be used during these times.

Children
Suitable for children at one-half the adult dosage.

Seniors
No special precautions are known.

Red Yeast Rice Extract

Used For

Elevated cholesterol levels
Effectiveness: A   Safety: D

General Information

The red yeast *(Monascus purpureus)* fermented on
rice has been used in China for its health-promoting
effects for over two thousand years. This yeast is the
source of a group of compounds known as monacolins that can lower cholesterol levels by blocking a
key enzyme in the liver. In fact, the cholesterol-
lowering prescription drug Mevacor is the trade
name for the compound lovastatin, also known as
monacolin K, one of the key monacolins in red yeast
rice extract.

The marketing of Cholestin (an extract of red yeast
fermented on rice, standardized for monacolin content) as a dietary supplement in the United States
has caused quite a controversy since 1997. Because
it contains a natural source of a prescription drug
the FDA and the maker of Mevacor, Merck, tried to
prohibit the sale of Cholestin and other red yeast
rice extracts as a dietary supplement. The FDA's rul-

ing against Cholestin was temporarily reversed in March 1999 but two years later the FDA's ruling was upheld. Nonetheless, many red yeast rice products remain on the market.

These products, like their prescription counterparts, clearly are effective in lowering cholesterol levels. Over twenty clinical trials conducted in China involving thousands of subjects have shown red yeast rice extract to effectively lower high blood cholesterol levels by roughly 20 percent while raising protective HDL cholesterol about 18 percent. A study conducted at the UCLA Center for Human Nutrition under the direction of David Heber, M.D., has also demonstrated positive results. The double-blind, placebo-controlled study consisted of eighty-three healthy subjects with a cholesterol level between 200 and 239 mg/dl. Subjects were treated with 2.4 g of red yeast rice extract (Cholestin) supplying 9.6 mg of monacolins per day or a placebo. Both groups were instructed to maintain a diet consisting of 30 percent fat with less than 10 percent saturated fat and less than 300 mg of cholesterol. On average, cholesterol decreased in the Cholestin group from 254 to 208 mg/dl by eight weeks, with no change in the placebo group.

Red yeast rice extract works by inhibiting the manufacture of cholesterol. Most of the body's supply of cholesterol (approximately 80 percent) is made in the liver. This process is rigorously controlled by biochemical feedback mechanisms. The amount of cholesterol produced by the liver is controlled by the enzyme HMG-CoA reductase. When the liver senses that more cholesterol is needed, the activity of this enzyme increases to raise cholesterol production. When the liver senses that there is enough cholesterol in your body, the activity of HMG-CoA reductase is decreased to lower cholesterol production. The essential feedback mechanism helps to keep cholesterol levels in balance. However, in many people this feedback system becomes faulty. By inhibiting HMG-CoA reductase activity, red yeast rice extract can help the body maintain normal cholesterol levels.

Available Forms

Red yeast rice extract is available in capsules and tablets.

Cautions and Warnings

Since lovastatin and related drugs are associated with some rare (among less than 1–2 percent of users) but serious side effects, including diseases of the liver and skeletal muscle, it is recommended that users of red yeast rice extract be supervised by a health care professional. Consult with your physician before using red yeast rice extract if you are taking any medication or if you are under physician supervision for cholesterol control.

Do not take red yeast rice extract under the following conditions:

• You are pregnant, expect to become pregnant, or are breast-feeding.
• You are at risk for liver disease or have active liver disease or any history of liver disease.
• You consume more than two alcoholic drinks per day.
• You have a serious infection.
• You have undergone an organ transplant.
• You have a serious disease or physical disorder or have recently undergone major surgery.

• You are taking a prescription medication that adversely affects lovastatin.
• You are under twenty years of age.

Stop the use of red yeast rice extract immediately if you experience unexplained muscle pain, tenderness, or weakness, especially if accompanied with flulike symptoms. Keep out of reach of children.

Possible Side Effects

Side effects are uncommon. The most frequent side effects reported in studies with red yeast rice extract were stomach irritation or abdominal discomfort (reported in 2.8 percent of subjects) and elevations in liver enzymes (reported in 3.4 percent of patients).

Drug Interactions

Lovastatin and related drugs (pravastatin, simvastatin, etc.) reduce blood levels of **coenzyme Q$_{10}$**. **Niacin** at a dosage of 500 mg three times per day potentiates the effects of lovastatin and probably exerts similar effects on red yeast rice extract. This potentiation by high doses of niacin may also increase the risk for side effects, including serious damage to the liver and skeletal muscle, and should therefore be used with caution.

Lovastatin, and therefore red yeast rice extract, may increase the effects of warfarin (a clot inhibitor) and digoxin (a heart medication). If you are taking these drugs, please consult your physician.

Several other drugs have been shown to produce potentially dangerous interactions, including the antifungal drug itraconazole (Sporanox); antibiotics such as cyclosporin and erythromycin; and other lipid-lowering drugs such as gemfibrozil. Consult with a physician before taking red yeast rice extract if you are taking any prescription medications.

Food and Nutrient Interactions

The absorption of lovastatin has been shown to be enhanced when taken with food, but it is reduced by fiber supplements. The absorption of the monacolins in red yeast rice extract may be greater than that of isolated lovastatin, as the extract contains fatty acids and other compounds that may enhance absorption. Nonetheless, taking red yeast rice extract with food is recommended as long as the food is not too high in fiber.

Usual Dosage

The dosage is based upon the content of monacolins in the red yeast rice extract. The typical recommendation is 4.8–9.6 mg of monacolins per day.

Overdosage

None reported.

Special Populations

Pregnant/breast-feeding women
Should not be used during pregnancy and lactation.

Children
Should not be used by persons under the age of twenty years.

Seniors
No special precautions are known.

Reishi *(Ganoderma lucidum)*

Used For

Fatigue
Effectiveness: C   Safety: C

Hepatitis
Effectiveness: B   Safety: C

Infections and immune enhancement
Effectiveness: C   Safety: B

General Information

The reishi mushroom has been used in traditional
Chinese medicine for more than four thousand years
for the treatment of general fatigue and weakness,
asthma, insomnia, and cough. The Chinese name,
ling zhi, translates as "mushroom of spiritual potency." It was also referred to as the "mushroom of
immortality." Despite this storied past, reishi has not
been subjected to significant scientific investigation.
Preliminary human research demonstrates that it
may boost some aspects of immune function, especially in cases of chronic hepatitis, but more research
is needed to document its effectiveness and safety.

Available Forms

Reishi mushroom is available as a food. The dried mushroom is available in bulk form and in capsules and tablets. It is also available in tincture and dry powdered extract form.

Cautions and Warnings

None known.

Possible Side Effects

With continuous use over a three- to six-month period, reishi may cause dryness of the mouth, throat, and nasal area, and gastrointestinal upset.

Drug Interactions

Theoretically, reishi may increase bleeding time, so it is not recommended for those taking anticoagulant medications such as warfarin (Coumadin).

Food and Nutrient Interactions

None known.

Usual Dosage

The typical recommendation is the equivalent of 3 to 9 g per day of the crude dried mushroom.

Overdosage

May cause diarrhea or intestinal pain.

Special Populations

Pregnant/breast-feeding women
As the effects of reishi preparations during pregnancy and lactation have not been sufficiently evaluated, it should not be used during these times.

Children
Suitable for use in children at one-half the adult dosage.

Seniors
No special precautions are known.

Resveratrol

Used For

Antioxidant effects
Effectiveness: A   Safety: B

General Information

Resveratrol is a compound found in grapes and red wine that acts as an antioxidant. It has also been shown to decrease the stickiness of blood platelets, which helps prevent clot formation and reduce the buildup of plaque on arteries. In addition to possibly reducing the risk for atherosclerosis (hardening of the arteries), animal studies demonstrate some anticancer effects and anti-inflammatory action. Whether these effects in animal studies translate to effectiveness in humans has not been investigated.

The amount used in animals to prevent cancer, however, would exceed 500 mg per human adult (far in excess of the usual dosage).

Available Forms

Resveratrol is available in capsules and tablets.

Cautions and Warnings

None known.

Possible Side Effects

None known.

Drug Interactions

None known.

Food and Nutrient Interactions

None known.

Usual Dosage

Resveratrol is generally recommended in the dosage range of 200–600 mcg per day. For comparative purposes, a glass of red wine or purple grape juice provides approximately 640 mcg of resveratrol.

Overdosage

None known.

Special Populations

Pregnant/breast-feeding women
As the effects of resveratrol supplementation during pregnancy and lactation have not been sufficiently evaluated, it should not be used during these times unless directed to do so by a physician.

Children
Suitable for use in children at one-half the adult dosage.

Seniors
No special precautions are known.

Royal Jelly

Used For

Elevated cholesterol levels
Effectiveness: A   Safety: D

General Information

Royal jelly is produced by worker bees to feed the queen bee. Between the sixth and twelfth days of the so-called nurse bees' lives, they mix honey and **bee pollen** with enzymes in the glands of their throats to produce a thick, milky substance that they then feed to the queen bee. Royal jelly is a concentrated food, as evidenced by the queen bee's superior size, astounding ovulation, stamina, and longevity. It contains all of the B vitamins, including

high concentrations of pantothenic acid (B_5) and
pyridoxine (B_6). Other nutritional qualities are similar to those of pollen. The scientific investigation
into the health-promoting properties of royal jelly
has focused on its ability to protect against atherosclerosis (hardening of the arteries).

Over the past thirty years various medical journals
have published animal and human studies showing
that royal jelly can significantly lower cholesterol
and triglyceride levels. Despite problems with study
design and lack of standardization of commercial
preparations used in the studies, there is evidence
that royal jelly can produce a significant reduction in
total serum lipids and cholesterol levels. Specifically, the human studies indicate that royal jelly at a
dosage of 50 to 100 mg per day decreases total cholesterol levels by about 14 percent in patients with
moderate to severe elevations in total cholesterol
(range 210–325 mg/dl).

Available Forms

Royal jelly is available in bulk (usually in jars), capsules, and tablets.

Cautions and Warnings

If you are allergic to bee pollen, honey, or conifer
and poplar trees, do not use royal jelly. Severe allergic reactions have been reported.

Possible Side Effects

Allergic reactions are the most common side effects
(see "Cautions and Warnings"). Allergic reactions
can range from very mild (e.g., mild gastrointestinal
upset) to more severe reactions including asthma,

anaphylaxis (shock), and even death in people who are extremely allergic to bee products. Use with caution.

Drug Interactions

None known.

Food and Nutrient Interactions

None known.

Usual Dosage

The typical dosage used in the cholesterol-lowering studies is 50 to 100 mg daily.

Overdosage

None known.

Special Populations

Pregnant/breast-feeding women
As the effects of royal jelly during pregnancy and lactation have not been sufficiently evaluated, it should not be used during these times unless directed to do so by a physician.

Children
Suitable for use in children at one-half the adult dosage.

Seniors
No special precautions are known.

Rutin (*see* Citrus Bioflavonoids)

General Information

Rutin is one of the chief citrus bioflavonoids.

S-adenosylmethionine (SAMe)

Used For

Depression
Effectiveness: A   Safety: A

Fibromyalgia
Effectiveness: A   Safety: A

Liver disorders
Effectiveness: A   Safety: A

Migraine headaches
Effectiveness: B   Safety: A

Osteoarthritis
Effectiveness: A   Safety: A

General Information

S-adenosylmethionine (SAMe) is formed in the body by combining the essential amino acid **methionine** to adenosine-triphosphate (ATP). It is involved in over forty biochemical reactions in the body. It functions closely with folic acid and vitamin

B_{12} in methylation reactions. Methylation is the process of adding a methyl group (three hydrogen atoms joined to a carbon atom) to another molecule. SAMe is many times more effective in transferring methyl groups than other methyl donors. Methylation reactions are critical in the manufacture of many body components, especially brain chemicals, as well as in detoxification reactions.

SAMe is also required in the manufacture of all sulfur-containing compounds in the human body, including **glutathione** and various cartilage components, including **chondroitin sulfate**.

The beneficial effects of SAMe supplementation are far-reaching due to its central role in so many metabolic processes. Currently, the main uses of SAMe are in the treatment of depression, fibromyalgia, liver disorders, migraine headaches, and osteoarthritis.

Depression

Based on results from a number of clinical studies, it appears that SAMe is perhaps the most effective natural antidepressant (although a strong argument could also be made for **St. John's wort** extract). In fact, in these studies SAMe has demonstrated better results than conventional antidepressant drugs and fewer side effects. In addition to generalized depression, SAMe has produced significant effects in relieving postpartum depression and to reduce the anxiety and depression associated with drug detoxification and rehabilitation.

SAMe's antidepressant effects are related to its ability to increase levels of important brain chemicals such as serotonin, dopamine, and phosphatidylserine. SAMe also leads to improved binding of serotonin and dopamine to their receptor sites.

Fibromyalgia

Fibromyalgia is a recently recognized disorder regarded as a common cause of chronic musculoskeletal pain and fatigue. SAMe has been shown in at least four clinical studies to produce excellent benefits in patients suffering from fibromyalgia. Improvements were indicated by a significant reduction in the number of trigger points and painful areas as well as improvements in mood.

Liver disorders

SAMe has been shown to be quite beneficial in several liver disorders, including cirrhosis, Gilbert's syndrome (see below), and oral-contraceptive-induced liver damage. Its benefits are related to its function as the major methyl donor in the liver and promotion of detoxification reactions.

One of the key functions of SAMe in the liver is the inactivation of estrogens. Clinical studies have shown that SAMe is quite useful in protecting the liver from damage and improving liver function in conditions associated with estrogen excess, namely, oral contraceptive use, pregnancy, and premenstrual syndrome.

SAMe has been shown to be quite helpful in the treatment of Gilbert's syndrome, a common condition characterized by a chronically elevated serum bilirubin level (1.2 to 3.0 mg/dl). Previously considered rare, this disorder is now known to affect as much as 5 percent of the general population. The condition is usually without symptoms, although some patients do complain about loss of appetite, malaise, and fatigue (typical symptoms of impaired liver function). SAMe supplementation produces a significant decrease in serum bilirubin in patients with Gilbert's syndrome.

SAMe has been shown to offer benefits in the treatment of more-severe liver disorders, including cirrhosis. One of the greatest risks of chronic liver diseases such as chronic hepatitis is liver cancer. Supplementation with SAMe appears to be very much indicated in these patients in the attempt to reduce the risk of liver cancer. Animal studies have shown a significant protective effect for supplemental SAMe against liver cancer in animals exposed to liver cancer.

Migraine headaches

SAMe has been shown to be of benefit in the treatment of migraine headaches. The benefit arises gradually, and long-term treatment is required for therapeutic effectiveness.

Osteoarthritis

SAMe has demonstrated impressive results in the treatment of osteoarthritis. A deficiency of SAMe in the joint tissue, just like a deficiency of **glucosamine,** leads to loss of the gel-like nature and shock-absorbing qualities of cartilage. As a result, osteoarthritis can develop.

SAMe has been studied in a total of 21,524 patients in detailed clinical trials. In these studies, SAMe has demonstrated reductions in pain scores and clinical symptoms similar to those achieved with non-steroidal anti-inflammatory drugs such as ibuprofen, indomethacin, naproxen, and piroxicam. While these drugs are associated with significant risk of toxicity, side effects, and actual promotion of the disease process in osteoarthritis, SAMe offers similar benefits without the same risks or side effects.

Available Forms

SAMe is available in capsules and tablets. It has been available commercially in Europe since 1975 and was introduced in the United States in 1998.

Cautions and Warnings

Individuals with bipolar disorder (manic-depression) should not take SAMe unless under strict medical supervision because SAMe's antidepressant activity may lead to the manic phase in these individuals.

Possible Side Effects

No significant side effects have been reported with oral SAMe other than occasional nausea and gastrointestinal disturbances.

Drug Interactions

None known.

Food and Nutrient Interactions

None known.

Usual Dosage

SAMe is usually recommended at a dosage of 200 to 400 mg twice daily.

Overdosage

None known.

Special Populations

Pregnant/breast-feeding women
Considered safe during pregnancy and lactation.

Children
Suitable for children at one-half the adult dosage.

Seniors
No special precautions are known.

Shark Cartilage

Used For

Cancer
Effectiveness: C   Safety: C

Osteoarthritis
Effectiveness: C   Safety: C

Rheumatoid arthritis
Effectiveness: C   Safety: C

General Information

Shark cartilage as well as other animal cartilage contain primarily **chondroitin sulfate** and may produce similar benefits in osteoarthritis. In addition to chondroitin sulfate, shark cartilage appears to contain a substance that strongly inhibits the growth of new blood vessels (angiogenesis). This antiangiogenic effect is thought to have potential in the treatment of cancer and rheumatoid arthritis, as the aggressiveness of tumor growth and the inflammation of rheumatoid arthritis are directly related to the number of new blood vessels to the tumor or area of inflammation.

Most of the studies on shark cartilage and cancer have been performed in test tubes and animals. In addition, injectable forms were often used. Human evidence on effectiveness is lacking. Preliminary studies indicate little, if any, positive effects in cancer patients.

Available Forms

Shark cartilage is available in powder, capsules, or tablets. Brand names available include BeneFin.

Cautions and Warnings

Due to the lack of human data on cancer treatment with shark cartilage, it should not be used as a primary therapy in cancer. Cancer is a potentially life-threatening disease that requires proper medical treatment.

Possible Side Effects

Shark cartilage is generally well tolerated. At higher dosages it can lead to a bad taste in the mouth, nausea, and constipation. There has been one case report of liver inflammation (elevated liver enzymes) with the use of shark cartilage.

Drug Interactions

None known.

Food and Nutrient Interactions

None known.

Usual Dosage

The dosage recommendation ranges from 500 to 5,000 mg one to six times daily.

Overdosage

None known.

Special Populations

Pregnant/breast-feeding women
As the effects of shark cartilage during pregnancy and lactation have not been sufficiently evaluated, it should not be used during these times.

Children
Suitable for use in children at one-half the adult dosage.

Seniors
No special precautions are known.

Shiitake *(Lentinus edodes)*

Used For

Low immunity and immune support
Effectiveness: B   Safety: C

General Information

The shiitake mushroom is a mainstay in the Japanese diet and is regarded as a protector against cancer. Scientific research has focused on the immune-enhancing and anticancer effects of shiitake polysaccharides (complex sugars). Lentinan, one of these components, is a highly purified complex sugar extracted from shiitake and used in Japan for cancer treatment. Lentinan must be injected because it is poorly absorbed orally. Animal studies have shown that lentinan does not suppress tumor growth in animals when it is given orally. However, KS-2, another shiitake polysaccharide, is absorbed orally in an active form. KS-2 is used by cancer patients in China and has been viewed as an oral alternative to lentinan.

Available Forms

Shiitake is available fresh or dried in many supermarkets. Commercial preparations use primarily LEM (Lentinus edodes mycelium extract), the mycelium of the mushroom (the form before the cap and stem grow). Extracts supplying KS-2 are also available. Shiitake extracts are most often available in capsules and tablets.

Cautions and Warnings

Shiitake mushrooms may produce an increase in blood eosinophil counts. Eosinophils are white blood cells associated with allergy.

Possible Side Effects

Shiitake has an excellent record of safety but has been known to induce temporary diarrhea and abdominal bloating when used in high dosages (above 15–20 g per day). Allergic reactions (e.g., eosinophilia) have been reported.

Drug Interactions

None known.

Food and Nutrient Interactions

None known. Shiitake preparations are typically recommended to be taken on an empty stomach.

Usual Dosage

The recommended dosage of the whole dried shiitake mushroom, in soups or as a decoction (a tea made by boiling the substance rather than steeping it), is 6 to 16 g per day in divided dosages. For LEM (see "Available Forms"), the recommendation is 1 to 3 g two to three times per day. For other forms, please follow label instructions.

Overdosage

None known.

Special Populations

Pregnant/breast-feeding women

Intake of shiitake as a food is generally regarded as safe during pregnancy and lactation. However, as the effects of shiitake extracts such as LEM during pregnancy and lactation have not been sufficiently evaluated, these forms should not be used during these times unless directed to do so by a physician.

Children
Suitable for use in children over six years of age at a level one-half the adult dosage.

Seniors
No special precautions are known.

Soy Isoflavones

Used For

Cancer prevention
Effectiveness: C   Safety: B

Cholesterol reduction
Effectiveness: B   Safety: B

Menopause
Effectiveness: B+   Safety: B

Osteoporosis
Effectiveness: B   Safety: B

General Information
The soy isoflavone compounds daidzein and genistein are often classified as phytoestrogens—naturally occurring plant compounds that bind to estrogen receptor sites in humans. One cup of soybeans provides about 300 mg of isoflavones. Diets

rich in isoflavones as well as studies using isolated isoflavones are showing promise in cancer prevention, cholesterol reduction, alleviation of menopausal symptoms, and prevention of osteoporosis.

Cancer prevention

The first clues soy isoflavones might provide protection from cancer came from population studies noting that Asian cultures eating a diet high in soy foods, such as tofu, demonstrated lower rates of several types of cancers. There is now considerable evidence from test tube, animal, and population-based studies indicating a possible anticancer effect of soy isoflavones, particularly in hormone-sensitive cancers such as breast and prostate cancer. However, the use of soy isoflavones in people with existing hormone-sensitive cancers remains controversial.

Cholesterol reduction

Soy-supplemented diets have been shown to significantly decrease total cholesterol (a 9.3 percent reduction), LDL cholesterol (a 12.9 percent decrease), and triglycerides (a 10.5 percent drop) while raising HDL cholesterol (an increase of 2.4 percent). Soy isoflavones are thought to play a major role in this effect. In addition, soy isoflavones have been shown to exert antioxidant effects in protecting LDL cholesterol from becoming oxidized (damaged).

Menopause

Soy isoflavones are often recommended to reduce the hot flashes and vaginal atrophy associated with menopause. There is some clinical evidence to support this recommendation. In one study of postmenopausal women, those women consuming enough soy foods to provide about 200 mg of soy isoflavones daily demonstrated signs of estrogenic activity when compared to a control group. Specifically, the women consuming the soy foods demonstrated an increase in the number of superficial cells that line the vagina. This increase offsets the vaginal drying and irritation that are common in postmenopausal women. Based upon scientific evidence, it is thought that 300 mg of soy isoflavones is equivalent in effect to about 0.45 mg of conjugated estrogens or one tablet of Premarin.

Osteoporosis

Soy isoflavones have been shown to enhance bone density in animal studies and in preliminary human studies. In one study in postmenopausal women, those taking 90 mg of soy isoflavones daily demonstrated significant increases in both bone mineral content and density in the lumbar spine. There were no changes in the placebo group or in the group receiving 56 mg/day.

Available Forms

Soy isoflavones are available in capsules, tablets, and powder. Brand names available include Estroven.

Cautions and Warnings

Due to the lack of human data, soy isoflavones should not be used by cancer patients (particularly women with estrogen-sensitive breast cancer) unless directed to do so by a physician.

Possible Side Effects

Soy isoflavones are generally well tolerated. Allergy is a possible side effect in people sensitive to soy products. Although most of the studies with dietary phytoestrogens, including soy isoflavones, are positive and show protective effects against breast cancer and other hormone-sensitive cancers, these compounds do work by binding to estrogen and progesterone receptors (they actually act as an antagonist to progesterone). Because of these effects, there is concern that they may encourage growth of breast cancers and uterine cancers.

Drug Interactions

Theoretically, because the soy isoflavones occupy estrogen receptors and are capable of producing antiestrogenic effects, the use of soy isoflavone supplements at higher dosages (e.g., greater than 120 mg per day) is not recommended in women taking birth control pills or other sources of estrogen (e.g., Premarin).

Food and Nutrient Interactions

None known.

Usual Dosage

The recommended dosage of soy isoflavones for the relief of menopausal symptoms, including protection against heart disease and osteoporosis, is 90 to 120 mg daily.

Overdosage

None known.

Special Populations

Pregnant/breast-feeding women
As the effects of soy isoflavones during pregnancy and lactation have not been sufficiently evaluated, they should not be used during these times unless directed to do so by a physician.

Children
There does not appear to be any suitable use for soy isoflavones in children at this time.

Seniors
No special precautions are known.

Spirulina

Used For

Anticancer effects
Effectiveness: B   Safety: C

Antioxidant
Effectiveness: B   Safety: C

Nutritional support
Effectiveness: B   Safety: C

Weight loss
Effectiveness: B   Safety: C

General Information

Spirulina is a blue-green algae that is particularly rich in protein, carotenoids, vitamins, minerals, and essential fatty acids. In addition to its excellent nutritional profile, test tube and animal studies of spirulina have demonstrated antioxidant, anticancer, and immune-enhancing effects. Although human studies have been limited and generally have been of lower quality, they do indicate some possible applications. For example, one study found that spirulina reversed precancerous lesions of the mouth (leukoplakia) in 45 percent of the group given 1 g per day for one year, compared with only 7 percent of the group receiving placebo. Another small study found that overweight individuals taking 8.4 g per day of spirulina lost an average of 3 pounds in four weeks, compared with 1.5 pounds when taking placebo.

Available Forms

Spirulina is available as a powder or in flakes as well as in capsules and tablets.

Cautions and Warnings

Be sure that the spirulina is certified to be free of heavy metals such as lead, mercury, and cadmium.

Possible Side Effects

Generally spirulina is not associated with any side effects, although there have been a few reports of allergylike reactions. Also, as spirulina and other algae can accumulate heavy metals such as lead, mercury, and cadmium, it is extremely important that manufacturers employ proper quality control steps to prevent such contamination.

Drug Interactions

None known.

Food and Nutrient Interactions

None known.

Usual Dosage

The typical recommended dosage range is 3,000 to 5,000 mg per day.

Overdosage

None known.

Special Populations

Pregnant/breast-feeding women

Because the effects of spirulina during pregnancy and lactation have not been sufficiently evaluated, and because there appear to be quality-control issues, it should not be used during these times unless directed to do so by a physician.

Children

Suitable for use in children at one-half the adult dosage.

Seniors

No special precautions are known.

Spleen Extracts

Used For

Low white blood cell count
Effectiveness: B   Safety: C

General Information

The spleen is a fist-sized, spongy, dark purple organ that lies in the upper left abdomen behind the lower ribs. Weighing about 7 ounces, the spleen is the largest mass of lymphatic tissue in the body. The spleen's functions include producing white blood cells, engulfing and destroying bacteria and cellular debris, and destroying worn-out red blood cells and platelets.

A series of case reports as early as the 1930s documented that orally administered beef (bovine) spleen extracts were able to raise white blood cell counts in individuals with extremely low counts, as well as being of some benefit in patients with malaria and typhoid fever. However, there do not appear to be any recent studies with these sorts of preparations. Most of the recent research with spleen extracts has focused on the use of injectable preparations (including porcine-derived spleen extract) or isolated proteins manufactured by the spleen, such as tuftsin and splenopentin. Although these preparations have been shown to enhance immune function, it is not known if the same benefits can be derived using commercially available oral preparations.

Available Forms

Spleen extracts derived from either bovine or porcine sources are available as nutritional supplements in capsules and tablets.

Cautions and Warnings

None known.

Possible Side Effects

None known.

Drug Interactions

None known.

Food and Nutrient Interactions

None known.

Usual Dosage

The recommended amount depends on the concentration, method of preparation, and quality of the extract. Follow the manufacturer's recommendation on the label.

Overdosage

None known.

Special Populations

Pregnant/breast-feeding women
Considered safe during pregnancy and lactation.

Children
Suitable for children at one-half the adult dosage.

Seniors
No special precautions are known.

Sulforaphane

Used For

Cancer prevention
Effectiveness: B   Safety: C

General Information

Sulforaphane was identified in broccoli sprouts by scientists at the Johns Hopkins University School of Medicine in Baltimore, Maryland. These researchers were investigating the anticancer compounds present in broccoli when they discovered that broccoli sprouts contain anywhere from thirty to fifty times the concentration of protective chemicals in mature broccoli plants. Sulforaphane is one of a class of chemicals called isothiocyanates. Sulforaphane and other isothiocyanates are antioxidants and potent stimulators of natural detoxifying enzymes in the body. These compounds are believed to be responsible for the lowered risk of cancer that is associated

with the consumption of broccoli and other cruciferous vegetables such as cauliflower, cabbage, and
kale.

Feeding sulforaphane-rich broccoli sprout extracts to laboratory rats exposed to a carcinogen
dramatically reduced the frequency, size, and number of tumors in the animals. Human studies with
sulforaphane and other cruciferous-vegetable components have shown that these compounds stimulate the body's production of detoxification enzymes
and exert antioxidant effects.

Preliminary studies suggest that in order to cut
the risk of cancer in half, the average person would
need to eat about two pounds of broccoli or other
cruciferous vegetables per week. Because the concentration of sulforaphane is much higher in broccoli sprouts than in mature broccoli, the same
reduction in risk theoretically might be had with a
weekly intake of just over an ounce of sprouts.

Available Forms

Sulforaphane is available from broccoli sprout extracts in capsules or tablets.

Cautions and Warnings

None known.

Possible Side Effects

None known.

Drug Interactions

There are no known drug interactions at recommended dosages. Theoretically, sulforaphane may

influence the way in which drugs are detoxified in the liver.

Food and Nutrient Interactions

None known.

Usual Dosage

The usual recommendation by manufacturers is 200 to 400 mcg of sulforaphane daily from broccoli sprout extracts.

Overdosage

None known.

Special Populations

Pregnant/breast-feeding women
As the effects of sulforaphane supplementation during pregnancy and lactation have not been sufficiently evaluated, it should not be used during these times.

Children
Can be used by children over the age of two years even at the full adult dosage.

Seniors
No special precautions are known.

Synephrine
(*see* Bitter Orange)

General Information

Synephrine is a compound in bitter orange that appears to have some of the same effects as ephedrine (see **ephedra**). However, since synephrine does not cross the blood-brain barrier, it does not produce the stimulatory effects of ephedrine. Synephrine is marketed as a replacement for ephedrine in thermogenic formulas (see **ephedrine-caffeine combinations**), but it is not known if synephrine produces the same sort of weight-loss effects as ephedrine.

Taurine

Used For

Congestive heart failure
Effectiveness: B   Safety: C

Epilepsy
Effectiveness: B   Safety: C

High blood pressure
Effectiveness: B   Safety: C

General Information

Taurine is an amino acid (one of the building blocks of protein) that regulates heartbeat, maintains cell membrane stability, and helps prevent brain cell overactivity. It has been shown in small double-blind studies to be effective in improving heart function in congestive heart failure, lowering blood pressure, and reducing seizures in people whose epilepsy is poorly controlled with antiseizure drugs. Larger studies are required to better assess the therapeutic potential of taurine.

Available Forms

Taurine is available in capsules, powder, and tablets.

Cautions and Warnings

None known.

Possible Side Effects

No significant side effects have been reported.

Drug Interactions

None known.

Food and Nutrient Interactions

None known.

Usual Dosage

The typical dosage is 2 g taken three times per day, for a total of 6 g per day.

Overdosage

None known.

Special Populations

Pregnant/breast-feeding women
As the effects of taurine supplementation during pregnancy and lactation have not been sufficiently evaluated, it should not be used during these times.

Children
Suitable for use in children at one-half the adult dosage.

Seniors
No special precautions are known.

Thymus Extracts

Used For

Allergies
Effectiveness: B   Safety: B

Cancer (prevention of side effects from radiation or chemotherapy)
Effectiveness: B   Safety: B

Enhancing immune function
Effectiveness: B+   Safety: B

Hepatitis
Effectiveness: B+   Safety: B

HIV infection
Effectiveness: B   Safety: B

General Information

The thymus is one of the major glands of our immune system. It is composed of two soft pinkish-gray lobes lying just below the thyroid gland and above the heart. To a large extent, the health of the thymus determines the health of the immune system. The thymus is responsible for many immune system functions, including the production of T lymphocytes, a type of white blood cell responsible for cell-mediated immunity—immune mechanisms not controlled or mediated by antibodies. Cell-mediated immunity is extremely important in resistance to infection by certain bacteria, yeast (including *Candida albicans*), fungi, parasites, and viruses (including herpes simplex, Epstein-Barr, and viruses that cause hepatitis). Cell-mediated immunity is also critical in protecting against the development of cancer, autoimmune disorders such as rheumatoid arthritis, and allergies. The thymus gland also releases several hormones, such as thymosin, thymopoietin, and serum thymic factor, that regulate many immune functions.

Allergies

The oral administration of Thymomodulin (a brand of calf thymus extract) has been shown in preliminary and double-blind clinical studies to improve the symptoms and course of hay fever, allergic rhinitis, asthma, eczema, and food allergies (in conjunction with an allergy elimination diet). Presumably this clinical improvement is the result of restoration of proper control over immune function.

Cancer

Thymomodulin (given orally or by injection) has been used in cancer patients to counteract the decline in white blood cell levels and activity that can result from chemotherapy or radiation. In test tube studies, Thymomodulin and other thymus extracts have been shown to exert a number of effects on white blood cells (increasing the production of white blood cells as well as increasing the cells' functional activity). However, it is not known if this effect can be achieved with use of oral thymus extracts.

Enhancing immune function

The ability of Thymomodulin to improve immune function and reduce the number of recurrent infections has been shown in double-blind studies of children and adults with a history of recurrent respiratory tract infections. Thymomodulin has also been shown in a double-blind study to improve immune function in cases of exercise-induced immune suppression, and in preliminary studies to improve immune function in diabetics and in elderly individuals. Extreme exercise, diabetes, and aging all are associated with suppression of immune function.

Hepatitis

Preliminary studies in patients with acute or chronic hepatitis suggest that supplementation with Thymomodulin may be helpful; however, additional studies are needed to confirm these preliminary findings.

HIV infection

In a preliminary study in patients with early-stage HIV infection, Thymomodulin improved several immune parameters, including an increase in the number of helper T cells, one of the goals in the treatment of HIV infection.

Available Forms

Thymus extracts used as nutritional supplements are most often derived from bovine sources (young calves). Thymomodulin is the brand name of a calf thymus extract specially prepared to concentrate small proteinlike molecules (polypeptides). It is the only scientifically studied orally administered thymus extract.

Thymus extracts are available in capsules and tablets. Those concentrated for polypeptides may offer the greatest benefits.

Cautions and Warnings

None known.

Possible Side Effects

None known.

Drug Interactions

None known.

Food and Nutrient Interactions

None known.

Usual Dosage

The recommended amount of thymus extract varies according to the type of preparation. Based on the clinical research with Thymomodulin, the daily amount should be equivalent to 120 mg pure polypeptides with molecular weights less than

10,000, or roughly 750 mg of the crude polypeptide fraction.

Overdosage

None known.

Special Populations

Pregnant/breast-feeding women
Considered safe during pregnancy and lactation.

Children
Suitable for children at one-half the adult dosage.

Seniors
No special precautions are known.

Thyroid Extracts

Used For

Hypothyroidism
Effectiveness: D   Safety: C

General Information

The hormones of the thyroid gland regulate metabolism in every cell of the body. The medical treatment of low thyroid hormone levels in the body (hypothyroidism) involves the use of either desiccated thyroid from animals or synthetic thyroid hormone. The difference between prescription desiccated thyroid and the thyroid extracts sold as nutritional supplements is that the latter are required by the FDA to be free of active thyroid hormones. The use of hormone-free thyroid preparations has not been evaluated in scientific studies, but it may provide some nutritional support to the thyroid gland or contain trace levels of other active hormones to provide gentle support for thyroid function.

Available Forms

Thyroid extracts (from bovine and porcine sources) are available as nutritional supplements in capsules and tablets.

Cautions and Warnings

None known.

Possible Side Effects

None known.

Drug Interactions

None known.

Food and Nutrient Interactions

None known.

Usual Dosage

The recommended intake is dependent upon the concentration, method of preparation, and quality of the thyroid extract. Follow the manufacturer's recommendation on the label.

Overdosage

None known.

Special Populations

Pregnant/breast-feeding women
Considered safe during pregnancy and lactation.

Children
Suitable for children at one-half the adult dosage.

Seniors
No special precautions are known.

Tocotrienols

Used For

Antioxidant
Effectiveness: A   Safety: A

Elevated cholesterol levels
Effectiveness: B+   Safety: A

Heart disease (atherosclerosis) prevention
Effectiveness: B   Safety: A

General Information

Tocotrienols are members of the vitamin E family. Like vitamin E, tocotrienols are antioxidants that protect against lipid peroxidation (the damaging of fats by oxidation). Human studies indicate that, in addition to their antioxidant function, tocotrienols have other important functions, especially in maintaining a healthy cardiovascular system. Test tube and animal studies indicate a possible role for tocotrienols in protection against cancer (particularly breast and skin cancer); however, these results need confirmation in human studies.

Elevated cholesterol levels

Although tocotrienols inhibited cholesterol synthesis in test tube studies, human studies have produced contradictory results. In one double-blind study, supplementation with 200 mg of gamma-tocotrienol reduced total cholesterol levels by 13 percent in four weeks, while there was no change in the group receiving the placebo. And, in another double-blind study, 200 mg of tocotrienols produced a 15 percent drop in total cholesterol and an 8 percent reduction in LDL levels, while there were no changes in these levels in the placebo group (P < 0.05). However, other studies have shown that tocotrienols failed to produce changes in total cholesterol, LDL cholesterol, or HDL cholesterol levels after four weeks of supplementation.

Heart disease (atherosclerosis) prevention

Like vitamin E, tocotrienols may offer protection against atherosclerosis (hardening of the arteries) by preventing oxidative damage to LDL cholesterol. (Oxidation of LDL cholesterol is believed to be one of the triggering factors for atherosclerosis.) In a

double-blind study in patients with severe atherosclerosis of the carotid artery—the main artery supplying blood to the head—tocotrienol administration
(200 mg/day) reduced the level of lipid peroxides in
the blood. Moreover, in seven of twenty-five patients receiving tocotrienols for twelve months, the
size of the atherosclerotic plaques became smaller;
in contrast, none of the twenty-five patients receiving the placebo showed an improvement in their
atherosclerosis.

Available Forms

Tocotrienols are found primarily in the oil of rice bran,
palm fruit, barley, and wheat germ. Supplemental
sources of tocotrienols are derived from rice bran oil
and palm oil distillates. Tocotrienol supplements are
available in capsules and tablets.

Cautions and Warnings

None known.

Possible Side Effects

None known.

Drug Interactions

In test tube studies tocotrienols were shown to enhance the anticancer effects of tamoxifen—an estro-
gen-receptor-blocking drug used in breast cancer
—via a mechanism that did not involve binding to estrogen receptors. It is not known whether this effect
occurs in humans. Individuals taking tamoxifen
should consult a doctor before using tocotrienols.

Food and Nutrient Interactions

Tocotrienols work very closely with vitamin E in the human body.

Usual Dosage

The typical recommendation is 140 to 360 mg daily. Most studies have used 200 mg daily.

Overdosage

None known.

Special Populations

Pregnant/breast-feeding women
Considered safe during pregnancy and lactation.

Children
Suitable for children at one-half the adult dosage.

Seniors
No special precautions are known.

Tyrosine

Used For

Depression
Effectiveness: B   Safety: C

Fatigue
Effectiveness: B   Safety: C

General Information

Tyrosine is an amino acid (a building block of protein) that is important to the structure of almost all
proteins in the body and is also converted into several neurotransmitters, including L-dopa, dopamine,
norepinephrine, and epinephrine. Tyrosine, through
its effect on neurotransmitters, may affect several
health conditions, including depression and fatigue.

Depression
   Low brain levels of dopamine, norepinephrine,
and epinephrine may contribute to depression.
Several double-blind studies have shown that tyrosine supplementation can help some people with
depression. At a dosage of 100 mg per kg (2.2
pounds) body weight, one double-blind study found
that tyrosine demonstrated a response rate (60–70
percent) typical of most major antidepressants, but
without the side effects.

Fatigue
   L-tyrosine supplementation may help in improving energy levels and is being investigated by the
U.S. military for that purpose. Study results indicate
that tyrosine supplementation is associated with a
significant drop in fatigue-related memory impairment and loss of hand-eye coordination. It also was
associated with a reduction in feelings of sleepiness
and intensity of other fatigue-related symptoms.
Unlike conventional stimulants, L-tyrosine exerted
absolutely no inhibition of sleep, elevation in blood
pressure and pulse, or other negative effects.

Available Forms

Tyrosine is available in capsules, tablets, and powder.

Cautions and Warnings

None known.

Possible Side Effects

None known.

Drug Interactions

None known.

Food and Nutrient Interactions

Tyrosine competes with other amino acids for absorption into the brain. For best results, take it on an empty stomach.

Usual Dosage

The dosage most often used in depression is 100 mg per kg (2.2 pounds) of body weight daily. For fatigue, the dosage is 75 mg per kg of body weight one to two times daily.

Overdosage

None known.

Special Populations

Pregnant/breast-feeding women
As the effects of tyrosine supplementation during pregnancy and lactation have not been sufficiently evaluated, it should not be used during these times.

Children
Suitable for children at one-half the adult dosage.

Seniors
No special precautions are known.

Whey Protein

Used For

Protein source
Effectiveness: A   Safety: A

General Information

Whey is a natural byproduct of the cheesemaking process. Cow's milk has about 6.25 percent protein. Of that protein, 80 percent is casein (another type of protein) and the remaining 20 percent is whey. Cheesemaking uses the casein molecules leaving whey. Whey protein is made via filtering off the other components of whey such as lactose, fats, and minerals.

Whey protein is a complete protein in that it contains all essential and nonessential amino acids and has the highest biological value of all proteins.

Biological value (BV) is used to rate protein based on how much of the protein consumed is actually absorbed, retained, and used in the body. One of the key reasons why the BV of whey protein is so high is that it has the highest concentrations of **glutamine** and branched chain amino acids (BCAAs) found in nature. Glutamine and branched chain amino acids are critical to cellular health, muscle growth, and protein synthesis.

Although the most popular use of whey protein is by body builders and athletes, whey protein can also be used to support recovery from surgery, to prevent the "wasting syndrome" of **AIDS**, and to off-set some of the negative effects of radiation therapy and chemotherapy.

Available Forms

You can find whey protein powder in a variety of flavors including vanilla, chocolate, and strawberry available in premeasured individual serving packets and bulk canisters. Protein powders are usually found in the "body building" section of a health food store. The highest quality is referred to as microfiltered, ion-exchanged whey protein.

Cautions and Warnings

Long-term, excessive protein intake may be associated with deteriorating kidney function and possibly osteoporosis.

Possible Side Effects

People who are allergic to milk and other dairy products could react to whey protein and should therefore avoid it.

Drug Interactions

None known.

Food Interactions

None known.

Usual Dosage

The typical recommendation to boost protein levels is 25 to 50 g daily. For prevention of the wasting syndrome of AIDS and the side effects of chemotherapy the dosage is generally up to 1 g per two pounds of body weight.

Overdosage

None known.

Special Populations

Pregnant/breast-feeding women

Whey protein is generally regarded as safe during pregnancy and lactation.

Children

For children under six years of age, the dosage should be no more than 1 g per four pounds of body weight. For children over the age of six years the dosage can be up to 1 g per two pounds of body weight.

Seniors

No special precautions are known.

Wobenzyme N
(see Pancreatin)

PART IV
Herbal Products

This section discusses not only crude herb preparations but also compounds composed of or derived from herbs and other medicinal plants. Herbal products are a major business in the United States, with estimated annual sales of $3 billion for 2000.

Commercial herbal preparations are available in several different forms: bulk herbs, tea bags, tinctures, fluid extracts, and tablets or capsules. It is important to understand the differences between these forms, as well as methods of expressing strengths of herbal products.

One of the major developments in the herb industry involves improvements in extraction and concentration processes. An extract is defined as a concentrated form of the herb obtained by mixing the crude herb with an appropriate solvent (such as alcohol and/or water).

When an herbal tea bag is steeped in hot water, it is actually a type of herbal extract known as an infusion. The water is serving as a solvent in removing some of the medicinal properties from the herb. If the herbal material is boiled in the water, the resulting tea is called a decoction. Most often, infusions are made with leaves and flowers, while decoctions are made from roots. Teas often are better sources of bioavailable compounds than the powdered herb, but they are relatively weak in action compared to tinctures, fluid extracts, and solid extracts. These forms are commonly used by herbal practitioners for medicinal effects.

Tinctures are typically made using an alcohol and

water mixture as the solvent. The herb is soaked in the solvent for a specified amount of time, depending on the herb. This soaking is usually from several hours to days; however, some herbs may be soaked for much longer periods of time. The solution is then pressed out, yielding the tincture.

Fluid extracts are more concentrated than tinctures. Although they are most often made from hydroalcoholic mixtures, other solvents may be used (vinegar, glycerine, propylene glycol, etc.). Commercial fluid extracts usually are made by distilling off some of the alcohol, typically by using methods that do not require elevated temperatures, such as vacuum distillation and countercurrent filtration.

A solid extract is produced by further concentration of the extract by the mechanisms described above, as well as by other techniques, such as thin-layer evaporation. The solvent is completely removed, leaving a viscous extract (soft solid extract) or a dry solid extract, depending upon the plant, portion of the plant, or solvent used or if a drying process was used. The dry solid extract, if not already in powdered form, can be ground into coarse granules or a fine powder. A solid extract also can be diluted with alcohol and water to form a fluid extract or tincture.

Strengths of Extracts

The potencies or strengths of herbal extracts are generally expressed in two ways. If they contain known active principles, their strengths are commonly expressed in terms of the content of these active principles. Otherwise, the strength is expressed in terms of their concentration. For example, tinctures are typically made at a 1:5 concentration. This means one part of the herb (in grams) is soaked in five parts liquid (in milliliters). This means that there is five times the amount of solvent (alcohol/water) in a tincture as there is herbal material.

A 4:1 concentration means that one part of the extract is equivalent to, or derived from, four parts of the crude herb. This is the typical concentration of a solid extract—1 g of a 4:1 extract is concentrated from 4 g of crude herb. However, some solid extracts are concentrated as high as 100:1.

Since a tincture is typically a 1:10 or 1:5 concentration, while a fluid extract is usually 1:1, a 4:1 solid extract is typically at least four times as potent when compared to an equal amount of fluid extract and as much as forty times as potent as a tincture if they are produced from the same quality of herb. Thus, 1 g of a 4:1 solid extract is equivalent to 4 ml of a fluid extract (⅛th of a fluid ounce) and 40 ml of a tincture (almost 1½ fluid ounces).

Quality Control and Herbal Products

In the past, the quality of the extract produced often was difficult to determine, as many of the active principles of the herbs were unknown. However, recent advances in extraction processes, coupled with improved analytical methods, have reduced this problem of quality control. The concentration method of expressing the strength of an extract does not accurately measure potency, since there may be great variation among manufacturing techniques and raw materials. By using a high-quality herb (an herb high in active compounds), it is possible to have a dried herb, tincture, or fluid extract that is more potent than a solid extract that was made from a lower-quality herb. Standardization is the solution to this problem.

Standardized herbal preparations are products

guaranteed to contain a certain level of active compounds or key biological markers. Stating the content of active compounds rather than the concentration ratio allows for more accurate dosages, thereby providing a more consistent clinical response. Standardization is possible only when research has identified the components responsible for the desired therapeutic effect.

Drug-Herb Interactions

One area of growing concern for pharmacists, physicians, and, of course, consumers is drug-herb interactions. The mechanisms responsible for these interactions are discussed in each entry. It is important to point out once again that if you are taking any prescription drug, it is essential to talk to your doctor about the use of any herbal product, to avoid any drug-herb interaction.

Alfalfa *(Medicago sativa)*

Used For

Arthritis
Effectiveness: D   Safety: A

Asthma
Effectiveness: D   Safety: A

Gastrointestinal tonic
Effectiveness: C   Safety: A

High cholesterol
Effectiveness: C   Safety: A

Menopause
Effectiveness: C   Safety: A

General Information

Alfalfa is a member of the pea family that is cultivated worldwide primarily as feed for livestock.
Alfalfa sprouts have become a popular food and are
rich in many nutrients, especially vitamins C, E, and
K, carotenes, trace minerals, and protein. Alfalfa
supplements are usually made from the dried leaves
of the plant.

As a good source of chlorophyll and fiber, alfalfa
supplements are often recommended as tonics for
the gastrointestinal tract. This modern use follows
quite closely alfalfa's historical use. Early Chinese
physicians used young alfalfa leaves to treat disorders of the digestive tract. In India, physicians prescribed the leaves and flowering tops for poor
digestion. And in the United States, physicians in

the late 1800s and early 1900s used alfalfa preparations as a tonic for indigestion.

The ability of alfalfa to lower blood cholesterol levels has been demonstrated in animal studies. This beneficial effect is due to the fiber and steroid-like components known as saponins binding to cholesterol and bile acids in the intestinal tract and promoting their excretion. Although these effects have not been studied in humans, similar fiber supplements have been shown to lower blood cholesterol levels in human clinical trials.

Since alfalfa is a very rich source of phytoestrogens, it is becoming an increasingly popular recommendation for menopausal complaints, but there are no human clinical studies to rely on to gauge effectiveness. There are, however, studies with other phytoestrogen sources (see **red clover**).

Available Forms

Dried alfalfa and alfalfa extracts are available in tablets, capsules, liquid extracts, and powders.

Cautions and Warnings

Alfalfa should not be used in patients taking warfarin (Coumadin) (see "Drug Interactions"). Persons with systemic lupus erythematosus (SLE) or a history of SLE should avoid alfalfa seeds and sprouts (see "Possible Side Effects").

Possible Side Effects

Alfalfa is categorized as Generally Regarded as Safe by the FDA. There have been a few case reports of persons having allergic reactions to alfalfa, and some people may experience diarrhea or stomach upset when taking alfalfa supplements.

It should be noted that in studies in monkeys, ingestion of large amounts of the seed and/or sprouts caused the development of systemic lupus erythematosus (SLE), a serious autoimmune illness that is characterized by inflamed joints and potential kidney damage. Experts believe that canavanine, a toxic derivative of the amino acid arginine, was responsible for this reaction. There have been a few human reports of an association with alfalfa seed consumption. Although these reports involved the ingestion of the seeds or sprouts, persons with SLE or with a history of SLE should avoid the use of alfalfa products.

Drug Interactions

Alfalfa sprouts interact with warfarin (Coumadin), a drug that is often given to patients with a history of heart attacks, transient ischemic attacks (ministrokes), and strokes because it blocks blood clotting. Warfarin works by interfering with the actions of vitamin K. Since alfalfa can be a good source of vitamin K, it is important for people taking warfarin to avoid vitamin K supplementation, including multivitamins containing vitamin K, as well as alfalfa and other green leafy vegetables such as kale and parsley.

Food and Nutrient Interactions

None known.

Usual Dosage

No therapeutic dose of alfalfa has been established for humans. Some experts recommend the equivalent of 500–1,000 mg of the dried leaf per day.

Overdosage

No overdosage has been reported.

Special Populations

Pregnant/breast-feeding women
Considered safe during pregnancy and lactation.

Children
Suitable for children at one-half the adult dosage.

Seniors
No special precautions are known.

Aloe Vera Gel

Used For

Asthma
Effectiveness: B   Safety: C

Diabetes
Effectiveness: B   Safety: C

Low immunity, immune support, and HIV infection
Effectiveness: B   Safety: C

Peptic ulcers
Effectiveness: B   Safety: C

General Information

Aloe vera is a well-known perennial plant with yellow flowers and tough, fleshy spearlike leaves arising in a rosette configuration. The leaves are up to 20 inches long and 5 inches across at the base, tapering to a point. The outer margin of the leaves are characterized by sawlike teeth. There may be as many as 30 leaves per plant.

The leaf is composed of three distinct layers: an outer layer of tough tissue, a corrugated lining just beneath the outer layer, and the inner layer (the major portion of the leaf), consisting of a semisolid, gelatinous transparent gel. The bitter latex of the corrugated layer protects the plants from predators. Should an animal bite the leaf, the sap causes irritation. The dried **aloe latex** (sap) derived from the corrugated layer is the source of the plant's laxative properties. The gel is the portion of the aloe plant referred to in this profile.

Aloe products, for both internal and external use, are widely used in the United States. Despite this widespread acceptance, there are very few controlled studies on *Aloe vera*. The use of aloe orally (other than for the well-accepted laxative effect of the latex) has not been fully studied. Preliminary and anecdotal studies indicate that when taken internally, *Aloe vera* products may be helpful in asthma, diabetes, immune system enhancement and HIV infection, and healing peptic ulcers.

Asthma

In one study the oral administration of an extract of *Aloe vera* gel for six months was shown to produce good results in the treatment of asthma in some individuals. However, the *Aloe vera* extract was not effective at all in patients with more severe asthma who were dependent upon corticosteroids (e.g., prednisone).

Diabetes

Aloe vera gel preparations have produced blood-sugar-lowering effects in animal and human experiments. In addition to being potentially effective on its own, aloe gel preparations have been shown to enhance the blood-sugar-lowering effects of the drug glyburide (Diabeta, Micronase). Individuals with diabetes who ingest aloe gel preparations will need to monitor their blood sugar levels and notify their physician of any significant changes, as insulin or drug dosages may need to be adjusted.

Low immunity, immune support, and HIV infection

A key polysaccharide component of *Aloe vera* gel, acemannan, has demonstrated significant immune-enhancing and antiviral activity in experimental studies. In fact, acemannan in injectable form is approved for veterinary use in fibrosarcomas (a type of cancer) and feline leukemia. Its action in feline leukemia is quite impressive. Feline leukemia is caused by a virus that is similar to human immunodeficiency virus (HIV), which causes AIDS. The feline leukemia virus is so lethal that once cats develop clinical symptoms they are usually put to sleep to avoid unnecessary suffering. However, acemannan therapy has been shown to be effective in roughly 70 percent of cases.

Preliminary studies indicate acemannan may be useful as a support to current conventional HIV and AIDS therapy in minimally affected HIV-infected individuals (i.e., those who have a T4 cell count greater than $150/mm^3$ and a p24 core antigen level of less than 300). Unfortunately, acemannan does not appear to be helpful at all in more advanced stages of HIV infection, based on the results of a comprehensive study that assessed the safety and efficacy of acemannan in sixty-three patients with advanced

HIV disease receiving zidovudine (AZT) or didanosine (ddI).

Peptic ulcers

The use of *Aloe vera* gel internally to treat peptic ulcers was first studied in 1963. Unfortunately, there has been little research since. In the 1963 study, twelve patients with X-ray-confirmed duodenal ulcers were given 1 tablespoon of an emulsion of *Aloe vera* gel in mineral oil once daily. At the end of one year, all patients demonstrated complete recovery and no recurrence. Based on experimental evidence, the healing effect was thought to be due to *Aloe vera* gel inhibiting the release of hydrochloric acid, as well as acting as an extremely good demulcent, which both heals and prevents irritants from reaching the sensitive ulcer.

Available Forms

Aloe vera is available as a gel, a concentrate, a juice, acemannan, a latex, and a powder.

Aloe vera *gel:* Naturally occurring, undiluted tissue obtained from the leaves of *Aloe vera.* The inner cells of the leaf produce a slightly viscous, clear gel or mucilage that is separated from the outer cells with care to avoid the laxative-containing latex. Aloe gel is 96 percent water with various polysaccharides (complex sugars), enzymes, minerals, and amino acids in solution. When frozen it becomes a red, gelatinous substance.

Aloe vera *concentrate: Aloe vera* gel from which the water has been removed.

Aloe vera *juice:* An ingestible product containing a minimum of 50 percent *Aloe vera* gel mixed with water.

Acemannan: A water-soluble, long-chain polysac-charide component of *Aloe vera.*

Aloe vera *latex:* A bitter yellow latex from the outer cells of the leaf that is dried to give a yellow to dark brown solid material (called aloes in many older pharmacy texts). This material is a strong laxative containing various anthraquinone com-pounds usually designated as aloin (see **Aloe Latex, Whole Leaf, and Aloin**).

Aloe vera *leaf powder:* Dried *Aloe vera* powder from the entire leaf. Contains dried gel and latex, in-cluding aloin.

Cautions and Warnings

As detailed information is currently lacking on *Aloe vera* preparations, it is recommended to follow the manufacturer's dosage recommendations.

Possible Side Effects

Preparations containing *Aloe vera* gel are generally well tolerated, with no known side effects.

Drug Interactions

Preparations containing *Aloe vera* gel may increase the effectiveness of drugs that lower blood sugar levels in the treatment of non-insulin-dependent di-abetes (type 2 diabetes) such as glyburide (Diabeta, Micronase). If taking this type of drug, please inform the prescribing physician that you are taking *Aloe vera* gel.

Food and Nutrient Interactions

None known.

Usual Dosage

Aloe vera *gel:* Typical dosage is 1 tablespoon twice daily.

Aloe vera *concentrates:* Typical dosage is the equivalent of 5 g of the gel one to three times daily.

Aloe vera *juice:* As detailed information is currently lacking as to the optimal dose of *Aloe vera* juice, it is recommended that no more than 1 quart be consumed in any one day.

Acemannan: Typical dosage is 800–1,600 mg per day.

Overdosage

There have been no reports of overdosage with preparations containing *Aloe vera* gel or juice.

Special Populations

Pregnant/breast-feeding women

Since the safety of *Aloe vera* preparations during pregnancy and lactation has not been fully determined, their use is not recommended during these times.

Children

Aloe vera gel preparations are suitable for children at one-half the adult dosage.

Seniors

No special precautions are known.

Aloe Latex, Whole Leaf, and Aloin

Used For

Constipation
Effectiveness: A   Safety: D

General Information

The outer cells of the leaf of **Aloe vera** produce a bitter yellow latex that contains aloin, the laxative component of the plant. Although an effective laxative, aloin-containing preparations produce more irritation and cramping than other stimulant laxatives. The use of aloin and aloe latex preparations as a laxative has been largely replaced by less irritating agents such as senna and cascara.

Cautions and Warnings

Preparations containing aloin should not be used during pregnancy or lactation. Nor should they be used in people experiencing unexplained abdominal pain, intestinal obstruction, or inflammatory conditions of the intestines (such as Crohn's disease and ulcerative colitis). *Aloe vera* latex preparations should not be used in children less than twelve years of age and should not be used for more than ten days.

Possible Side Effects

Preparations containing aloin can produce excessive bowel activity (griping, bloody diarrhea, nau-

sea), and in very high doses possible kidney damage and potassium loss. Use of these preparations
for long periods of time (e.g., nine to twelve months)
may produce pseudomelanosis coli, a condition in
which the lining of the colon turns black. This condition is generally reversible within four to fifteen
months after discontinuation of the laxative.

Drug Interactions

Preparations containing aloin should not be used in
conjunction with other laxative agents. Aloin and
other stimulant laxatives may decrease the absorption of other drugs that pass through the gastrointestinal tract. If you are currently taking an oral
medication, talk to your pharmacist or doctor before
self-medicating with aloin.

Aloin may potentiate the action of digoxin and
other heart medications due to potassium depletion.
The use of aloin with thiazide diuretics and corticosteroids may further decrease potassium levels.

Food and Nutrient Interactions

None known.

Usual Dosage

Dosage is based upon the level of aloin, 50 to 200
mg daily. For example, the dosage of an aloe product containing 25 percent aloin would be 200 to 800
mg daily.

Overdosage

Overdosage with preparations containing *Aloe vera*
latex can lead to severe diarrhea and electrolyte dis-

turbances. As little as 1,000 mg taken daily for several days can be fatal.

Special Populations

Pregnant/breast-feeding women
Preparations containing aloin should not be used during pregnancy, as aloin may stimulate uterine muscle activity and possibly cause uterine contractions. Preparations containing aloin should also be avoided during lactation, as they may be secreted in breast milk and produce a laxative effect in the nursing child.

Children
Aloin preparations should not be used in children under twelve years of age.

Seniors
No special precautions are known.

Andrographis paniculata

Used For

Common cold
Effectiveness: B+   Safety: C

General Information

Andrographis paniculata is a shrub native to India and China. Several double-blind studies using a standardized extract (Kan Jang) have shown that, taken daily at the onset of cold or flu, Kan Jang is effective at reducing headache pain, fever, nasal irritation, congestion, and fatigue associated with the common cold. Kan Jang was also shown to be protective against developing the common cold in another double-blind study. In this study, the relative risk of catching a cold was 33 percent lower for the Kan Jang group.

Available Forms

A standardized extract, Kan Jang, is available in tablets. Other forms of products containing *Andrographis paniculata* include liquid extracts, capsules, and tablets.

Cautions and Warnings

None known.

Possible Side Effects

None known.

Drug Interactions

None known.

Food and Nutrient Interactions

None known.

Usual Dosage

The usual dosage for Kan Jang is one tablet (300 mg) four times daily. Other forms should approximate this dosage.

Overdosage

None known.

Special Populations

Pregnant/breast-feeding women

As the effects of Kan Jang or other forms of *Andrographis paniculata* during pregnancy and lactation have not been sufficiently evaluated, it should not be used during these times.

Children

Suitable for children at one-half the adult dosage.

Seniors

No special precautions are known.

Artichoke *(Cynara scolymus)*

Used For

Digestive disturbances
Effectiveness: B   Safety: C

High cholesterol levels
Effectiveness: B   Safety: C

General Information

The modern use of artichoke as a medicine utilizes extracts of the leaves of the plant standardized for key components known as caffeoylquinic acids. Artichoke extract acts as a choleretic, a substance that increases the formation and flow of bile to and from the liver.

Bile is a thick, yellowish green fluid excreted from the liver, stored in the gallbladder, and released into the intestine to aid in the digestion and absorption of fats. Bile plays an important role in making the stool soft by promoting the incorporation of water into the stool. Without enough bile, the stool can become quite hard and difficult to pass. Bile also helps to keep the small intestine free from harmful microorganisms.

Digestive disorders

Decreased bile flow is a common cause of digestive disturbance, including the inability to absorb fat (fat malabsorption), excessive flatulence (gas), bloating after eating, and constipation or diarrhea. Artichoke extract has increased the flow of bile by 90 to 150 percent in human and animal experiments.

The improvement in bile flow can improve digestion in people with various digestive disorders. Studies in patients with abdominal pain, bloating, constipation, lack of appetite, and nausea have demonstrated that artichoke extract can produce improvements in 65 to 72 percent of patients after one week and 80 to 92 percent after six weeks.

High cholesterol levels

Artichoke extract has been shown to exert a dual effect on cholesterol metabolism: (1) it decreases the manufacture of cholesterol in the liver, and (2) it increases the conversion of cholesterol to bile acids. Artichoke extract has been shown to produce an 11.5 percent reduction in total blood cholesterol and a 12.5 percent reduction in triglyceride levels after six weeks of therapy.

Available Forms

Artichoke extract is available in capsules as the dried powdered extract. For greater reliability and proper dosage, look for products that note the level of caffeoylquinic acids on the label. Brand names available include Cynara-SL.

Cautions and Warnings

Should not be used by people who are allergic to artichokes or who have blockage of bile flow due to the presence of gallstones.

Possible Side Effects

Since artichoke extract can increase the output of bile, some people may experience looser stools and/or a transient increase in flatulence. Generally artichoke extracts are well tolerated, with no side effects reported. In a large safety study, only one out of a hundred subjects reported side effects, and these were mild (e.g., transient increase in flatulence).

Drug Interactions

None known.

Food and Nutrient Interactions

Increasing the intake of high-fiber foods may reduce the likelihood of experiencing loose stools or diarrhea when using artichoke extracts.

Usual Dosage

The usual dosage is based upon the level of caffeoylquinic acids. The typical dosage is 20 to 60 mg of caffeoylquinic acids three times daily with meals. For the extract standardized to contain 13–18 percent caffeoylquinic acids, the corresponding dosage is 160 to 320 mg three times daily with meals.

Overdosage

Overdosage may produce gastrointestinal discomfort, excessive flatulence, and loose stools.

Special Populations

Pregnant/breast-feeding women
Considered safe during pregnancy and lactation.

Children
Suitable for children at one-half the adult dosage.

Seniors
No special precautions are known.

Astragalus membranaceus

Used For

Common cold
Effectiveness: B   Safety: A

Low immunity and immune support
Effectiveness: B   Safety: C

General Information

Astragalus root *(Astragalus membranaceus)* is a traditional Chinese medicine used to treat viral infections including the common cold. Clinical studies in China have shown it to be effective when used as a preventive measure against the common cold. It has also been shown to reduce the duration and severity of symptoms in acute treatment of the common cold, as well as raise white blood cell counts in chronic leukopenia (a condition characterized by low white blood cell levels).

Research in animals indicates that astragalus works by stimulating several factors of the immune system. In particular, it appears to stimulate white blood cells to engulf and destroy invading organisms and cellular debris, and it also seems to enhance the production of interferon (a key natural compound produced by the body to fight viruses).

Astragalus appears particularly useful in cases where the immune system has been damaged by chemicals or radiation (e.g., in patients undergoing chemotherapy and/or radiation treatment).

Available Forms

Astragalus root is available in bulk as the dried root, in tea bags, as a tincture, as a fluid extract, and as the dry powdered root or extract in capsules and tablets.

Cautions and Warnings

Since astragalus can enhance immune function, it must not be used in people who have had organ transplants or who are taking drugs such as cyclophosphamide to purposely suppress the immune system.

Possible Side Effects

Astragalus has no known side effects at recommended levels.

Drug Interactions

Astragalus can interfere with drugs that are purposely used to suppress the immune system, such as cyclophosphamide, which is used in patients who have had organ transplants to prevent the body from rejecting the transplanted organ.

Food and Nutrient Interactions

None known.

Usual Dosage

Dried root (or as a decoction, or as a powder in capsules or tablets): 1–2 g three times daily
Tincture (1:5): 2–4 ml three times daily

Fluid extract (1:1): 1–2 ml three times daily
Solid extract (standardized to contain 0.5 percent
    4-hydroxy-3-methoxy/isoflavone): 100–150 mg
    three times daily

Overdosage

None known.

Special Populations

Pregnant/breast-feeding women

As the effects of astragalus during pregnancy and
lactation have not been sufficiently evaluated, it
should not be used during these times.

Children

Suitable for children at one-half the adult dosage.

Seniors

No special precautions are known.

Barberry *(Berberis vulgaris)*

General Information

The common barberry is a deciduous spiny shrub
native to Europe and Asia that has been naturalized
in eastern North America. The parts used are the
bark of the stem and of the root. Barberry shares
similar indications and effects with other **berberine-
containing plants** such as goldenseal and Oregon
grape root.

Berberine-Containing Plants

Used For

Antibiotic and immune enhancement
Effectiveness: B+   Safety: B

Infectious diarrhea
Effectiveness: B+   Safety: B

Psoriasis
Effectiveness: C   Safety: B

General Information

The medicinal value of goldenseal *(Hydrastis canadensis)*, barberry *(Berberis vulgaris)*, Oregon grape root *(Berberis aquifolium)*, and coptis *(Coptis chinensis)* (also called goldthread) is thought to be due to their high content of alkaloids, of which berberine has been the most widely studied. Berberine has demonstrated significant antibiotic and immune-enhancing effects in both experimental and clinical settings.

Antibiotic effect and immune enhancement

Berberine exhibits a broad spectrum of antibiotic activity. Berberine has shown antibiotic activity against bacteria, protozoa, and fungi. Berberine has also been shown to inhibit the adherence of bacteria to human cells, so that the bacteria cannot infect the cells. The primary immune-enhancing action of berberine is the activation of white blood cells known as macrophages. These cells are responsible for engulfing and destroying bacteria, viruses, tumor cells, and other particulate matter. Historically, berberine-containing plants, especially coptis, have been used to bring down fevers. Berberine has produced in rats an antipyretic effect three times as potent as that of aspirin. However, while aspirin suppresses fever through its action on prostaglandins, berberine appears to lower fever by enhancing the immune system's ability to handle fever-producing compounds (pyrogens) produced by microorganisms.

Infectious diarrhea

Berberine has shown significant success in the treatment of acute diarrhea in several clinical studies. It has been found effective against diarrheas caused by *Klebsiella, Escherichia coli* (traveler's diarrhea), *Shigella dysenteriae* (shigellosis), *Salmonella paratyphi* (food poisoning), *Giardia lamblia* (giardiasis), and even *Vibrio cholerae* (cholera). However, despite positive clinical results, the best approach may be to use berberine-containing plants along with standard antibiotic therapy, because of the serious consequences if infectious diarrhea is not treated effectively.

Psoriasis

Berberine-containing plants, particularly **Oregon grape root,** have a long history of use in psoriasis, both orally and topically.

Available Forms

Goldenseal root, barberry bark, Oregon grape root, and coptis (goldthread) are available in bulk, as capsules, and as tablets, as well as in tinctures, fluid extracts, and solid extracts. Extracts stating the concentration of alkaloids are preferred by most experts.

Cautions and Warnings

Do not use berberine-containing preparations during pregnancy or lactation.

Although most acute cases of diarrhea are self-limiting, if any of the following apply, a physician should be consulted immediately: diarrhea in a child under six years of age, severe or bloody diarrhea, diarrhea that lasts more than three days, or significant signs of dehydration (sunken eyes, severe dry mouth, strong body odor, etc.).

Possible Side Effects

Berberine-containing plants are generally without side effect when used at recommended dosages. However, higher amounts may lead to gastrointestinal distress and possible cardiovascular or nervous system effects.

Drug Interactions

Do not take berberine-containing plants with tetracycline antibiotics. One double-blind study found that giving 100 mg of berberine at the same time as 500 mg of tetracycline four times daily in people with cholera led to a reduction of the efficacy of tetracycline. Although this effect was not confirmed in another study, berberine-containing plants should not be taken simultaneously with tetracycline until more studies are completed to clarify this issue.

Food and Nutrient Interactions

None known.

Usual Dosage

The usual dosage depends upon the form. One of the following forms can be taken three times a day:

Dried root (or bark for barberry) or in an *infusion* (tea): 1,000 to 2,000 mg
Tincture (1:5): 4–8 ml (1–2 teaspoons)
Fluid extract (1:1): 2–4 ml (½ to 1 teaspoon)
Solid extract (4:1 or 8–12 percent alkaloid content): 250–500 mg

Overdosage

Overdosage is unlikely. But do the following in case of accidental overdose: If the victim is unconscious or having convulsions, call for an ambulance immediately. If you take the victim to an emergency room, be sure to bring the bottle or container with you. If the victim is conscious, call your local poison control center or a health care professional. The poison control center may suggest inducing vomiting with ipecac syrup (available without a prescription at any pharmacy). *Do not* induce vomiting unless specifically instructed to do so.

Special Populations

Pregnant/breast-feeding women
Berberine-containing plants are not recommended during pregnancy and lactation.

Children
Suitable for children over the age of two years at one-half the adult dosage.

Seniors
No special precautions are known.

Bilberry *(Vaccinium myrtillus)*

Used For

Capillary fragility and easy bruising
Effectiveness: A   Safety: A

Cataracts
Effectiveness: B+   Safety: A

Macular degeneration and other retinal disorders
Effectiveness: B+   Safety: A

Varicose veins
Effectiveness: B+   Safety: A

General Information

Bilberry, also known as European blueberry, is a shrubby perennial plant that grows in the woods and forest meadows of Europe. Bilberry differs from the American blueberry in that the meat of the fruit is also purple, while the American variety has a cream- or white-colored interior.

Bilberries have, of course, been used as food. Interest in the medicinal use of bilberry was first aroused when it was observed during World War II that British Royal Air Force pilots reported improved nighttime visual acuity on bombing raids after consuming bilberries. Subsequent studies showed that administration of bilberry extracts to healthy subjects resulted in improved nighttime visual acuity, quicker adjustment to darkness, and faster restoration of visual acuity after exposure to glare.

The most active compounds of bilberries are flavonoid compounds known as anthocyanidins. The concentration of anthocyanidins in the fresh fruit is approximately 0.1 to 0.25 percent, whereas concentrated extracts of bilberry yield an anthocyanidin content of 25 percent.

The anthocyanidins of bilberry extracts have been shown to be potent antioxidants. In addition, they improve the integrity and function of small blood vessels. Bilberry's benefit to the eyes presumably is through its ability to improve the delivery of oxygen and blood to that organ.

Capillary fragility and easy bruising

When capillaries (small blood vessels) become too "leaky," it leads to easy bruising and possibly signs of broken blood vessels. Bilberry extracts have been shown to produce a substantial drop in capillary leakage in human studies. Bilberry accomplishes this effect by stabilizing the membranes of capillaries via its antioxidant effect, along with increasing the integrity of the protective sheath of connective tissue surrounding the blood vessels.

Cataracts

Bilberry extracts may offer significant protection against the development of cataracts because of their antioxidant effects. In one human study, bilberry extract plus vitamin E stopped progression of cataract formation in forty-eight out of fifty patients with age-related cataracts.

Macular degeneration and other retinal disorders

Light passing through the lens of the eye is focused on the retina. The macula is the portion of the retina responsible for fine (central) vision. Degeneration of the macula and other parts of the retina (primarily due to diabetes) is a leading cause of severe vision loss. Bilberry extracts may offer significant protection against the development of macular and/or retinal degeneration because of their antioxidant effects. This use is supported by a few clinical studies showing benefits in patients with various types of retinal degeneration (twenty with diabetic retinopathy, five with retinitis pigmentosa, four with macular degeneration, and two with hemorrhagic retinopathy due to anticoagulant therapy).

Varicose veins

Bilberry extracts are helpful in varicose veins because of their ability to strengthen the vein wall and improve vein function. Clinical studies have shown that bilberry extracts reduce swelling, feelings of heaviness, paresthesia (pins-and-needles sensation), pain, and skin changes in patients with varicose veins.

Available Forms

Bilberry extracts are available in capsules and tablets. Products noting the concentrations of anthocyanidins are recommended to ensure proper dosage. *Note:* Because bilberry anthocyanidins are not stable in alcohol, alcohol-based fluid extracts may not offer the same benefits as dried bilberry extracts.

Brands available include MirtoSelect and Strix.

Cautions and Warnings

None known.

Possible Side Effects

No side effects for bilberry extracts have been reported.

Drug Interactions

Bilberry extract may counteract the capillary fragility, hemorrhagic tendencies, and easy bruising caused by warfarin (Coumadin)—a drug used to inhibit blood clot formation.

Food and Nutrient Interactions

None known.

Usual Dosage

The standard dose for bilberry extract is based on its anthocyanoside content, as calculated by its anthocyanidin percentage. The typical dosage is 20–40 mg of anthocyanidin three times daily. For bilberry extracts with a 25 percent anthocyanidin content, this translates to 80–160 mg three times daily.

Overdosage

Extensive toxicity tests in animals confirm that bilberry extracts have absolutely no toxic effects. Rats administered doses as high as 400 mg per kg (2.2 pounds) showed no apparent side effects, and excess levels were quickly excreted through the urine and bile.

Special Populations

Pregnant/breast-feeding women
Considered safe during pregnancy and lactation.

Children
Suitable for children at one-half the adult dosage.

Seniors
No special precautions are known.

Bitter Melon
(Momardica charantia)

Used For

Diabetes
Effectiveness: B+   Safety: B

General Information

Bitter melon, also known as balsam pear, is a tropical fruit widely cultivated in Asia, Africa, and South America. A green cucumber-shaped fruit covered with gourdlike bumps, bitter melon looks like an ugly cucumber. In addition to the unripe fruit being eaten as a vegetable, it has been used extensively in folk medicine as a remedy for diabetes. The fresh juice of the unripe fruit and an extract derived from that juice, as well as the dried fruit or seeds, have demonstrated blood-sugar-lowering effects. Several active compounds have been identified, including an insulinlike substance known as p-insulin (the *p* is for *plant).*

The blood-sugar-lowering action of the fresh juice or extract has been clearly established in human clinical trials as well as experimental models. In one study, blood sugar control was improved in 73 percent of type 2 diabetics given 2 fluid ounces of the juice. In another study, 15 g of the water-soluble extract of bitter melon produced a 54 percent decrease in after-meal blood sugar level after three weeks of use and a 17 percent reduction in glycosylated hemoglobin (an indicator of average blood sugar levels over time) after seven weeks of use.

Available Forms

Unripe bitter melon is available primarily at Asian grocery stores. An extract of unripe bitter melon is also available in capsules and tablets.

Cautions and Warnings

Blood sugar levels must be monitored carefully while taking bitter melon, particularly if you are on insulin or have poorly controlled diabetes. Home glucose monitoring and the glycosylated hemoglobin (HgB A1c) test are the best measures to monitor progress. It is important to recognize that bitter melon usage may require adjustments in dosages of insulin and other drugs. Under no circumstances should a person suddenly stop a medication for diabetes, especially insulin, without direct medical supervision.

Possible Side Effects

None known.

Drug Interactions

Bitter melon usage may require adjustment of dosages of insulin or other diabetes drugs.

Food and Nutrient Interactions

None known.

Usual Dosage

The usual dosage is 2 fluid ounces of the juice of unripe bitter melon once or twice daily. The dosage of other forms should approximate this dose. Most labels will provide equivalencies.

Overdosage

None known.

Special Populations

Pregnant/breast-feeding women
Considered safe during pregnancy and lactation.

Children
Suitable for children at one-half the adult dosage.

Seniors
No special precautions are known.

Bitter Orange
(Citrus aurantium)

Used For

Weight loss
Effectiveness: C   Safety: C

General Information

Bitter orange contains trace amounts of a substance known as **synephrine** as well as similar compounds such as octopamine. Some of the actions of synephrine appear to be similar to those of **ephedrine,** but since synephrine does not cross the blood-brain barrier, it does not produce the stimulatory effects of ephedrine. However, there have been no published clinical studies with bitter orange extract or synephrine for any application. Synephrine and bitter orange are marketed as replacements for ephedrine in thermogenic formulas (see **ephedrine-caffeine combinations**), but it is not known if synephrine produces the same sort of weight-loss effects as ephedrine.

Available Forms

Bitter orange peel extract and purified synephrine are available primarily in capsules and tablets.

Cautions and Warnings

None known.

Possible Side Effects

None known.

Drug Interactions

None known.

Food and Nutrient Interactions

None known.

Usual Dosage

The usual dosage for the extract of bitter orange standardized to contain 6 percent synephrine is 300 to 500 mg three times per day. This dosage translates to 18 to 30 mg of synephrine three times daily.

Overdosage

None known.

Special Populations

Pregnant/breast-feeding women

As the effects of bitter orange extract and synephrine during pregnancy and lactation have not been sufficiently evaluated, they should not be used during these times.

Children

There does not appear to be any appropriate use of bitter orange extract or synephrine in children.

Seniors
No special precautions are known.

Black Cohosh
(Cimicifuga racemosa)

Used For

Menopause
Effectiveness: A   Safety: A

General Information

Black cohosh is a perennial herb native to North America. It is used primarily in the treatment of menopausal symptoms. A special extract of black cohosh, **Remifemin,** has been shown in double-blind studies to produce better results than conjugated estrogens (i.e., Premarin) in relieving common menopausal symptoms such as hot flashes, vaginal atrophy, depression, and anxiety. For example, in one study, eighty patients were given either Remifemin (2 tablets twice daily, providing 4 mg 27-deoxyacteine daily), conjugated estrogens (0.625 mg daily), or placebo for twelve weeks. Remifemin produced better results for all menopausal symptoms. The number of hot flashes experienced each day dropped from an average of five to less than one in the Remifemin group. In comparison, the estrogen group dropped from five only to three and a half. Even more impressive was the effect of Remifemin on the vaginal lining. While conjugated estrogens as well as the placebo produced little effect, a dramatic increase in the number of superficial cells was noted in the Remifemin group.

The current data indicate that black cohosh (specifically, Remifemin) offers a suitable natural alternative to hormone replacement therapy for menopause, especially where hormone replacement therapy is contraindicated, such as in women with a history of estrogen-dependent cancer, unexplained uterine bleeding, liver or gallbladder disease, pancreatitis, endometriosis, uterine fibroids, or fibrocystic breast disease.

Black cohosh is thought to work as a result of complex actions of its key ingredients, triterpenes and flavone derivatives. These compounds act on a number of regulatory centers such as the hypothalamus and vasomotor centers. An estrogenic effect was noted in some early animal studies, but more recent studies with black cohosh extracts and Remifemin demonstrated no estrogenic activity. In studies with various types of breast cancer cells, Remifemin has shown no stimulatory effects, making it suitable for use in women with a history of breast cancer.

Available Forms

The rhizome is the portion of black cohosh used for medicinal purposes. The crude rhizome is available in bulk, capsules, and tablets; also available are tinctures, fluid extracts, and dry extract in tablets and capsules. Brand names available include Remifemin.

Cautions and Warnings

None known.

Possible Side Effects

No serious side effects have ever been reported. The most common mild side effects reported include headache and stomach irritation.

Drug Interactions

Remifemin was shown to potentiate tamoxifen's inhibitory effects on breast cancer development in an in vitro study.

Food and Nutrient Interactions

None known.

Usual Dosage

The dosage of black cohosh is usually based on its content of 27-deoxyactein, which serves as an important biochemical marker to indicate therapeutic effect. The dosage of the black cohosh extract used in the majority of clinical studies, Remifemin, provides 1 or 2 mg of 27-deoxyacteine twice daily. Here are the approximate dosage recommendations using other forms (nonstandardized) of black cohosh:

Powdered rhizome: 1 to 2 g
Tincture (1:5): 4–6 ml
Fluid extract (1:1): 3–4 ml (1 teaspoon)
Solid extract (4:1): 250–500 mg

Based on currently available data, black cohosh is appropriate for long-term, continued use.

Overdosage

Overdosage may cause dizziness, headache, or tremors due to lowered blood pressure.

Special Populations

Pregnant/breast-feeding women
As the effects of black cohosh during pregnancy and lactation have not been sufficiently evaluated, it should not be used during these times.

Children
There does not appear to be any appropriate use for black cohosh in children.

Seniors
No special precautions are known.

Boswellic Acids
(Boswellia serrata)

Used For

Asthma
Effectiveness: B+   Safety: B

Crohn's disease and ulcerative colitis
Effectiveness: A   Safety: B

Osteoarthritis
Effectiveness: B+   Safety: B

Rheumatoid arthritis
Effectiveness: B- Safety: B

General Information

Boswellia serrata is a large branching tree native to India. It yields an exudative gum resin known as salai guggul. Although salai guggul has been used for centuries, newer preparations concentrated for the active components (boswellic acids) are apparently giving better results.

Boswellic acid extracts have demonstrated anti-inflammatory and other beneficial effects in treating arthritis in a variety of animal models. However, there have not been many clinical trials. Uncontrolled case studies along with its historical use suggest possible benefits in osteoarthritis and rheumatoid arthritis as well as in asthma. Although a double-blind study failed to show any benefit in rheumatoid arthritis, positive results were found in a double-blind study in asthma, as 70 percent of patients showed significant improvement in asthma symptoms compared to only 27 percent of patients receiving the placebo. Double-blind studies have now confirmed the benefit of *Boswellia serrata* in the treatment of Crohn's disease and ulcerative colitis.

Available Forms

Salai guggul (the gum resin of *Boswellia serrata*) and alcohol extracts of gum resin are available usually in tablets or capsules. Preparations that state the level of boswellic acids are recommended to ensure proper dosage. Brand names available include Boswellin.

Cautions and Warnings

None known.

Possible Side Effects

No significant side effects have been reported.

Drug Interactions

None known.

Food and Nutrient Interactions

None known.

Usual Dosage

The dosage should be based upon the level of boswellic acids in the resin or extract. A dosage of 200–400 mg of boswellic acids two to three times daily is typical. Since the gum resin typically contains approximately 30 percent boswellic acids, the dosage of this form of *Boswellia serrata* would be 650 to 1,300 mg per day. Some extracts of the resin may contain up to 65 percent boswellic acids. Typically, these stronger preparations will list the boswellic acid content, making it easy to calculate how much is needed to reach the recommended dosage levels.

Overdosage

None known.

Special Populations

Pregnant/breast-feeding women
Considered safe during pregnancy and lactation.

Children
Suitable for children at one-half the adult dosage.

Seniors
No special precautions are known.

Bromelain (from Pineapple, *Ananas comosus*)

Used For

Antibiotic potentiation
Effectiveness: A   Safety: A

Arthritis
Effectiveness: B+   Safety: A

Cancer
Effectiveness: C   Safety: A

Digestive aid
Effectiveness: B+   Safety: A

Inflammation
Effectiveness: A   Safety: A

Painful menstruation (dysmenorrhea)
Effectiveness: B   Safety: A

Sports injuries
Effectiveness: B+   Safety: A

Recovery from surgery
Effectiveness: A   Safety: A

Respiratory tract infections
Effectiveness: A   Safety: A

Thrombophlebitis
Effectiveness: A   Safety: A

General Information

The term *bromelain* refers to a group of sulfur-containing proteolytic enzymes or proteases (enzymes that digest protein) obtained from the pineapple plant *(Ananas comosus).* Commercial bromelain is usually derived from the stem, which differs from the bromelain derived from the fruit. Commercial bromelain contains a mixture of several proteases, small amounts of several other enzymes, and organically bound calcium. Bromelain was introduced as a therapeutic agent in 1957, and since that time more than two hundred scientific papers on its therapeutic applications have appeared in the medical literature.

Bromelain is one of the most popular natural agents in use. Because of its ability to impact many aspects of inflammation, it is used predominantly in cases of injury, sprains, strains, arthritis, recovery from surgery, and other inflammatory conditions. However, it is also used as a digestive aid and in infections (particularly respiratory tract infections), thrombophlebitis, and dysmenorrhea, and as an adjunct in cancer therapy.

Bromelain's ability to reduce inflammation has been documented in a variety of experimental models and clinical studies. Bromelain is thought to work primarily by stimulating the production of plasmin, a compound that blocks the formation of pro-inflammatory compounds as well as breaks down fibrin—a substance that promotes swelling, inflammation, and scar formation. Via a separate mechanism, bromelain has also been shown to reduce the production of compounds known as kinins. These compounds cause much inflammation, swelling, and pain after traumatic injuries (such as sports injuries).

Antibiotic potentiation

According to the results from several studies, bromelain has been shown to increase levels of a variety of antibiotics (including amoxycillin, tetracycline, and penicillin) in many different body fluids and tissues (cerebrospinal fluid, sputum, mucus, blood, urine; uterus, vagina, ovary, gallbladder, appendix, skin). This effect makes bromelain a valuable supportive therapy whenever antibiotics are used. In these studies the researchers also concluded that bromelain itself possesses significant effects in helping fight infections. However, bromelain should not be used as a sole therapy for any infection unless under direct medical supervision.

Arthritis

Bromelain is useful in both rheumatoid arthritis and osteoarthritis. Its use in rheumatoid arthritis may allow a reduction in the dosage of prednisone (a corticosteroid often used in severe inflammatory diseases), a drug that carries with it significant side effects.

Cancer

Bromelain has shown anticancer effects in test tube and animal studies. Human research indicates that it may augment standard chemotherapy treatment. Unfortunately, the few studies that do exist are small and uncontrolled. For example, in one study conducted in France, twelve patients with ovarian or breast cancer fared significantly better with standard therapy plus bromelain use compared to standard therapy alone. Further studies are necessary in this application.

Digestive aid

Bromelain is a suitable alternative to **pancreatin** in the treatment of pancreatic insufficiency. Since it is a plant-based enzyme, many vegetarians prefer to use bromelain as a digestive aid rather than the animal-based pancreatin.

Painful menstruation (dysmenorrhea)

Bromelain and papain have been used successfully in the treatment of dysmenorrhea (painful menstruation). Bromelain is believed to be a smooth-muscle relaxant, since it decreases uterine spasms in these patients.

Sports injuries

Bromelain has been shown to be effective in a variety of sports-related injuries. One of the most interesting studies was a 1960 study involving boxers. The group receiving the bromelain experienced quicker resolution of their facial injuries. Fifty-eight of seventy-four boxers receiving bromelain reported that all signs of bruising had cleared completely within four days. Of the remaining sixteen, complete clearance took eight to ten days. In contrast, of the seventy-two controls, only ten had complete clearance of their bruises at the end of four days, with the remainder taking seven to fourteen days.

Recovery from surgery

The ability of bromelain to reduce swelling, bruising, healing time, and pain following surgical procedures has been demonstrated in several clinical studies. Some studies have shown that the best results are obtained if bromelain is given both before and after surgery. However, at this time there are insufficient studies to evaluate possible adverse effects or interactions during surgery. Therefore, it is recommended that bromelain be used only after surgery.

Respiratory tract infections

Bromelain exerts several beneficial effects in respiratory tract infections such as sinusitis, bronchitis, and even pneumonia. For example, in addition to its antibiotic activity, bromelain suppresses coughs and reduces the viscosity of sputum. Patients with chronic bronchitis showed increased lung capacity and function after bromelain treatment, believed to be the results of bromelain's decongestant effect. Bromelain is also helpful in acute sinusitis.

Thrombophlebitis

In acute thrombophlebitis (inflammation of a vein), bromelain has been shown to reduce all the symptoms of inflammation: pain, edema, redness, tenderness, elevated skin temperature, and disability. Apparently higher doses (e.g., 500–750 mg) are needed to achieve consistent results for thrombophlebitis.

Available Forms

Bromelain is available primarily in tablets and capsules. The activity of bromelain is expressed in a variety of enzyme units. The Food Chemistry Codex (FCC) officially recognizes the use of milk clotting units (MCUs). The gelatin digesting unit (GDU) is another enzyme unit that is acceptable and equal in numerical value to the MCU. Different grades of bromelain are available on the basis of the MCU or GDU. For most indications the recommended MCU or GDU range is 1,200 to 1,800.

Cautions and Warnings

If you are allergic to pineapple, do not use bromelain.

Possible Side Effects

Very large single doses of bromelain (nearly 2 g) have been given with no side effects. However, allergic reactions may occur (as with most therapeutic agents). Other possible, but unconfirmed, reactions include nausea, vomiting, diarrhea, and increased menstrual blood flow.

Drug Interactions

As noted above, bromelain can enhance the effectiveness of antibiotics.

Food and Nutrient Interactions

Copper and iron deactivate bromelain, while magnesium and cysteine (a sulfur-containing amino acid) activate bromelain. If using bromelain other than as a digestive aid it is recommended that it be taken away from food.

Usual Dosage

Unless bromelain is being used as a digestive aid, it should be taken on an empty stomach between meals. If it is being used as a digestive aid, it should be taken just before meals.

The dosage depends largely on the potency of the bromelain preparation. Most currently available bromelain is in the 1,200- to 1,800-MCU range, with the typical dosage for most conditions being 250 to 750 mg three times per day between meals.

Overdosage

Bromelain is virtually nontoxic. Animal studies show that dosages of up to 10 g per kg (2.2 pounds) of body weight were not associated with any deaths.

Special Populations

Pregnant/breast-feeding women
Considered safe during pregnancy and lactation.

Children
Suitable for children at one-half the adult dosage.

Seniors
No special precautions are known.

Butcher's Broom
(Ruscus aculeatus)

Used For

Hemorrhoids
Effectiveness: B+   Safety: A

Lymphedema
Effectiveness: B+   Safety: B

Varicose veins
Effectiveness: A   Safety: B

General Information

Butcher's broom is a subshrub of the lily family that grows in the Mediterranean region. The rhizome of butcher's broom has a long history of use in treating venous disorders such as hemorrhoids and varicose veins. There is clinical research showing support for these applications as well as in lymphedema (swelling due to blockage in lymphatic flow). The active ingredients in butcher's broom are compounds known as ruscogenins, which have demonstrated a wide range of pharmacological actions useful in strengthening veins and capillaries (small blood vessels) as well as improving lymphatic drainage.

Hemorrhoids

Hemorrhoids are varicose veins of the rectum. See "Varicose veins," below.

Lymphedema

Lymphedema is an accumulation of lymphatic fluid causing swelling of a limb. Lymphatic fluid resides outside blood vessels in the intercellular spaces of body tissues and is collected in the lymphatic system to be filtered and put back into the bloodstream. If lymphatic vessels are blocked or are removed through surgery, it can lead to lymphedema. One of the leading causes of lymphedema, for example, is a complete (radical) mastectomy. The lymph flow from the arm is blocked because of removal of lymph nodes and vessels. Butcher's broom extract appears useful in any type of lymphedema because of its ability to improve capillary function and promote improved lymphatic flow. In a study in women with lymphedema after mastectomy, butcher's broom extract combined with massage led to a significant reduction in the volume of arm edema compared to massage alone. The significance of this improvement could be sufficient to prevent loss of function in the limb.

Varicose veins

Veins are fairly fragile structures that are at significant risk for damage to their structural integrity. Varicose veins occur in most individuals mostly due to a combination of poor structural integrity in a vein coupled with increased stress on the vein. When an individual stands for long periods of time, the pressure within the veins of the leg can increase up to ten times. Individuals with occupations that require long periods of standing are at greatest risk for developing varicose veins. If there are defects in the wall of a vein, or if the vein's structural integrity is weakened, the vein may dilate, damaging the valves. When the valves become damaged, the increased pressure within the vein results in the formation of a varicose vein.

Butcher's broom extracts have been shown in numerous clinical trials to be very effective in improving blood flow through a varicose vein as well as relieving symptoms such as fatigue, aching discomfort, feelings of heaviness, or pain in the legs. Butcher's broom extract has also been shown to be helpful in hemorrhoids (varicose veins of the rectum). The extract improves capillary and lymphatic function, increases the integrity of supportive connective tissue within the vein, and improves the tone and function of the diseased vein. Results are usually noticeable within the first month of therapy. Maintenance of the results usually requires continued use.

Available Forms

The rhizome of butcher's broom is the portion of the plant used for medicinal purposes. The crude rhizome is available in bulk and in capsules, and tablets; also available are tinctures, fluid extracts, and solid extracts in tablets and capsules. Dry extracts standardized for ruscogenin content are the preferred form for therapeutic use.

Brands available include Sanhelios CircuVeg.

Cautions and Warnings

None known.

Possible Side Effects

Butcher's broom extracts have been well tolerated, with no significant reports of side effects.

Drug Interactions

None known.

Food and Nutrient Interactions

None known.

Usual Dosage

The dosage of butcher's broom extract for therapeutic use should be based on the ruscogenin content. The dosage of ruscogenins should be in the range of 16.5 to 33 mg of ruscogenins three times daily. Standardized extracts are preferred for therapeutic use because they allow for more accurate dosages. Recommendations for other forms of butcher's broom are as follows:

Dried rhizome in capsules, tablets, or tea: 500 to 1,000 mg three times daily
Tincture (1:5): 2–4 ml three times daily
Fluid extract (1:1): 1–2 ml three times daily

Overdosage

None known.

Special Populations

Pregnant/breast-feeding women
As the effects of taking butcher's broom during pregnancy and lactation have not been sufficiently evaluated, it should not be used during these times.

Children
Suitable for children at one-half the adult dosage.

Seniors
No special precautions are known.

Caffeine

Used For

Asthma
Effectiveness: B+   Safety: C

Central nervous system stimulant
Effectiveness: A   Safety: C

Diuretic
Effectiveness: C   Safety: C

Weight loss aid
Effectiveness: B+   Safety: C

General Information

Caffeine is a compound found in many plants, such as coffee *(Coffea arabica)*, cola nuts *(Cola nitida)*, guarana *(Paullinia cupana)*, maté *(Illex paraguariensis)*, tea *(Camellia sinensis)*, and cacao *(Theobroma cacao)*. Caffeine is a member of the methylxanthine alkaloid family along with two related compounds, theophylline and theobromine. These compounds are very similar chemically, differing only in the position of methyl groups, but they have different biochemical effects and are present in different ratios in caffeine-containing plants.

The effects of caffeine are well known. It increases the blood pressure, stimulates the central nervous system, promotes urine formation, and stimulates the action of the heart and lungs. Caffeine is used in treating migraine, increases the potency of analgesics such as aspirin, and can relieve asthma by widening the bronchial airways.

Purified caffeine is produced commercially chiefly as a byproduct in the making of decaffeinated coffee. Purified caffeine can be found in a variety of over-the-counter products, including preparations to fight off sleep and increase mental alertness and in combination with acetaminophen or aspirin to treat headache or the fluid retention that can accompany menstruation.

Caffeine-containing herbs can be used for these same purposes. In fact, due to their mild stimulatory action, many caffeine-containing herbs have historically been used to sustain people during long journeys or long hours of work in virtually every culture in the world. For example, cola nuts are used in West Africa; guarana is used by the natives of South America; coffee was originally used by East Africans and later by other cultures; tea is used by Asian cultures. Western societies seem to have adopted coffee as their herbal stimulant.

Caffeine and caffeine-containing herbs appear to be helpful in asthma, as regular caffeine consumption was found to be associated with a reduction in asthma symptoms. Numerous studies have shown that caffeine and theophylline (found in tea) are effective as mild bronchodilators. Also, a single cup of coffee was shown to offer a 29 percent reduced risk for adult-onset asthma. The public health implications of this may be important, as asthma is quite common in adults.

Currently, perhaps the most popular use of caffeine-containing herbs is as ingredients in thermogenic formulas used in the promotion of weight loss (see **ephedrine-caffeine combinations**). Although caffeine, as well as caffeine-containing herbs such as guarana, tea, and maté, has been shown to increase the metabolic rate, combining it with ephedrine greatly increases this effect.

Available Forms

Caffeine is available in purified form in a variety of over-the-counter products. It is also a component in many plants, such as coffee *(Coffea arabica)*, cola nuts *(Cola nitida)*, guarana *(Paullinia cupana)*, maté *(Ilex paraguariensis)*, tea *(Camellia sinensis)*, and cacao *(Theobroma cacao)*. These plants are available in crude, bulk form as well as in tea bags, ground or powdered in tablets and capsules, as liquid extracts, and as dry powdered extracts, including standardized extracts in tablets and capsules. Brands available include No-Doz and Vivarin.

Cautions and Warnings

Do not exceed the recommended dosage of caffeine or caffeine-containing herbs, especially if combined with other plant stimulants such as ephedrine.

Caffeine may have the potential to cause cardiac arrhythmia (irregular heartbeat). As a precaution, it is recommended that caffeine be avoided by individuals with a history of arrhythmia and/or palpitations and during the first month after suffering a heart attack.

Chronic caffeine consumption can lead to physical and psychological dependence. If caffeine intake is stopped abruptly, physical signs of withdrawal may occur. The most common symptoms of caffeine withdrawal are fatigue and headache. These symptoms usually begin twelve to twenty-four hours after caffeine intake is stopped and may last as long as a week.

Possible Side Effects

Caffeine can produce anxiety, irritability, and insomnia, especially in people sensitive to these effects or already experiencing some degree of these difficulties. Other possible side effects include light-headedness, headache, nausea, gastric irritation, and vomiting.

Drug Interactions

The breakdown of caffeine is inhibited by the following drugs: birth control pills, estrogen (e.g., Premarin), mexiletine, cimetidine (Tagamet), and various antibiotics (e.g., norfloxacin, enoxacin, and ciprofloxacin). Tricyclic antidepressant drugs, ephedrine, and theophylline (used in asthma) all potentiate the effects of caffeine.

Food and Nutrient Interactions

Alcohol inhibits the breakdown of caffeine.

To avoid the potential danger of caffeine overdose, be aware of your consumption of caffeine-containing foods and beverages.

Caffeine Content of Coffee and Tea

Drip	115–175 mg per 7 fluid ounces
Brewed	80–135 mg per 7 fluid ounces
Espresso	100 mg per 1.5–2 fluid ounces
Instant	65–100 mg per 7 fluid ounces
Decaf, brewed	3–4 mg per 7 fluid ounces
Decaf, instant	2–3 mg per 7 fluid ounces
Tea	30–70 mg per 7 fluid ounces

Note: The variability in the amount of caffeine in a cup of coffee or tea is relatively large even if prepared by the same person using the same equipment and ingredients day after day.

Caffeine Content of Soft Drinks (mg per 12 fluid ounces)

Diet brands contain virtually the same amount of caffeine as the regular soft drink of the same name.

Jolt	71.2
Mountain Dew	55.0
Kick	54
Mello Yello	52.8
Surge	51.0
Tab	46.8
Coca-Cola	45.6
Shasta Cola	44.4
Mr. Pibb	40.8
Dr Pepper	39.6
Pepsi Cola	37.2
RC Cola	36.0
Canada Dry Cola	30.0
7-Up	0

Usual Dosage

The typical dosage of caffeine as a stimulant is 100 to 200 mg no more than once every four hours and no less than six hours before bedtime. The dosage for the various herbal sources of caffeine is based upon supplying an equivalent amount of caffeine.

The caffeine content of the various medicinal plants is as follows:

Cola nut	35–50 mg per 1,000 mg crude nut
Guarana	26–70 mg per 1,000 mg crude herb
Maté	15–30 mg per 1,000 mg crude herb
Tea (including green tea)	30–50 mg per 1,000 mg crude herb

Extracts can have higher concentrations of caffeine. Dosages for these preparations are based upon their caffeine content (often the level will be stated on the label).

Overdosage

Doses of caffeine over 250 mg can produce definite signs of toxicity, such as stomach pain, nervousness, increased heart rate, elevation in blood pressure, frequent urination, and disordered thought and speech. More serious symptoms include arrhythmia (irregular heartbeat) and seizures. In the case of severe symptoms seek emergency treatment.

Special Populations

Pregnant/breast-feeding women

Caffeine is to be avoided during pregnancy and lactation. Caffeine has long been suspected of causing malformations in the fetus, although this is controversial. The dosage required for this effect is probably quite large, and the data are scant, as experimentation on humans is not feasible. Caffeine has been shown to cause malformations in rats when ingested at rates comparable to seventy cups a day for humans. In humans, daily doses of 300 mg per day or more in pregnant women have been linked to slowed growth and low birth weight of the infant.

Caffeine passes into breast milk and may cause wakefulness and irritability in nursing infants.

Children

There does not appear to be any appropriate use of caffeine or caffeine-containing beverages in children. The adverse effects of caffeine are usually more severe in children because their breakdown of caffeine is slower than that of adults.

Seniors

Seniors are often more sensitive to caffeine's stimulant effects and may be more likely to experience nervousness, anxiety, and insomnia. Seniors are also more likely to be taking drugs that interact with caffeine.

Carob (Ceratonia siliqua)

Used For

Diarrhea
Effectiveness: B+   Safety: A

General Information

Carob is a dome-shaped evergreen tree originally from the Mediterranean region and the western part

of Asia. These trees produce fruit in the form of pods
that can grow up to a foot in length. John the Baptist
is believed to have eaten carob, and thus it is sometimes called St. John's bread. Carob powder is a
popular substitute for chocolate in health food products.

Carob pods and the powder (flour) produced from
them have been used to treat diarrhea for centuries.
Since the early 1950s, there have been several reports in the medical literature that carob powder
and other carob preparations are effective and without side effects in the treatment of acute-onset diarrhea. The best method of administration appears to
be mixing carob powder with oral rehydration solution (e.g., Pedialyte). In these studies, recovery was
much quicker in the subjects given carob compared
to those receiving oral rehydration solution only.

Carob is rich in dietary fiber (26 percent) and
polyphenols (21 percent). These components are
thought to be responsible for the beneficial effects
in helping control diarrhea.

Available Forms

Carob powder (flour) is available in bulk at most
health food stores.

Cautions and Warnings

Although most acute cases of diarrhea resolve on
their own without medical attention, if any of the following apply, a physician should be consulted immediately:

• Diarrhea in a child under six years of age
• Severe or bloody diarrhea
• Diarrhea that lasts more than three days

• Significant signs of dehydration (sunken eyes, severe dry mouth, strong body odor, etc.)

Possible Side Effects

Consumption of carob can be constipating for the same reasons it is an effective antidiarrheal agent. Rare cases of allergy to carob have also been reported.

Drug Interactions

None known.

Food and Nutrient Interactions

None known.

Usual Dosage

In the treatment of diarrhea, carob powder at a dosage of 1.5 g per kg (2.2 pounds) body weight per day can be given. For best results, the carob powder should be dissolved in an oral rehydration solution.

Overdosage

None known.

Special Populations

Pregnant/breast-feeding women
Considered safe during pregnancy and lactation.

Children

Suitable for children at the same dosage as adults, since dosage in the treatment of diarrhea is based upon body weight.

Seniors

No special precautions are known.

Cascara sagrada and Casanthranol

Used For

Constipation
Effectiveness: A   Safety: C

General Information

Cascara sagrada is a stimulant laxative made from the dried bark of the buckthorn tree *(Rhamnus pur-shiana).* The laxative components are compounds known as anthraquinones. Casanthranol is the isolated, purified anthraquinones of cascara. It produces its laxative effect by increasing the strength of contraction of the intestinal muscles. Like other stimulant laxatives, cascara has its place in clinical medicine. Its use should be limited, as tolerance and dependence can develop. Long-term use of cascara may increase the risk for colon cancer.

Available Forms

Cascara is available in fluid extract, tablet, and capsule form. Casanthranol preparations are usually in tablets or capsules. Brands available include Nature's Remedy.

Cautions and Warnings

Do not use cascara for more than seven days unless directed by your doctor.

Stimulant laxatives should not be used in patients with abdominal pain, nausea or vomiting, intestinal obstruction, inflammatory bowel disease, appendicitis, pregnancy, or during lactation.

Do not take more than the recommended amount. Excessive laxative use or inadequate fluid intake may lead to significant fluid and electrolyte imbalance.

Possible Side Effects

Stimulant laxatives such as cascara are likely to cause abdominal cramping, nausea, and increased mucus secretion. Less common side effects are associated with chronic use and are usually related to loss of potassium and other electrolytes (e.g., muscle spasms, weakness, and fatigue). Call your doctor right away if you have any of these side effects: a sudden change in bowel habits that persists over a period of two weeks, rectal bleeding, or failure to have a bowel movement after use.

A benign blackish brown pigmentation of the colonic mucosa (pseudomelanosis coli) may occur with prolonged use (at least four months) of cascara, due to the anthraquinones. This condition is generally reversible within four to fifteen months after discontinuing the substance.

Drug Interactions

Cascara and other stimulant laxatives may decrease the absorption of other drugs that pass through the gastrointestinal tract. If you are currently taking an oral medication, talk to your pharmacist or doctor before self-medicating with cascara.

Cascara may potentiate the action of digoxin and other heart medications due to potassium depletion. The use of cascara with thiazide diuretics and corticosteroids may further decrease potassium levels.

Food and Nutrient Interactions

Generally, cascara is recommended on an empty stomach. Drink six to eight glasses of liquid daily while taking this laxative.

Usual Dosage

Follow the manufacturer's instructions on the label. The usual dosage recommendation for crude dried bark preparations in capsules or tablets for adults is 300–1,000 mg at bedtime; for the fluid extract it is 2–6 ml at bedtime. The dosage for casanthranol is 30–90 mg at bedtime.

Overdosage

Symptoms of overdosage include persistent diarrhea and dehydration. In severe cases of accidental overdose do the following: If the victim is unconscious or having convulsions, call for an ambulance immediately. If you take the victim to an emergency room, be sure to bring the bottle or container with you. If the victim is conscious, call your local poison control center or a health care professional. The poison control center may suggest inducing vomiting with ipecac syrup (available without a prescription at any pharmacy). *Do not* induce vomiting unless specifically instructed to do so.

Special Populations

Pregnant/breast-feeding women

Cascara and other stimulant laxatives should be avoided during pregnancy. Only bulk-forming laxatives or stool softeners are recommended for pregnant women.

Check with your doctor before using cascara if you are breast-feeding. Cascara anthraquinones pass into the breast milk, but the concentration is usually insufficient to affect the infant. Nonetheless, there have been reported cases of infants experiencing diarrhea after breast-feeding from a mother who had taken cascara.

Children

In general, stimulant laxatives should be avoided in children less than six years of age unless prescribed by a physician. Cascara is suitable for children older than six years of age at one-half of the adult dosage.

Seniors

Seniors commonly experience constipation and are most susceptible to becoming dependent on laxatives. Seniors are most likely to experience the more serious side effects of long-term use because of the potassium-depleting effects of cascara and other stimulant laxatives. Bulk-forming laxatives are usually preferred for seniors.

Cat's Claw
(Uncaria tomentosa)

Used For

AIDS and HIV
Effectiveness: B   Safety: C

Asthma and hay fever
Effectiveness: B   Safety: C

Cancer
Effectiveness: B   Safety: C

Common cold
Effectiveness: B   Safety: C

Low immunity and immune support
Effectiveness: B   Safety: C

Rheumatoid arthritis and other autoimmune disorders
Effectiveness: B   Safety: C

General Information

Cat's claw is an interesting medicinal plant from South America. The Spanish called the plant *uña de gato* (cat's claw) because the plant's hooks resemble a cat's claw. In traditional Peruvian medicine, the root of cat's claw has been used for a variety of ailments and applications, including arthritis, asthma, cancer, peptic ulcers, infections, and wound healing. Preliminary studies seem to support this traditional use.

Most of the recent scientific research on cat's claw has focused on the effects of various pentacyclic alkaloids and other constituents on the immune system and immune-system-related conditions. Some of the effects noted in test tube studies with pentacyclic alkaloids include a powerful effect on phagocytosis, the process by which certain white blood cells engulf and destroy foreign particles, including bacteria, viruses, cancer cells, and cellular debris.

AIDS and HIV infection

Saventaro, a brand of cat's claw, has een the subject of several preliminary studies in people with HIV infection. The initial data is promising: Some of the test subjects taking Saventaro demonstrated a significant increase in helper T cells and a reduction in viral load. They also reported increased well-being and vitality, a better tolerance of anti-HIV drug therapy, and fewer opportunistic infections. These results will need to be confirmed in larger, better-designed trials.

Asthma and hay fever

Although there are no clinical studies with cat's claw in allergic disorders, there have been a number of individual case reports with Saventaro indicating potential benefit in asthma and hay fever.

Cancer

Given the seriousness of cancer and the lack of scientific studies on cat's claw, it cannot be recommended as a primary therapy for cancer. It appears, however, that it can be used as a supportive therapy in individuals undergoing conventional anticancer therapies. Cat's claw does not appear to interfere with the action of chemotherapy agents or radiation. Physicians in Austria have reported that use of Saventaro results in a marked increase in quality of life and better tolerance of radiation and chemotherapy. In particular, they report a reduction in chemotherapy-induced nausea, a reduction in the fall in blood pressure values following treatment sessions, shortening of the recovery phase between individual treatment cycles, and a reduction in susceptibility to infection.

Common cold and low immunity

Saventaro has been shown to boost immune function in people who have a tendency toward recurrent colds and flulike infections (especially the elderly) and in people who suffer from genital herpes outbreaks.

Rheumatoid arthritis

Saventaro was shown to produce significant improvement in rheumatoid arthritis in a double-blind study. Specifically, the number of tender joints and the blood measurement of rheumatoid factor was significantly lower in the Saventaro group than in the placebo group. These results are encouraging but need to be confirmed in a larger study.

Available Forms

The bark of the root is the portion of cat's claw used for medicinal purposes. The crude herb is available in bulk, tea bags, capsules, and tablets; also available are tinctures, fluid extracts, and dry extracts in tablets and capsules. The majority of scientific studies on cat's claw have been done on Saventaro.

Cautions and Warnings

Cat's claw preparations should be avoided in people scheduled for an organ transplant or skin graft, as it may activate the immune system and lead to rejection of the transplanted organ or cells.

Possible Side Effects

Cat's claw is generally regarded as being quite safe. Toxicity studies in animals have confirmed this safety.

Drug Interactions

None known.

Food and Nutrient Interactions

Cat's claw is generally recommended to be taken on an empty stomach.

Usual Dosage

The dosage of Saventaro is one 20 mg capsule three times daily for the first ten days and one capsule daily thereafter.

The dosage recommendation for dried bark is usually 250 to 1,000 mg daily (providing 10 to 30 mg total alkaloids).

For the decoction of cat's claw, the typical recommendation is to mix 30 g (about 1 ounce) of powder to 800–850 ml (approximately 24 fluid ounces) of water. Allow the mixture to simmer on the stove for about forty-five minutes or until 500 milliliters (15 fluid ounces) of liquid is left. When the decoction has cooled, strain it through filter paper and store refrigerated in an airtight container in a refrigerator. The adult dose based on traditional use is approximately 60 ml (2 fluid ounces) of the decoction on an empty stomach in the morning.

Overdosage

None known.

Special Populations

Pregnant/breast-feeding women

Because the effects of cat's claw during pregnancy and lactation have not been sufficiently studied, it should not be taken by women who are pregnant or breast-feeding.

Children

Because the effects of cat's claw usage in children has not been sufficiently studied, it is generally advised that it not be taken by children unless recommended by a physician.

Seniors

No special precautions are known.

Cayenne Pepper
(Capsicum frutescens)

Used For

Heart disease (atherosclerosis) prevention
Effectiveness: B   Safety: A

Weight loss
Effectiveness: B+   Safety: A

General Information

Cayenne pepper (also known as chili or hot pepper) is the fruit of *Capsicum frutescens,* a shrubby tropical plant. The fruit is technically a berry. Paprika and red or green bell peppers are milder and sweeter-tasting fruit produced from different species in the genus *Capsicum.* Although cayenne pepper is native to tropical America, it is now cultivated in tropical locations throughout the world and has found its way into the cuisines of many parts of the world, particularly Southeast Asia, China, southern Italy, and Mexico.

Capsaicin is the active component of cayenne pepper. It is also the component responsible for the pungent and irritating effects of cayenne pepper. Typically, cayenne pepper contains about 1.5 percent capsaicin and related principals.

The folk use of cayenne pepper is quite extensive. It has been used to treat asthma, fevers, sore throats, and other respiratory tract infections, digestive disturbances, and cancers. The modern medicinal use of cayenne pepper is primarily in the form of topical preparations containing capsaicin. Oral preparations are used primarily to protect against atherosclerosis (hardening of the arteries) and to promote weight loss.

Interestingly, although many people complain that eating spicy foods irritates their stomach, research indicates that consumption of cayenne pepper actually protects against ulcers. Population studies indicate that people who consume the highest level of hot peppers have the lowest rate of peptic ulcer. Capsaicin has been shown to inhibit the growth of the bacterium *Helicobacter pylori*—a suspected causative agent in ulcer formation. Other studies have shown that cayenne pepper can protect the stomach against ulcer formation.

Heart disease (atherosclerosis) prevention

Cayenne pepper exerts a number of beneficial effects on the cardiovascular system. In addition to containing antioxidant compounds, studies have shown that cayenne pepper reduces the likelihood of developing atherosclerosis by reducing blood cholesterol and triglyceride levels; it also reduces the likelihood of blood clot formation, which can lead to a stroke or heart attack. Cultures consuming large amounts of cayenne pepper have a much lower rate of cardiovascular disease.

Weight loss

Recent studies have shown that increasing the intake of cayenne pepper may be an effective alternative to stimulant-containing thermogenic formulas (see **ephedrine-caffeine combinations**) in promoting weight loss. In one study, the addition of 10 g of cayenne pepper to meals significantly increased diet-induced thermogenesis and the burning of fat. In another study, subjects who consumed 10 g of red pepper at breakfast demonstrated significant increases in metabolic markers that represent a thermogenic effect.

Available Forms

The fruit (pepper) is the portion of the plant used for medicinal purposes. Cayenne pepper is available in bulk (ground or flaked), capsules, and tablets as well as in the form of tinctures, fluid extracts, and dry extracts in tablets and capsules).

Cautions and Warnings

Cayenne pepper preparations are extremely irritating to mucous membranes, especially the eyes. Avoid any contact between cayenne and the eyes or other mucous membranes. Wash hands immediately after touching any cayenne pepper preparation to avoid irritation.

Possible Side Effects

In rare cases allergic reactions (hives) have been reported.

Drug Interactions

Cayenne pepper has been shown to block the ulcer-producing effects of aspirin and may also protect against ulcers caused by other NSAIDs. No other drug interactions are known.

Food and Nutrient Interactions

None known.

Usual Dosage

Cayenne pepper is usually taken in one of the following forms three times daily:

Crude powder or flakes: 10 g
Tincture (1:5): 2–4 ml (½–1 teaspoon)
Fluid extract: 1–2 ml (¼–½ teaspoon)
Dry extract (standardized to contain 0.8–1.1 percent ligustilide): 150–200 mg

Overdosage

Gastrointestinal irritation, heartburn, nausea, and/or diarrhea are the most common symptoms of overdosage.

Special Populations

Pregnant/breast-feeding women
Considered safe during pregnancy and lactation.

Children
Suitable for children at one-half the adult dosage.

Seniors
No special precautions are known.

Cellasene

Used For

Cellulite
Effectiveness: C   Safety: C

General Information

Cellasene is a proprietary formula that features a blend of natural herbal extracts (bladderwrack, grape seed, sweet clover, and *Ginkgo biloba)* that is promoted as helping reduce cellulite, the lumpy, irregular fatty deposits that appear as dimpled skin around the hips, buttocks, and thighs, mostly in women.

The marketing materials claim that Cellasene is a safe, clinically studied formula, but none of the studies has been published for review. It is also claimed that the herbal extracts in Cellasene work to increase blood circulation, reduce fluid buildup, stimulate metabolism, and reduce localized fats. These claims have not been verified.

Available Forms

Cellasene is provided in soft gelatin capsules.

Cautions and Warnings

Bladderwrack extract contains iodine, and total iodine intake may exceed recommended levels when taking this product. If you suffer from a thyroid condition or if you are taking blood-thinning drugs or other medications, consult your health care professional before using this product. Cellasene should not be taken when pregnant or nursing.

Possible Side Effects

None known.

Drug Interactions

Because of the iodine content in the bladderwrack extract, use of Cellasene may interfere with or enhance the effects of thyroid hormone.

Food and Nutrient Interactions

Generally recommended to be taken after meals.

Overdosage

None known.

Special Populations

Pregnant/breast-feeding women
Cellasene should not be taken when pregnant or nursing.

Children
There does not appear to be any appropriate use of Cellasene in children.

Seniors
No special precautions are known.

Cernilton

Used For

Benign prostatic hyperplasia (prostate enlargement)
Effectiveness: A   Safety: A

Prostatitis
Effectiveness: B+   Safety: A

General Information

Cernilton is an extract of flower pollen that has been used in Europe to treat prostatitis (inflammation of the prostate) and benign prostatic hyperplasia (BPH) for more than thirty-five years. Numerous double-blind clinical trials have validated its use in BPH. In the most recent study, 85 percent of the test subjects experienced benefit after one year of use: 11 percent reporting "excellent," 39 percent reporting "good," 35 percent reporting "satisfactory," and 15 percent reporting "poor" as a description of their outcome. Patients who respond typically experience a 70 percent reduction in the number of nighttime and daytime urinations as well as significant improvements in complete voiding of the bladder.

In prostatitis, the results from several small studies demonstrate that Cernilton can improve symptoms of increased urinary frequency as well as normalize urinary analyses after prostatic massage (i.e., Cernilton eliminates the presence of urinary sediment, bacteria, or white blood cells) in roughly 70 percent of cases.

The extract has been shown to exert some anti-inflammatory action within the prostate and to produce a contractile effect on the bladder while relaxing the urethra. In addition, Cernilton contains a substance that inhibits the growth of prostate cells.

Available Forms

Each Cernilton tablet contains 60 mg of Cernitin T60 water-soluble pollen extract concentrate and 3 mg of Cernitin GBX fat-soluble pollen extract concentrate. It is also available in a triple-strength (Cernilton TS) capsule.

Cautions and Warnings

None known.

Possible Side Effects

None known. No side effects have been reported in the clinical studies.

Drug Interactions

None known.

Food and Nutrient Interactions

None known.

Usual Dosage

For use in prostate disorders, Cernilton: 6 tablets daily; Cernilton TS: 2 capsules daily.

Overdosage

None known.

Special Populations

Pregnant/breast-feeding women

Because the effects of using Cernilton during pregnancy and lactation have not been sufficiently studied, it should not be taken by pregnant or breast-feeding women.

Children

There does not appear to be any appropriate use of Cernilton in children.

Seniors

No special precautions are known.

Chamomile
(Matricaria chamomilla)

Used For

Infantile colic
Effectiveness: B+   Safety: C

Insomnia
Effectiveness: C   Safety: C

Irritable bowel syndrome
Effectiveness: C   Safety: C

General Information

Chamomile is a fragrant, low-growing annual herb. The dried yellow flower heads are the portion of the plant commonly used. In addition to its use orally, it is widely used in topical preparations. The primary use orally has been in the treatment of gastrointestinal complaints and as a mild sedative. Although chamomile has a long folk history of use, there are few scientific studies to document effectiveness. In one of the few studies, the gastrointestinal effects of a chamomile-containing tea marketed in Italy (Calma-Bebi) was confirmed in the treatment of infantile colic. The clinical effect was thought to be due to the ability of chamomile to relax spastic intestinal muscles. However, in addition to chamomile (Matricaria chamomilla), the tea also contained vervain (Verbena officinalis), licorice (Glycyrrhiza glabra), fennel (Foeniculum vulgare), and balm (Melissa officinalis), so the possibility of one of the other components producing the effect could not be ruled out.

Available Forms

Chamomile is available as the crude herb in bulk, capsules, and tablets; also available are tinctures, fluid extracts, and solid extracts in tablets and capsules.

Cautions and Warnings

None known.

Possible Side Effects

Chamomile is thought to be extremely safe, with no side effects known. Allergic reactions are possible in people allergic to plants of the *Compositae* (daisy) family.

Drug Interactions

None known.

Food and Nutrient Interactions

None known.

Usual Dosage

Dried flower heads: 1–2 g
Tincture (1:5): 4–6 ml
Fluid extract (1:1): 2–4 ml (1 teaspoon)
Solid extract (4:1): 250–500 mg

Overdosage

None known.

Special Populations

Pregnant/breast-feeding women
Chamomile tea is considered safe during pregnancy and lactation.

Children
Suitable for children, even infants, at one-half the adult dosage.

Seniors
No special precautions are known.

Chaparral *(Larrea tridentata)*

Used For

Cancer
Effectiveness: D   Safety: F

General Information

Chaparral, also known as creosote bush, is an evergreen desert shrub that has been used by Native Americans for a variety of purposes for thousands of years. It was employed primarily in tea form to help with cramping pains, joint pains, and allergic problems as well as to eliminate parasites. Applied to the skin, it was used to relieve pain and inflammation and to treat minor wounds.

Interest in chaparral as a possible treatment for cancer developed in 1969 when an eighty-five-year-old man refused medical treatment for a documented malignant melanoma of the right cheek that had metastasized to the jaw. Over the course of one year, he medicated himself with 2–3 cups daily of a tea made from the dried leaves and stems of chaparral. Without any other medical treatment during the year, the facial lesion shrank significantly and the jaw lesion completely disappeared.

This case history led to some scientific investigation. The antioxidant compound nordihydroguaiaretic acid (NDGA) was identified as the key component. A follow-up clinical study showed that of forty-five patients treated with this substance, four had significant tumor regression. However, in a significant number of cases there appeared to have been tumor stimulation. Later test tube studies with NDGA have shown stimulation of tumor cell growth at lower concentrations and inhibition at higher levels. Until NDGA's effects are better understood, cancer patients should avoid use of chaparral tea.

Available Forms

Chaparral is available in crude form, powdered in capsules and tablets, and as a fluid extract.

Cautions and Warnings

Do not use chaparral, as it has demonstrated no benefit but shown significant toxicity.

Chaparral may cause hepatitis. Between 1992 and 1994 the FDA received eighteen reports of illnesses associated with the ingestion of chaparral, including thirteen cases of liver damage. The toxicity occurred anywhere from three to fifty-two weeks after the ingestion of chaparral was started, and it resolved in most individuals one to seventeen weeks after stopping intake of chaparral. In four individuals there was

progression to cirrhosis; in two individuals liver failure occurred and liver transplants were necessary.
  Chaparral may stimulate tumor growth.

Possible Side Effects

Liver damage.

Drug Interactions

None known.

Food and Nutrient Interactions

None known.

Usual Dosage

The use of chaparral is not indicated at this time.

Overdosage

None known.

Special Populations

Pregnant/breast-feeding women
  Chaparral must not be used during pregnancy and lactation.

Children
  Chaparral is not suitable for children.

Seniors
  The elderly may be more susceptible to the toxicity of chaparral.

Chaste Berry
(Vitex agnus-castus)

Used For

Menstrual cycle irregularities
Effectiveness: B+   Safety: C

Premenstrual syndrome
Effectiveness: A   Safety: C

General Information

The chaste tree is native to the Mediterranean. Its berries have long been used for female complaints. As its name signifies, chaste berries were once believed to suppress the libido. In Germany, chaste berry extract is the most popular herbal approach to premenstrual syndrome (PMS) and menstrual irregularities. In two surveys of gynecological practices in Germany, physicians graded chaste berry extract as good or very good in the treatment of PMS. More than 1,500 women participated in the studies. One-third of the women experienced complete resolution of their symptoms, while another 57 percent reported significant improvement. In another more recent study, 170 women with PMS were given chaste berry extract or placebo daily for three consecutive menstrual cycles. The chaste berry group experienced significant improvements in irritability, mood alteration, anger, headache, breast fullness, bloating, and other menstrual symptoms.

Chaste berry extract appears to be particularly useful in the treatment of amenorrhea (absence of menstruation), oligomenorrhea (infrequent menstruation), and menorrhagia (heavy menstruation) due to excess production of the hormone prolactin or insufficient output of hormones by the ovaries after ovulation. But don't expect immediate results; it usually takes about three months for chaste berry extract to normalize hormone levels.

Chaste berry extract exerts its beneficial effects in PMS and menstrual irregularities by normalizing the release of hormones from the pituitary that control the function of the ovaries.

Available Forms

Chaste berry extract is available in liquid and dry powdered form.

Cautions and Warnings

None known.

Possible Side Effects

Side effects of using chaste berry are rare. Minor gastrointestinal upset and a mild skin rash with itching have been reported in less than 2 percent of the women monitored while taking it.

Drug Interactions

None known.

Food and Nutrient Interactions

None known.

Usual Dosage

The usual dosage of chaste berry extract (often standardized to contain 0.5 percent agnuside) in tablet or
capsule form is 175 to 225 mg daily. If using the liquid extract, the typical dosage is 2 ml daily.

Overdosage

None known.

Special Populations

Pregnant/breast-feeding women

As the effects of chaste berry during pregnancy
and lactation have not been sufficiently evaluated, it
should not be used during these times.

Children

There does not appear to be any appropriate use
of chaste berry in children.

Seniors

No special precautions are known.

Cola Nut (Cola nitida)

General Information

The cola nut is native to West Africa, where it has
historically been used to sustain people during long
journeys or long hours of work. Although the cola
nut contains many compounds, it is the **caffeine**

component that has brought about the most attention. Cola nuts contain approximately 3.5 percent caffeine and less than 1 percent theobromine, a compound related to caffeine. The cola nut's principal use in recent times is in the manufacture of cola beverages.

Comfrey
(Symphytum officinale)

General Information

Comfrey has a long history of use internally as a digestive aid and in the treatment of wounds, ulcers, and sprains. It was also used to treat broken bones, hence the name knit-bone. While comfrey preparations are still suitable as topical preparations, the use of comfrey internally is no longer recommended by most experts, as it contains pyrrolizidine alkaloids, potentially dangerous compounds that can cause serious liver damage. Even though the pyrrolizidine alkaloids are found almost exclusively in the roots, it is prudent to avoid even the use of comfrey leaves for internal use until more is known about the toxicity.

Cautions and Warnings

Comfrey is not recommended for oral use.

Coptis *(Coptis chinensis)*

General Information

Coptis (also called goldthread) is a perennial herb native to China. The part used is the root. Coptis shares indications and effects with other **berberine-containing plants** such as goldenseal and barberry.

Cranberry *(Vaccinium macrocarpon)*

Used For

Bladder infections
Effectiveness: A   Safety: A

General Information

Cranberry juice and cranberry extracts have shown benefit in preventing and treating urinary tract infections in several double-blind studies. For example, in one study of 153 women with active urinary tract infections, 16 fluid ounces of Ocean Spray cranberry drink per day produced beneficial effects in 73 percent of the subjects. When the cranberry juice was withdrawn, 61 percent of the women experienced a recurrence of their bladder infection.

Many believe that the action of cranberry juice is due to acidifying the urine and to the antibacterial effects of hippuric acid, a component of cranberries.

However, in order to acidify the urine, at least 1 quart of cranberry juice would have to be consumed at one sitting, and even then the concentration of hippuric acid in the urine as a result of drinking cranberry juice is insufficient to inhibit bacteria.

Recent studies have shown that components of cranberry juice, probably the proanthocyanidin flavonoids, reduce the ability of bacteria such as *E. coli* to adhere to the lining of the bladder and urethra. In order for bacteria to infect, they must first adhere to this mucosal lining. By interfering with adherence, cranberry juice or extracts greatly reduce the likelihood of infection and allow the body to marshal its own defenses.

Available Forms

Dehydrated cranberry juice and cranberry extracts are available in capsules and tablets. Brand names available include CranActin.

Cautions and Warnings

Consult a physician if you have symptoms suggestive of a bladder infection, such as pain or burning on urination, increased urinary frequency, or cloudy, foul-smelling, or dark urine.

Possible Side Effects

None known.

Drug Interactions

None known.

Food and Nutrient Interactions

None known.

Usual Dosage

The typical dosage for cranberry extract in treatment of a bladder infection is 400 mg four times per day. The dosage for prevention is 400 mg twice daily.

Overdosage

None known.

Special Populations

Pregnant/breast-feeding women
Considered safe during pregnancy and lactation.

Children
Suitable for children at one-half the adult dosage.

Seniors
No special precautions are known.

Curcumin *(Curcuma longa)*

Used For

Antioxidant effects
Effectiveness: A   Safety: A

Cancer prevention and treatment
Effectiveness: A   Safety: A

Heart disease (atherosclerosis) prevention
Effectiveness: A   Safety: A

Inflammatory conditions (arthritis, sports injuries, trauma, etc.)
Effectiveness: A   Safety: A

General Information

Curcumin is the yellow pigment of turmeric *(Curcuma longa),* the chief ingredient in curry powder. It has demonstrated significant activity in many experimental and clinical studies. Many of its beneficial effects are attributed to its antioxidant and anti-inflammatory effects.

Antioxidant effects
The antioxidant activity of curcumin is comparable to standard antioxidants such as vitamins C and E, butylated hydroxyanisole (BHA), and butylated hydroxytoluene (BHT). Because of its bright yellow color and antioxidant properties, curcumin is used in butter, margarine, cheese, and other food products. The advantage of curcumin over vitamin C and E is that while vitamin C is effective against only water-soluble pro-oxidants and vitamin E is effective against only fat-soluble pro-oxidants, curcumin is effective against both.

Cancer prevention and treatment
The anticancer effects of turmeric and curcumin have been demonstrated at all steps of cancer formation: initiation, promotion, and progression. Data obtained from several studies suggest that, in

addition to inhibiting the development of cancer, curcumin can also promote cancer regression when cancer is present. The protective effects of curcumin are only partially explained by its direct antioxidant effect. Other anticancer effects noted include the ability to inhibit the formation of cancer-causing nitrosamines, enhance the body's levels of anticancer compounds such as glutathione, and promote the proper detoxification of cancer-causing compounds by the liver. Curcumin may prove to be a useful antioxidant supplement for smokers. Cigarette smokers receiving curcumin demonstrate a significant reduction in the level of urinary-excreted mutagens—an indication of the ability of the body to rid itself of cancer-causing compounds via detoxification mechanisms.

Heart disease (atherosclerosis) prevention

Curcumin prevents LDL cholesterol from becoming oxidized and damaging arteries. In addition, it exerts other atherosclerosis-preventing effects, including lowering cholesterol levels, preventing plaque formation, and inhibiting the formation of blood clots by inhibiting platelet aggregation.

Inflammatory conditions (arthritis, sports injuries, trauma, etc.)

Turmeric has long been used in India, both topically and internally, in the treatment of sprains and inflammation. This use has been substantiated in experimental studies in animals as well as in studies in humans. In the treatment of rheumatoid arthritis, curcumin (1,200 mg/day) was shown to be comparable to drug therapy (phenylbutazone, 300 mg/day) in improving morning stiffness, walking time, and joint swelling. In a study in men undergoing hernia repair, curcumin was again shown to exert an anti-inflammatory action comparable to that of anti-inflammatory drugs. However, curcumin does not possess direct pain-relieving action.

Available Forms

Curcumin and concentrated turmeric extracts are available primarily in capsules and tablets. Because the absorption of orally administered curcumin may be limited, curcumin is often formulated in conjunction with an equal amount of **bromelain,** which may possibly enhance absorption as well as exert anti-inflammatory effects of its own. Combining curcumin with an oil base such as lecithin, fish oils, or essential fatty acids may also increase absorption.

Cautions and Warnings

None known.

Possible Side Effects

Used in the recommended amounts, curcumin and turmeric extracts are generally safe and without side effects.

Drug Interactions

None known.

Food and Nutrient Interactions

If taking a curcumin-bromelain combination, it is best to take it on an empty stomach, twenty minutes before meals or between meals. In other forms, including in combination with oils in a soft gelatin capsule, taking it with meals may increase its absorption.

Usual Dosage

The recommended dosage for curcumin as an anti-inflammatory is 200 to 400 mg three times a day.

Overdosage

Overdosage may induce mild to severe gastric distress. At high doses (e.g., 100 mg per kg [2.2 pounds] body weight), curcumin caused ulcers in rats.

Special Populations

Pregnant/breast-feeding women

Although turmeric is widely consumed as a spice in many parts of the world and animal studies demonstrate safety during pregnancy, the effects of supplementary curcumin during pregnancy and lactation have not been sufficiently evaluated, so it should not be used during these times.

Children

Suitable for children at one-half the adult dosage.

Seniors

No special precautions are known.

Damiana *(Turnera diffusa)*

Used For

Aphrodisiac
Effectiveness: C   Safety: C

General Information

Damiana is a small shrub native to the southwest United States, Mexico, South America, and the Caribbean. Damiana leaves have been used in the United States since 1874 as an aphrodisiac and to improve sexual ability. Although there are no clinical studies to support this claim, damiana use is very popular. Damiana is thought to slightly irritate the urethra, thereby producing increased sensitivity in the penis or clitoris. Damiana is seldom used alone; most often it is combined with other herbs in commercial preparations.

Available Forms

The dried leaves are the portion of the plant used for medicinal purposes. Dried damiana leaves are available in bulk, capsules, and tablets; also available are tinctures and fluid extracts.

Cautions and Warnings

None known.

Possible Side Effects

None known.

Drug Interactions

None known.

Food and Nutrient Interactions

None known.

Usual Dosage

Damiana is usually taken once daily in one of the following forms:
Dried leaves or in tea: 1–2 g
Tincture (1:5): 2–4 ml (½ –1 teaspoon)
Fluid extract: 1–2 ml (¼ – ½ teaspoon)
Dry extract (4:1): 250–500 mg

Overdosage

None known.

Special Populations

Pregnant/breast-feeding women
As the effects of damiana during pregnancy and lactation have not been sufficiently evaluated, it should not be used during these times.

Children
Damiana is not recommended for children.

Seniors
No special precautions are known.

Dandelion
(Taraxacum officinale)

Used For

Root

Liver tonic
Effectiveness: B   Safety: A

Leaves

Diuretic
Effectiveness: C   Safety: A

General Information

While the common dandelion is regarded by many as a weed, it is revered by herbalists for its medicinal effects. Generally regarded as a liver remedy, dandelion has a long history of folk use. In Europe, dandelion was used in the treatment of fevers, boils, eye problems, diarrhea, fluid retention, liver congestion, heartburn, and various skin problems. In China, dandelion has been used to treat breast problems (cancer, inflammation, lack of milk flow, etc.), liver diseases, appendicitis, and digestive ailments. Dandelion's use in India, Russia, and most other parts of the world revolved primarily around its action on the liver.

The portion of the plant that is most commonly used is the root; however, the leaves and whole plant can also be used. The primary therapeutic actions of dandelion are believed to be due to a bitter component known as taraxacin, **choline,** and its excellent nutritional profile (many studies show that dandelion is a rich source of vitamins and minerals).

Liver tonic

Studies in humans and laboratory animals show that dandelion root enhances the flow of bile by causing an increase in bile production and flow to the gallbladder (choleretic effect). It also exerts a direct effect on the gallbladder, causing contraction and release of stored bile (cholagogue effect). This ability to promote bile flow is thought to be the primary reason why dandelion improves liver function. Small clinical studies in patients with hepatitis have demonstrated improvements in appetite, energy, and jaundice with the use of dandelion.

Diuretic

In addition to its historical use as a diuretic, dandelion leaves have shown diuretic activity in animal studies. In one study in mice, an extract of dandelion leaves exerted diuretic activity comparable to that of the drug furosemide (Lasix). Because dandelion replaces potassium lost through increased urination, it does not have the potential side effects of furosemide, such as hepatic coma and circulatory collapse. The only drawback is that the dosage given to the mice (8 ml of the aqueous fluid extract of the leaf per kg [2.2 pounds] body weight) would be difficult to reach in humans.

Available Forms

The root and leaves are the portions of the plant used for medicinal purposes. The crude herb is available in bulk, capsules, and tablets; also available are tinctures, fluid extracts, and dry extracts in tablets and capsules.

Cautions and Warnings

None known.

Possible Side Effects

None known.

Drug Interactions

None known.

Food and Nutrient Interactions

None known.

Usual Dosage

As a mild liver tonic, the root can be used at the following dosages three times daily:

Dried root: 2–8 g by infusion or decoction

Fluid extract (1:1): 4–8 ml (1–2 teaspoons)

Tincture: alcohol-based tinctures of dandelion are not recommended because of the extremely high dosage required

Juice of fresh root: 4–8 ml (1–2 teaspoons)

Powdered solid extract (4:1): 250–500 mg

Preparations of the leaves can be used as a mild diuretic and weight loss agent at the following dosages three times daily:

Dried leaf: 4–10 g by infusion (tea)

Fluid extract (1:1): 4–10 ml

Dandelion leaves and root can also be consumed as a food and beverage. Tender leaves are used raw in salads and sandwiches, or lightly cooked as a vegetable. Tea is made from the leaves, coffee substitute from the roots, and wine and schnapps from the flowers.

Overdosage

None known.

Special Populations

Pregnant/breast-feeding women
Considered safe during pregnancy and lactation.

Children
Suitable for children at one-half the adult dosage.

Seniors
No special precautions are known.

Deglycyrrhizinated Licorice (DGL)

Used For

Canker sores
Effectiveness: B   Safety: A

Duodenal ulcer
Effectiveness: A   Safety: A

Gastric ulcer
Effectiveness: A   Safety: A

Gastroesophageal reflux disease
Effectiveness: B   Safety: A

General Information

Licorice has historically been regarded as an excellent medicine for peptic ulcer. However, due to the side effects of one of licorice's components, glycyrrhetinic acid (it causes elevations in blood pressure in some cases; see **licorice** for more information), a procedure was developed to remove this compound from licorice and form deglycyrrhizinated licorice (DGL).

Numerous studies over the years have found DGL to be an effective antiulcer medication. In several head-to-head studies, DGL has been shown to be more effective than not only a placebo but also standard drugs such as cimetidine (Tagamet), ranitidine (Zantac), and antacids in both short-term treatment of and maintenance therapy for gastric and duodenal ulcers. DGL has also been shown to be helpful in healing canker sores.

The proposed mechanism by which DGL protects against ulcer formation is increasing the number of cells that produce mucin—the slimy, protective coating of the stomach and intestines—thereby increasing the quality and amount of mucin. DGL can protect against gastric bleeding and ulcers caused by aspirin and other nonsteroidal anti-inflammatory drugs, and prednisone.

Available Forms

It appears that in order to be effective in healing peptic ulcers, DGL must mix with saliva. DGL may promote the release of salivary compounds that stimulate the growth and regeneration of stomach and intestinal cells. DGL in capsule form has not been shown to be effective. DGL in powder form or in chewable tablets is the preferred form.

Cautions and Warnings

Individuals experiencing any symptoms of a peptic (gastric or duodenal) ulcer need competent medical care. Peptic ulcer complications such as hemorrhage, perforation, and obstruction represent medical emergencies that require immediate hospitalization. Individuals with a peptic ulcer must be monitored by a physician.

Possible Side Effects

There is a small amount of glycyrrhetinic acid retained in the DGL extract. It is possible that in some rare instances DGL may produce elevations in blood pressure.

Drug Interactions

As DGL has been shown to reduce the gastric bleeding caused by aspirin, DGL is strongly indicated for the prevention of gastric ulcers in patients requiring long-term treatment with ulcer-causing drugs such as aspirin, other NSAIDs (e.g., ibuprofen, piroxicam, indomethacin, and diclofenac), and corticosteroids (e.g., prednisone).

Food and Nutrient Interactions

None known, although DGL is usually recommended to be taken on an empty stomach between or before meals.

Usual Dosage

The standard dosage for DGL in acute cases is two to four 380 mg chewable tablets between meals or twenty minutes before a meal. For canker sores, milder chronic ulcer symptoms, or maintenance, the dosage is one or two tablets twenty minutes before meals. Taking DGL after meals is associated with poor results. DGL therapy should be continued for at least eight to sixteen weeks after there is a full therapeutic response.

Overdosage

Overdosage may possibly result in elevation of blood pressure. The amount of glycyrrhetinic acid in an entire bottle of DGL is unlikely to produce the other side effects associated with licorice toxicity (see **licorice**).

Special Populations

Pregnant/breast-feeding women
Considered safe during pregnancy and lactation.

Children
Suitable for children at one-half the adult dosage. Do not self-diagnose an ulcer in children. Consult a physician for proper diagnosis and monitoring.

Seniors
No special precautions are known.

Devil's Claw
(Harpagophytum procumbens)

Used For

Digestive tonic
Effectiveness: C   Safety: C

Gout
Effectiveness: B   Safety: C

Low back pain
Effectiveness: B   Safety: C

Osteoarthritis
Effectiveness: B   Safety: C

General Information

Devil's claw is a plant native to Africa. The name was derived from the plant's unusual fruits, which seem to be covered with numerous small hooks. Devil's claw has a long history of use in the treatment of digestive disturbances, arthritis, inflammation, and pain. Recent clinical studies indicate that it may be helpful in patients with gout, low back pain, and osteoarthritis.

In the treatment of gout, devil's claw has been shown to reduce joint pain as well as reduce uric acid levels. In the treatment of low back pain, double-blind studies indicate that using devil's claw extracts can reduce the need for stronger medication.

In osteoarthritis, devil's claw use was associated with significant improvements in "sign and symptoms" (pain) in a double-blind study comparing it to a standard arthritis drug.

Available Forms

The root is the portion of the plant used for medicinal purposes. Devil's claw root is available in bulk, capsules, and tablets as well as in tinctures, fluid extracts, and dry powder extracts (for use in tablets and capsules). Dry powder extracts standardized for harpagoside content are the preferred form because of the tremendous variability of harpagoside content with other forms.

Cautions and Warnings

Do not use devil's claw if you are taking anticoagulant drugs such as warfarin (Coumadin).

Possible Side Effects

Since devil's claw may promote the secretion of stomach acid, it may produce mild gastric irritation and probably should not be used by people with gastric or duodenal ulcers.

Drug Interactions

May reduce the need for pain-relieving medications such as tramadol in cases of low back pain.

May increase the effectiveness of anticoagulant drugs such as warfarin (Coumadin), leading to excessive bleeding.

May increase the bleeding tendency in patients taking antiplatelet drugs such as ticlopidine (Ticlid).

Food and Nutrient Interactions

None known, but devil's claw is generally recommended to be taken on an empty stomach.

Usual Dosage

The usual dosage is the equivalent of 3 to 6 g daily
of the dried root between meals. This dosage corresponds to 6 to 12 ml daily of a fluid extract or 15 to
30 ml daily of a tincture. For the standardized extract, the dosage is based upon delivering 50 to 100
mg of harpagoside daily.

Overdosage

None known.

Special Populations

Pregnant/breast-feeding women
As the effects of taking devil's claw during pregnancy and lactation have not been sufficiently evaluated, it should not be used during these times.

Children
Suitable for children at one-half the adult dosage.

Seniors
No special precautions are known.

Dong Quai *(Angelica sinensis)*

Used For

Allergies
Effectiveness: C   Safety: C

Menopause
Effectiveness: C   Safety: C

Menstrual cramps
Effectiveness: C   Safety: C

General Information

The authentic and original dong quai is *Angelica sinensis.* While at least nine other angelica species are available, dong quai is by far the most highly regarded. For several thousand years, dong quai has been cultivated for medicinal use in the treatment of a wide variety of disorders, in particular those of women. It is often referred to as the "female ginseng." Besides being grown for their medicinal action, in the United States and Europe angelica species are cultivated for use as a flavoring agent. With all species, the root is the most extensively used portion of the plant.

Angelica species have been used throughout the world in the treatment of a wide variety of conditions. At this time dong quai appears most potentially useful in the treatment of painful menstrual cramps, menopausal symptoms such as hot flashes, and allergies. Further human research is needed to document the degree of clinical efficacy and safety of dong quai. One double-blind study of the relief of menopausal symptoms with dong quai failed to show any benefit.

Available Forms

The root is the portion of dong quai used for medicinal purposes. The crude root is available in bulk, capsules, and tablets; other forms available include tinctures, fluid extracts, and dry extracts in tablets and capsules.

Cautions and Warnings

Dong quai should not be used by people on the anticoagulant drug warfarin (Coumadin).

Possible Side Effects

Dong quai is generally considered to be of extremely low toxicity, and side effects are rare. However, it does contain many substances that can react with sunlight to cause a rash or sunburn, so theoretically this could be a possible side effect. There has also been one case report of a man who developed gynecomastia (breast enlargement) after taking a concentrated extract of dong quai.

Drug Interactions

Dong quai has been shown to potentiate the anticoagulant effect of the drug warfarin (Coumadin), leading to increased bleeding time. It should not be used by people taking this drug.

Food and Nutrient Interactions

None known.

Usual Dosage

Dong quai is usually taken in one of the following forms three times daily:

Powdered root or as tea: 1–2 g
Tincture (1:5): 2–4 ml (½ –1 teaspoon)
Fluid extract: 1–2 ml (¼ – ½ teaspoon)
Dry extract (standardized to contain 0.8–1.1 percent
    ligustilide): 150–200 mg

Overdosage

None known.

Special Populations

Pregnant/breast-feeding women
As the effects of dong quai during pregnancy and lactation have not been sufficiently evaluated, it should not be used during these times.

Children
Suitable for children at one-half the adult dosage.

Seniors
No special precautions are known.

Echinacea *(Echinacea spp.)*

Used For

Common cold
Effectiveness: B+   Safety: A

Infections and enhancing the immune system
Effectiveness: B+   Safety: A

General Description

Echinacea (purple coneflower) is a perennial herb native to midwestern North America, from Saskatchewan to Texas. Of the nine echinacea species, *E. angustifolia, E. purpurea,* and *E. pallida* are the most commonly used. Although studies have shown certain echinacea species (or components found in higher concentrations in those species) to be more effective than others, each commercial species has its advantages and disadvantages. There is no clear-cut best species at this time, nor is it known if preparations from the root are better than preparations derived from the aboveground (aerial) portion.

Echinacea has been the subject of over 350 scientific studies examining its immune-enhancing and infection-fighting properties. The overwhelming majority of the clinical studies have utilized **EchinaGuard,** an extract of the juice of the aerial portion of *E. purpurea* along with 22 percent ethanol (for preservation), or **Esberitox,** an extract from the roots of *E. purpurea* and *E. pallida* along with extracts of *Baptisia tinctoria* root and *Thuja occidentalis* leaves. In these studies, both preparations have demonstrated significant immune-enhancing and wound-healing properties. Echinacea components have also been shown to activate white blood cells and promote enhanced function. Clinical studies have demonstrated effectiveness in a number of infectious conditions. In general, echinacea appears to offer benefit for all infectious conditions, especially the common cold and upper respiratory tract infections.

Although not all studies with echinacea preparations in the treatment of the common cold have had positive results, the majority have suggested that echinacea displays an ability to reduce the duration and severity of symptoms. More controversial is the ability of echinacea to prevent the common cold. The research in this application is split; some studies show benefit, others do not. The most recent studies suggest that echinacea is not effective for the prevention of colds and flu in most healthy individuals. The people most likely to benefit from echinacea as a preventive measure are those with weaker immune systems who are more prone to infection.

Available Forms

Echinacea products are available in many different forms: crude plant in either ground or powdered form, freeze-dried, alcohol-based tinctures and liquid extracts, aqueous tinctures and liquid extracts, and dry powdered extracts. Although there is no consensus, many experts consider the fresh-pressed juice of *E. purpurea* the best preparation because it provides the greatest range of active compounds and has the greatest level of clinical support.

Brands on which research has been done include EchinaGuard, Esberitox, and Echinamide.

Cautions and Warnings

Echinacea should not be used by people with AIDS or HIV infection until more research has been done, as echinacea use may stimulate replication of the virus.

Allergic reactions have been reported in people who are allergic to other members of plants in the *Compositae* family (daisies, ragweed, marigolds, etc.)

Since echinacea can enhance immune function, it must not be used in people who have had organ transplants or who are taking drugs such as cyclophosphamide to purposely suppress the immune system.

People with autoimmune diseases such as rheumatoid arthritis, lupus, and multiple sclerosis should avoid long-term use of echinacea.

Possible Side Effects

Echinacea use is usually without side effects; however, allergic reactions have been reported in people who are allergic to other members of plants in the *Compositae* family.

Drug Interactions

Theoretically, echinacea may interfere with drugs that are purposely used to suppress the immune system, such as cyclophosphamide, which is used in patients who have had organ transplants to prevent the immune system from rejecting the transplanted organ.

Food and Nutrient Interactions

Generally recommended to be taken on an empty stomach.

Usual Dosage

The following recommendations are for the use of echinacea as a general immune stimulant during infection. Dosages should be given three times daily:

Dried root (or as tea): 1–2 g
Freeze-dried plant: 325–650 mg
Juice of aerial portion of E. purpurea *stabilized in 22 percent ethanol:* 2–3 ml (½ – ¾ teaspoon)
Tincture (1:5): 3–4 ml (¾ –1 teaspoon)

Fluid extract (1:1): 1–2 ml (¼ – ½ teaspoon)
Solid extract (6.5:1 or 3.5 percent echinacosides): 300 mg

The question of whether echinacea should be used on a long-term or continual basis has not been adequately answered. The usual recommendation for long-term use is eight weeks on followed by one week off.

Overdosage

None known.

Special Populations

Pregnant/breast-feeding women
Considered safe during pregnancy and lactation.

Children
Suitable for children at one-half the adult dosage.

Seniors
No special precautions are known.

EchinaGuard (*see* Echinacea)

General Information

EchinaGuard is perhaps the world's best-selling and most extensively researched echinacea product. It is made from the freshly pressed juice of the aboveground portion of *Echinacea purpurea.* It is among the oldest echinacea products in the world, having been developed by the German physician Gerhard Madaus in the 1930s. EchinaGuard has been the subject of over two hundred scientific studies and has been the product used in the vast majority of chemical, scientific, and clinical studies on single echinacea preparations. EchinaGuard is available in liquid form as well as capsules and tablets.

Elderberry *(Sambucus nigra)*

Used For

Common cold
Effectiveness: B+   Safety: A

Infections and enhancing the immune system
Effectiveness: B+   Safety: A

General Information

Numerous species of elderberry grow in Europe and North America, but only those with blue-black berries are medicinal because of their particular flavonoid components. Elderberry has been a popular flu and common cold remedy since the time of the Romans. Recent research has demonstrated that elderberry juice not only stimulates the immune system but also directly inhibits the influenza virus. In clinical trials, patients with influenza who took elderberry juice syrup (Sambucol) reported faster termination of symptoms. Twenty percent reported significant improvement within twenty-four hours, 70 percent felt better by forty-eight hours, and 90 percent claimed a complete cure after three days. Patients receiving the placebo required six days for recovery. Researchers found that the patients who took the elderberry preparation also had higher levels of antibodies against the flu virus.

Available Forms

Elderberry extracts and syrups are available in liquid form, tablets, and capsules. Brand names available include Sambucol. Elderberry flowers and dried berries are also available in bulk to make tea.

Cautions and Warnings

None known.

Possible Side Effects

None known.

Drug Interactions

None known.

Food and Nutrient Interactions

None known.

Usual Dosage

Liquid elderberry extract (e.g., Sambucol) is taken in amounts of 5 ml (for children) to 10 ml (for adults) twice per day. A tea made from 3–5 g of the dried flowers steeped in 250 ml (1 cup) boiling water for ten to fifteen minutes may also be drunk three times per day.

Overdosage

None known.

Special Populations

Pregnant/breast-feeding women
Considered safe during pregnancy and lactation.

Children
Suitable for children at one-half the adult dosage.

Seniors
No special precautions are known.

Ephedra *(Ephedra sinica)*

Used For

Asthma and hay fever
Effectiveness: B+   Safety: D

Weight loss aid
Effectiveness: B+   Safety: D

General Information

Ephedra species are erect, branching shrubs found in desert or arid regions throughout the world.

Ephedra sinica (Chinese ephedra or ma huang) is found in Asia; *Ephedra distacha* (European ephedra) is found in Europe; *Ephedra trifurca* or *Ephedra viridis* (desert tea), *Ephedra nevadensis* (Mormon tea), and *Ephedra americana* (American ephedra) are found in North America; and *Ephedra gerardiana* (Pakistani ephedra) is found primarily in India and Pakistan. The portion of the plant typically used for medicinal effects is the aboveground (aerial) portion.

The most popular ephedra species is *Ephedra sinica* (ma huang). Its medicinal use in China began before 2800 B.C. The pharmacology of ephedra centers on its content of alkaloids such as ephedrine and pseudoephedrine. Ephedrine and pseudoephedrine have been extensively investigated and are widely used in prescription and over-the-counter medications for asthma, hay fever, and the common cold.

Ephedrine's basic action is similar to that of epinephrine (adrenaline), although ephedrine is much less active. Like epinephrine, ephedrine will also increase heart rate and blood pressure as well as increase heart, brain, and muscle blood flow at the expense of blood flow to the kidneys and intestines. Ephedrine also differs from epinephrine in its ability to be absorbed orally, its longer duration of action, and its more pronounced effect on the brain. The effects of ephedrine on the brain are similar to those of amphetamines, but again much less potent. Pseudoephedrine is more popular than ephedrine now in OTC preparations because its effects on the brain and cardiovascular system are much less stimulatory than those of ephedrine.

Preparations containing ephedra provide naturally occurring ephedrine and pseudoephedrine. In *Ephedra sinica* the total alkaloid content is typically 1–3 percent, composed primarily of ephedrine, pseudoephedrine, and norpseudoephedrine. Interestingly, Mormon tea or *Ephedra nevadensis* contains no ephedrine.

Ephedra is used alone or in combination with other herbs in the treatment of asthma, hay fever, and the common cold, and as a weight loss aid.

Asthma and hay fever

Ephedrine is an effective treatment for mild to moderate asthma and hay fever. It is effective because it promotes the relaxation of bronchial muscles and the inhibition of the allergic response. The peak effect of ephedrine occurs one hour after administration and lasts about five hours total. The old-time herbal treatment of asthma involves the use of ephedra in combination with herbal expectorants. Expectorants modify the quality and quantity of secretions from the respiratory tract, allowing the user to cough up the secretions and ultimately improving respiratory tract function. Examples of commonly used expectorants include licorice *(Glycyrrhiza glabra)*, grindelia *(Grindelia camporum)*, euphorbia *(Euphorbia hirta)*, sundew *(Drosera rotundifolia)*, and senega *(Polygala senega)*.

Weight loss aid

Ephedra may be useful as a weight loss aid on its own, but it is usually combined with natural sources of caffeine. Ephedrine suppresses appetite, but its main mechanism for promoting weight loss appears to be by increasing the metabolic rate of adipose (fat) tissue. Its weight-reducing effects are greatest in those individuals with a low basal metabolic rate and/or decreased diet-induced thermogenesis. (See **ephedra-caffeine combinations**.)

Available Forms

Ephedra is available as the crude herb, tea bags, fluid extracts, and dry extracts. Since the optimal dosage of ephedra depends on the ephedrine content, preparations standardized for ephedrine may produce more dependable results. These preparations are usually available in tablets or capsules.

Cautions and Warnings

The U.S. Food and Drug Administration advisory review panel on nonprescription drugs has recommended that ephedrine not be taken by patients with heart disease, high blood pressure, thyroid disease, diabetes, or difficulty in urination due to enlargement of the prostate gland, or by those taking blood pressure medications or antidepressant drugs. These warnings are appropriate for ephedra preparations as well.

Possible Side Effects

Ephedra can produce the same side effects as ephedrine: increased blood pressure, increased heart rate, insomnia, and anxiety. It is recommended that individuals using ephedrine-containing herbal formulas monitor their heart rate (pulse) along with their blood pressure and discontinue use if there is an increase in blood pressure (the normal value is 120/80 mm Hg) or resting pulse (the normal value is 72 beats per minute).

Drug Interactions

Ephedrine should not be used with monoamine oxidase inhibitors (MAOIs) such as furazolidone, isocarboxazid, moclobemide, nialamide, pargyline, phenelzine, selegiline, or tranylcypromide. Also, it should not be used during the first fourteen days after the discontinuation of an MAOI. Acetazolamide, dichlorphenamide, and sodium bicarbonate may cause increased blood levels of ephedrine, thereby potentiating its effect.

Ephedrine should not be used along with halothane or cyclopropane, as it may induce cardiac arrhythmia.

Ephedrine will block the blood-pressure-lowering effect of bethanidine, guanethidine, and possibly other blood-pressure-lowering drugs.

Clonidine, midodrine, caffeine, and theophylline increase ephedrine's blood-pressure-elevating effects.

Reserpine decreases the effectiveness of ephedrine.

Food and Nutrient Interactions

None known.

Usual Dosage

The optimal dosage of ephedra depends on the alkaloid content in the form used. The average total alkaloid content of *Ephedra sinica* is 1–3 percent. When used in the treatment of asthma or as a weight loss aid, the ephedra dose should have an ephedrine content of 12.5–25.0 mg and be taken two to three times daily. For the crude herb, a dosage equal to this ephedrine content would be 500–1,000 mg two to three times per day.

Overdosage

Do the following in case of accidental overdose: If the victim is unconscious or having convulsions, call for an ambulance immediately. If you take the victim to an emergency room, be sure to bring the bottle or container with you. If the victim is conscious, call your local poison control center or a health care professional. The poison control center may suggest inducing vomiting with ipecac syrup (available without a prescription at any pharmacy). *Do not* induce vomiting unless specifically instructed to do so.

Special Populations

Pregnant/breast-feeding women
Not recommended during pregnancy and lactation.

Children
Children under twelve years of age should not use ephedra without medical supervision.

Seniors
No special precautions are known.

Ephedrine (*see* Ephedra [*Ephedra sinica*])

General Information

Ephedrine is the chief alkaloid of ephedra (*Ephedra sinica,* also known as ma huang). Western medicine's

interest in ephedrine and its sister compound, pseudoephedrine, began in 1923 when it was discovered
to possess a number of useful effects in the treatment of asthma, allergies, and the common cold.
Ephedrine was first synthesized in 1927, and since
this time both ephedrine and pseudoephedrine
have been used extensively in over-the-counter cold
and allergy medications. Preparations containing
ephedra provide naturally occurring ephedrine and
pseudoephedrine.

Ephedrine-Caffeine Combinations

Used For

Weight loss
Effectiveness: A   Safety: D

General Information

Ephedrine in combination with caffeine-containing
herbs is a very popular herbal supplement to promote weight loss. The combination produces better
results than either substance can produce on its
own. Ephedrine is found in *Ephedra sinica* (ma
huang); caffeine sources include coffee *(Coffea arabica),* tea *(Camellia sinensis),* cola nut *(Cola nitida),*
and guarana *(Paullinea cupana).*

Ephedrine-caffeine combinations work to promote weight loss by stimulating thermogenesis. A
certain amount of ingested food is converted immediately to heat. This process is known as diet-

induced thermogenesis. The activity of diet-induced thermogenesis is thought to play a major role in determining whether an individual is likely to be lean or obese. In lean individuals, a meal may stimulate up to a 40 percent increase in thermogenesis. In contrast, obese individuals often display a 10 percent or less increase in thermogenesis, as the food energy is stored instead of converted to heat. On their own, ephedrine and caffeine can increase the metabolic rate and thermogenesis, but when they are combined there is an additive effect.

Numerous double-blind studies have documented the thermogenic and weight-loss-promoting effects of ephedrine-caffeine combinations. In one of the largest studies, 180 overweight patients were treated by diet and either an ephedrine-caffeine combination (20mg/200mg), ephedrine (20 mg), caffeine (200 mg), or placebo three times a day for twenty-four weeks. Mean weight losses were significantly greater in the group given the ephedrine-caffeine combination. The ephedrine-caffeine group lost a total of thirty-six pounds in twenty-four weeks, compared to twenty-nine pounds for the placebo group. In the groups receiving ephedrine or caffeine only, weight loss was similar to that of the placebo group. Other studies have shown that ephedrine-caffeine combinations are able to promote the beneficial effect of reducing body fat stores while preserving lean body tissue (muscle).

The effectiveness of ephedrine-caffeine combinations in promoting weight is offset by potential problems with safety and side effects. At appropriate dosages, ephedrine-caffeine combinations can be used safely by most people, but they should not be used at higher dosages unless directly supervised by a physician. Nor should they be used in conditions where ephedrine and caffeine are not

indicated (see "Cautions and Warnings"), or by anyone who is overly sensitive to stimulants.

Available Forms

Herbal preparations containing ephedrine and caffeine are available in various forms—crude mixtures, teas, fluid extracts, and solid extracts. Since
the optimal dosage of the crude plant preparation or
extract depends on the content of active ingredient,
preparations standardized for ephedrine and caffeine may produce more dependable results. These
preparations are usually available in tablets or capsules.

Brand names available include Metabolife 356.

Cautions and Warnings

The U.S. Food and Drug Administration advisory review panel on nonprescription drugs has recommended that ephedrine not be taken by patients
with heart disease, high blood pressure, thyroid disease, diabetes, or difficulty in urination due to enlargement of the prostate gland. Nor should they be
taken by anyone on antihypertensive or antidepressant drugs. These warnings are appropriate for
ephedra preparations as well.

Possible Side Effects

Anxiety, nervousness, nausea, heart palpitations,
sweating, increased blood pressure, increased heart
rate, dizziness, and difficulty falling asleep are common side effects. It is recommended that individuals
using ephedrine-containing herbal formulas monitor their heart rate (pulse) along with their blood

pressure and discontinue use if there is an increase in blood pressure (the normal value is 120/80 mm Hg) or resting pulse (the normal value is 72 beats per minute).

Drug Interactions

The same drug interactions noted for ephedrine and caffeine are important with ephedrine-caffeine combinations. Ephedrine-caffeine combinations should not be used along with monoamine oxidase inhibitors (MAOIs) such as furazolidone, isocarboxazid, moclobemide, nialamide, pargyline, phenelzine, selegiline, or tranylcypromide. Nor should they be used during the first fourteen days after the discontinuation of an MAOI.

Acetazolamide, dichlorphenamide, and sodium bicarbonate may cause increased blood levels of ephedrine, thereby potentiating its effect.

Ephedrine-caffeine combinations should not be used along with halothane or cyclopropane, as they may induce cardiac arrhythmias.

Ephedrine-caffeine combinations will block the blood-pressure-lowering effect of bethanidine, guanethidine, and possibly other blood pressure-lowering drugs.

The blood-pressure-elevating effects of ephedrine-caffeine combinations are increased by clonidine, midodrine, and oxilofrine.

Reserpine decreases the effectiveness of ephedrine-caffeine combinations.

Food and Nutrient Interactions

None known.

Usual Dosage

Although some studies have used a daily dosage of 60 mg of ephedrine and 600 mg of caffeine, these high dosages may not be necessary. A daily dosage of 22 mg ephedrine and 80 mg of caffeine has been shown to produce equally good results with fewer side effects and is deemed by many authorities to be a more appropriate dosage for unsupervised use.

Overdosage

Do the following in case of accidental overdose: If the victim is unconscious or having convulsions, call for an ambulance immediately. If you take the victim to an emergency room, be sure to bring the bottle or container with you. If the victim is conscious, call your local poison control center or a health care professional. The poison control center may suggest inducing vomiting with ipecac syrup (available without a prescription at any pharmacy). *Do not* induce vomiting unless specifically instructed to do so.

Special Populations

Pregnant/breast-feeding women
Not recommended during pregnancy and lactation.

Children
As the effects of ephedrine-caffeine combinations in children have not been sufficiently evaluated, they should not be used by children under twelve years of age without medical supervision.

Seniors
No special precautions are known.

Esberitox

Used For

Common cold
Effectiveness: A   Safety: A

Enhancement of immune system
Effectiveness: A   Safety: A

General Information

Esberitox contains standardized extracts of the roots from two species of echinacea *(E. purpurea and E. pallida)* and extracts of *Thuja occidentalis* and *Baptisia tinctoria*—two other herbal medicines valued for their immune-enhancing activity. Esberitox has solid scientific studies showing it to be beneficial during infections, including the common cold.

In one of the studies researchers noted that Esberitox not only reduced the duration and severity of the common cold but also provided prophylaxis against recurrences. In the double-blind study, fifty patients were treated with Esberitox (two tablets three times daily) and fifty patients were given placebo. After three days, patients treated with Esberitox showed a significant improvement in all major symptoms (exhaustion, nasal congestion, and sore throat), while the placebo group experienced a slight worsening of symptoms. While twelve patients in the placebo group experienced a relapse, only three patients taking Esberitox experienced a relapse.

In addition to positive studies in adults, clinical studies have shown Esberitox to be quite effective in preventing colds, flu, and ear infections in children in day care.

Available Forms

Esberitox is available in small chewable tablets.

Cautions and Warnings

None known.

Possible Side Effects

None known.

Drug Interactions

Esberitox has been shown to enhance the effects of antibiotic therapy in eliminating infections by preventing antibiotic-induced suppression of the immune system.

Food and Nutrient Interactions

None known.

Usual Dosage

Adults and children over six years of age: two or three tablets three times daily. Children two to six years of age: one or two tablets three times daily. For children less than two years of age: one tablet three times daily.

Overdosage

None known.

Special Populations

Pregnant/breast-feeding women
Considered safe during pregnancy and lactation.

Children
Suitable for children at one-half the adult dosage.

Seniors
No special precautions are known.

Essic

Used For

Cancer
Effectiveness: C   Safety: C

General Information

Essic is a powdered mixture of burdock root *(Arctium lappa)*, turkey rhubarb root *(Saxifraga peltata)*, sheep sorrel *(Rumex acetosella)*, and slippery elm bark *(Ulmus fulva)* made popular by the Canadian nurse René Caisse *(Essic* is *Caisse* spelled backward). The formula for the herbal remedy was given to Caisse in 1922 by a hospital patient whose breast cancer had been healed by an Ontario Indian medicine man. Caisse reportedly used the formula to successfully treat thousands of cancer patients from the 1920s until her death in 1978 at the age of ninety. However, despite the formula's popularity, there have been no formal clinical trials. Essic was reportedly tested in animals at both Memorial Sloan-Kettering Cancer Center and the U.S. National Cancer Institute and was found to have no significant activity.

Available Forms

Essiac is available in powder form in plastic bottles.

Cautions and Warnings

Cancer is a serious disease. If you are being treated for cancer, do not self-medicate with Essiac or any other substance without informing your supervising physician.

Possible Side Effects

None known.

Drug Interactions

None known.

Food and Nutrient Interactions

Generally recommended to be taken on an empty stomach.

Usual Dosage

The recommended dosage of the tea made from Essiac is 60 ml (approximately 2 fluid ounces) morning and evening for fourteen days. Thereafter, take 30 ml (approximately 1 fluid ounce) morning and evening. After three months, the dosage may be dropped to 1 fluid ounce daily or every other day.

Here are the guidelines for making the tea:

1. Add 1 bottle of powder to 1.6 liters (approximately 56 fluid ounces) of water in a covered vessel. Bottled, distilled, and tap water are equally acceptable.
2. Bring to a boil and keep at a gentle boil for ten minutes, stirring occasionally.
3. Remove from heat, keep covered, and let stand for four hours.
4. Gently boil again for five minutes in the covered vessel, stirring occasionally.
5. Remove from heat and let stand overnight in the refrigerator in a tall narrow vessel, so that the sediment can settle out.
6. Carefully pour off the liquid into a clean glass or plastic container and store in the refrigerator. A small amount of sediment may be present in the final product.
7. Shake gently before use.

Overdosage

None known.

Special Populations

Pregnant/breast-feeding women
Not recommended during pregnancy and lactation.

Children
Suitable for children at one-half the adult dosage.

Seniors
No special precautions are known.

Fenugreek Seed Powder
(Trigonella foenum-graecum)

Used For

Diabetes
Effectiveness: B+   Safety: C

Elevated cholesterol levels
Effectiveness: B+   Safety: C

General Information

Fenugreek seeds *(Trigonella foenum-graecum)* are a rich source of fiber (50 percent), especially gel-forming fiber (20 percent). Like other **fiber** sources, defatted fenugreek seed powder has demonstrated significant effects in lowering blood cholesterol, triglycerides, and blood sugar. However, nonfiber components such as saponins and amino acids are thought to contribute to these effects as well. Defatted fenugreek seed powder given to diabetics has produced 25 percent drops in fasting blood sugar measurements in clinical trials; given to people with elevated blood lipids, it has shown the ability to lower total cholesterol levels by 24 percent, LDL cholesterol by 32 percent, and triglyceride levels by 37 percent.

Available Forms

Defatted fenugreek seed powder is available as a powder, similar to other sources of fiber.

Cautions and Warnings

If you·are a diabetic taking insulin or oral drugs to control blood sugar levels, taking defatted fenugreek seed powder may result in the need to change your dosage. Consult your physician.

Possible Side Effects

None known.

Drug Interactions

Fenugreek seed powder may interact with insulin or oral drugs to control blood sugar levels because of its ability to improve blood sugar levels in diabetics. Monitoring of blood sugar levels is recommended if taking fenugreek seed powder. Consult your physician if you are on insulin or an oral hypoglycemic drug such as metformin (Glucophage) or glyburide (Micronase, Diabeta).

Food and Nutrient Interactions

Fenugreek seed powder and other fiber supplements may reduce the absorption of minerals, including calcium, magnesium, zinc, and copper. Take fenugreek seed powder several hours before or after mineral supplements.

Usual Dosage

The dosages typically used in the studies with defatted fenugreek seed powder have been 25 to 50 mg twice daily.

Overdosage

None known.

Special Populations

Pregnant/breast-feeding women
Considered safe during pregnancy and lactation.

Children
Suitable for children at one-half the adult dosage.

Seniors
No special precautions are known.

Feverfew
(Tanacetum parthenium)

Used For

Migraine headaches
Effectiveness: B-   Safety: B

Rheumatoid arthritis
Effectiveness: C   Safety: B

General Information

Feverfew is a member of the sunflower family that grows in flower gardens throughout Europe and the United States. Its name is a corruption of the word *febrifuge*—the term given to a substance that can lower a fever. Feverfew has been used for centuries not only as a febrifuge, but also in the treatment of migraines and rheumatoid arthritis. Only the use in migraine headaches shows much promise.

Migraine headache

Feverfew appears to work in the treatment and prevention of migraine headaches by inhibiting the release of blood-vessel-dilating substances from platelets (serotonin and histamine), inhibiting the production of inflammatory substances (leukotrienes, serine proteases, etc.), and reestablishing proper blood vessel tone. Results from clinical studies show mostly a positive effect in preventing migraine attacks, but there is some controversy regarding the most effective form (discussed below). Treatment with feverfew has been associated with a reduction in the mean number and severity of attacks and in the degree of vomiting.

Rheumatoid arthritis

Feverfew has historically been used in the treatment of rheumatoid arthritis. While there are some experimental studies in animals that indicate a potential benefit in humans with rheumatoid arthritis, there is no clinical study to date that shows any real benefit with feverfew. In fact, in one double-blind study there was no apparent benefit from oral feverfew in the treatment of rheumatoid arthritis. However, this study has been criticized because the dosage used was extremely small (76 mg of dried powdered feverfew leaf per day), the level of parthenolide (a key component of feverfew) was not determined in the product, and the patients continued to take their medications (nonsteroidal anti-inflammatory drugs such as aspirin, ibuprofen, piroxicam, etc.) even though it has been suggested that this reduces the efficacy of feverfew. Therefore,

it is safe to conclude that the benefit of feverfew in
rheumatoid arthritis has not yet been determined
one way or another.

Available Forms

The leaves are the portions of the plant used for medicinal purposes. Dried feverfew leaves are available
in bulk, capsules, and tablets; also available are tinctures, fluid extracts, and dry extracts in tablets and
capsules. Freeze-dried feverfew leaves are also
available in capsules and tablets.

The effectiveness of feverfew may be greater if fresh
or freeze-dried preparations are used. Also, the product should provide adequate levels of parthenolide, the
active principle. The majority of the products on the
market may not be effective. A study conducted by the
Canadian government indicated that more than thirty-
five different commercial preparations varied widely in
the amount of parthenolide, with the majority of products containing no parthenolide or only traces.

Cautions and Warnings

None known.

Possible Side Effects

No side effects have been reported from the clinical
studies with feverfew in pill form. However, chewing
the leaves may result in aphthous ulcerations
(canker sores).

Drug Interactions

None known.

Food and Nutrient Interactions

None known.

Usual Dosage

Studies suggest that the effective daily dosage of parthenolide for prevention of migraine headache is roughly 0.25–0.5 mg. A higher dose (1–2 g) is necessary during an acute attack.

Overdosage

None known.

Special Populations

Pregnant/breast-feeding women
The effects of feverfew during pregnancy and lactation have not been sufficiently evaluated, so it should not be used during these times.

Children
Suitable for children at one-half the adult dosage.

Seniors
No special precautions are known.

Garcinia *(Garcinia cambogia)*

Used For

Weight loss
Effectiveness: D   Safety: B

General Information

Garcinia fruit, also known as the Malabar tamarind or Brindall berry, is yellowish and about the size of an orange, with a thin skin and deep furrows similar to an acorn squash. It is native to south India, where it is dried and used extensively in curries. It has also been used historically in the Ayurvedic system of medicine for the treatment of obesity. The active component is hydroxycitric acid (HCA). Typically, the dried fruit contains 20 to 30 percent HCA, while most commercial preparations are extracts that contain about 50 percent HCA.

Although preliminary research suggested that HCA could promote weight loss, the most recent double-blind study demonstrated that a garcinia extract containing 50 percent HCA at a dosage of 1,000 mg three times daily did not demonstrate any weight-loss-promoting effect.

Available Forms

Garcinia extract is available in tablet, capsule, and powder form. Brand names available include Citri-Max.

Cautions and Warnings

None known at this time.

Possible Side Effects

None known.

Drug Interactions

None known.

Food and Nutrient Interactions

None known.

Usual Dosage

Typically the dosage recommended for the 50 percent HCA garcinia extract is 1,000 mg three times daily.

Overdosage

None known.

Special Populations

Pregnant/breast-feeding women

As the effects of garcinia during pregnancy and lactation have not been sufficiently evaluated, it should not be used during these times.

Children

The use of garcinia in children has not been established, although historical use suggests that it is safe and suitable for children at one-half the adult dosage.

Seniors
No special precautions are known.

Garlic (Allium sativum)

Used For

Cancer prevention
Effectiveness: B   Safety: A

High blood pressure
Effectiveness: A   Safety: A

High cholesterol
Effectiveness: A   Safety: A

Infection
Effectiveness: B   Safety: A

Inhibition of platelet aggregation
Effectiveness: A   Safety: A

General Information

Garlic is well known to all for its culinary and medicinal qualities. The pungent odor of garlic is caused mainly by allicin, which is formed when the enzyme alliinase reacts with the compound alliin. The essential oil of garlic yields approximately 60 percent of its weight in allicin after exposure to alliinase. Because the enzyme is inactivated by heat, cooked garlic produces less odor than raw garlic

and is not nearly as powerful in its medicinal effects.
Some manufacturers have developed highly sophisticated methods in an effort to provide the full benefits of garlic—they provide "odorless" garlic
products concentrated for alliin because alliin is relatively odorless until it is converted to allicin in the
body.

Cancer prevention

Human population studies show that regular garlic consumption is associated with a reduced risk of
certain cancers (e.g., esophageal, stomach, and
colon cancer). Animal and test tube studies also
show that garlic and its sulfur compounds inhibit
the formation of cancer-causing compounds and tumors. Additional research is needed to confirm
these effects in humans.

High blood pressure

Results from eight double-blind studies with a
commercial preparation (Kwai) that is standardized
to contain 1.3 percent alliin demonstrated a reduction in blood pressure at a dosage of 900 mg per
day—about 11 mm Hg for the systolic measure and
5 mm Hg for the diastolic measure.

High cholesterol

According to the results of numerous double-
blind studies in patients with initial cholesterol levels greater than 200 mg/dl, supplementation with
900 mg per day of a commercial preparation (Kwai)
standardized to contain 1.3 percent alliin can lower
total serum cholesterol levels by about 10 to 12 percent. In addition, LDL cholesterol will decrease by
about 15 percent, HDL cholesterol levels will usually
increase by about 10 percent, and triglyceride levels
will typically drop 15 percent.

Infection

Garlic exerts broad-spectrum antimicrobial activity against many species of bacteria, virus, worms, and fungi. It also displays some immune-enhancing effects. These findings seem to support the historical use of garlic in the treatment of a variety of infectious conditions, but there is little in the area of clinical research in this area.

Inhibition of platelet aggregation

Excessive platelet aggregation (clumping) is linked very strongly to atherosclerosis, heart disease, and strokes. Garlic preparations standardized for alliin content, as well as garlic oil, have been shown to inhibit platelet aggregation. In one study, 120 patients with increased platelet aggregation were given either 900 mg per day of a commercial garlic preparation standardized to contain 1.3 percent alliin (Kwai) or a placebo for four weeks. In the garlic group, spontaneous platelet aggregation disappeared and microcirculation in the skin increased by 47.6 percent—a sign of improved blood flow.

Available Forms

Garlic preparations are available in many different forms. It appears that preparations standardized for alliin content or total allicin potential provide the greatest assurance of quality. The majority of studies showing a positive effect of garlic and garlic preparations have used products that deliver a sufficient dosage of allicin. Studies using inferior garlic preparations and garlic oil rarely show the benefits noted with high-quality garlic preparations.

Since allicin is the component in garlic that is responsible for its odor, some manufacturers have de-

veloped highly sophisticated methods in an effort to
provide the full benefits of garlic—they provide
"odorless" garlic products concentrated for alliin,
because alliin is relatively odorless until it is converted to allicin in the body. Products concentrated
for alliin and other sulfur components provide all of
the benefits of fresh garlic but are more socially acceptable. The commercial product should provide a
daily dose of at least 8 mg of alliin or a total allicin
potential of 4,000 mcg. This amount is equal to approximately 1 clove (4 g) of fresh garlic.

Brand names available include Kwai, Garlique,
and Garlicin.

Cautions and Warnings

Do not use garlic for at least three days prior to any
surgical procedure, as it can inhibit platelet aggregation and lead to increased postoperative bleeding.

Possible Side Effects

Garlic preparations taken orally, even "odorless"
products, can produce a garlic odor on the breath
and through the skin. Gastrointestinal irritation and
nausea are the most frequent side effects.

Drug Interactions

Theoretically, garlic preparations may potentiate
the effects of the blood-thinning drug warfarin
(Coumadin) as well as enhance the antiplatelet effects of drugs such as aspirin and ticlopidine (Ticlid).

Garlic may increase the effectiveness of drugs that
lower blood sugar levels in the treatment of non-
insulin-dependent diabetes (type 2 diabetes) such as

glyburide (Diabeta, Micronase). Consult a physician to discuss proper monitoring of blood sugar levels before taking a garlic product.

Food and Nutrient Interactions

None known.

Usual Dosage

Based on a great deal of clinical research, a daily dose of at least 8 mg alliin or a total allicin potential of 4,000 mcg is needed to produce meaningful reductions in cholesterol and blood pressure. This dosage equates to roughly one to four cloves of fresh garlic.

Overdosage

Prolonged feeding of large amounts of raw garlic to rats results in anemia, weight loss, and failure to grow. Although the exact toxicity of garlic has yet to be definitively determined, side effects are rare at the dosage recommended above.

Special Populations

Pregnant/breast-feeding women
Considered safe during pregnancy and lactation at recommended dosage levels.

Children
Suitable for children at one-half the adult dosage.

Seniors
No special precautions are known.

Ginger *(Zingiber officinale)*

Used For

Arthritis
Effectiveness: B   Safety: A

Migraine headaches
Effectiveness: B   Safety: A

Motion sickness
Effectiveness: B+   Safety: A

Nausea and vomiting
Effectiveness: B–   Safety: A

Nausea and vomiting during pregnancy
Effectiveness: B+   Safety: B

General Information

The rhizome of ginger is widely used as a condiment for its unique flavor, but it has important medicinal effects as well. Like many other culinary herbs and spices such as garlic and onions, ginger provides many health-promoting effects. Historically, the majority of complaints for which ginger was used concerned the gastrointestinal system. This historical use has been validated by recent studies demonstrating positive effects in the treatment of motion sickness, nausea and vomiting during pregnancy, and drug-induced and postoperative nausea and vomiting. Preliminary human studies have also shown a positive effect in arthritis and migraine headaches.

In experimental studies, ginger and various ginger components have been shown to have numerous

beneficial properties, the most relevant being antioxidant effects, inhibition of the production of compounds that mediate inflammation, and cholesterol-
lowering action. It also has a number of effects on the
gastrointestinal system, including improving the output of bile and helping improve the tone and function
of the small and large intestines.

Migraine headaches

There have been a few case reports of ginger
being helpful in migraine headaches, but this application has not been supported by a formal clinical
trial.

Motion sickness

Ginger was first shown to be effective in treating
motion sickness in a 1982 article that appeared
in the respected medical journal *The Lancet.* Since
this time there have been several follow-up studies
showing positive effects. Unlike anti-motion-
sickness drugs that act primarily on the brain and
inner ear, ginger appears to exert its effects primarily by partially inhibiting the excessive stomach
motility (churning) characteristic of motion sickness.
Although the overall effectiveness of ginger in motion sickness has yet to be determined, it is certainly
a safe recommendation, with some evidence of effectiveness.

Nausea and vomiting

Ginger appears to be somewhat useful in the
treatment of drug-induced and postoperative nausea and vomiting. Conflicting results have been obtained from double-blind studies. In postoperative
nausea, some comparative studies report statistically significant improvement in symptoms compared to placebo and similar efficacy compared to

the drug metoclopramide, although one study reported lack of efficacy (this study, however, also failed to show benefit with the drug droperidol). It appears that ginger is at least as effective as commonly prescribed drugs.

In the relief of drug-induced nausea and vomiting, preliminary results are quite promising. For example, in a small study of eleven cancer patients undergoing chemotherapy, 1,590 mg of dried ginger root powder taken thirty minutes prior to chemotherapy treatment reduced the degree of nausea experienced by at least two-thirds.

Nausea and vomiting during pregnancy

Ginger's ability to help with nausea and vomiting during pregnancy was demonstrated in a study of women with hyperemesis gravidum, the most severe form of nausea and vomiting during pregnancy. This condition usually requires hospitalization. In the study, 250 mg of dried ginger root powder administered four times a day brought about a significant reduction in both the severity of the nausea and the number of attacks of vomiting in nineteen of twenty-seven cases studied during early pregnancy (less than twenty weeks). These preliminary clinical results, along with ginger's safety and the relatively small dose required, support the use of ginger to treat in nausea and vomiting in pregnancy. Ginger is becoming a well-accepted prescription even in orthodox obstetrical practices.

Available Forms

Ginger is available dried, freeze-dried, as a tincture, and as various extracts, mostly in capsule or tablet form. Although most studies have used powdered ginger root, fresh (or possibly freeze-dried) ginger root or extracts may yield even better results because they may deliver higher levels of active components.

Cautions and Warnings

None known.

Possible Side Effects

Ginger is usually well tolerated at recommended dosages. At higher dosages (single dosages of 6,000 mg or more) powdered dried ginger has been shown to irritate the lining of the stomach. This action may cause some gastric distress and ultimately could lead to ulcer formation. Therefore, it is recommended that dosages on an empty stomach be less than 6,000 mg.

Drug Interactions

Ginger has been shown in some studies to lessen nausea due to chemotherapy drugs and anesthesia.

Food and Nutrient Interactions

None known.

Usual Dosage

In the treatment of nausea and vomiting due to motion sickness, nausea and vomiting during pregnancy, or other causes, the typical dosage has been 1 to 2 g of powdered dried ginger. This dosage would be equivalent to approximately 10 g (⅓ ounce) of fresh ginger root, roughly a ¼-inch slice. For ginger extracts standardized to contain 20 percent gingerol and shogaol, an equivalent dosage in treating motion sickness or nausea and vomiting would be 100–200 mg. In the treatment of arthritis and migraine headaches, the dosage recommended is usually double that used for the treatment of nausea and vomiting.

Overdosage

None known.

Special Populations

Pregnant/breast-feeding women
Considered safe during pregnancy and lactation.

Children
Suitable for children at one-half the adult dosage.

Seniors
No special precautions are known.

Ginkgo Biloba

Used For

Cerebral vascular insufficiency (insufficient blood flow to the brain)
Effectiveness: A   Safety: A

Dementia and Alzheimer's disease
Effectiveness: A   Safety: A

Depression
Effectiveness: B+   Safety: A

Impotence
Effectiveness: B+   Safety: A

Inner ear dysfunction (vertigo, tinnitus)
Effectiveness: B   Safety: A

Peripheral vascular insufficiency (intermittent claudication, Raynaud's phenomenon)
Effectiveness: A   Safety: A

Premenstrual syndrome
Effectiveness: B   Safety: A

Retinopathy (macular degeneration, diabetic retinopathy)
Effectiveness: B   Safety: A

General Information

Ginkgo biloba is a deciduous tree that lives as long as a thousand years and may grow to a height of more than 120 feet and a diameter of as much as 4 feet. Ginkgo trees have been on the earth for more than two hundred million years—for this reason ginkgo is often referred to as a "living fossil."

Extracts made from ginkgo leaves are perhaps the most popular herbal products in the world. The key components of *Ginkgo biloba* extract (GBE) are flavonoids and terpenes (ginkgolides and bilobalides) unique to ginkgo. The most widely studied GBE (and the gold standard to which all other ginkgo extracts are compared) is EGB-761, a GBE standardized to contain 24 percent flavone glycosides and 6 percent terpenenoids. The brand Ginkgold contains this extract.

Cerebral vascular insufficiency (insufficient blood flow to the brain)

Cerebral vascular insufficiency is extremely common among the elderly in developed countries, owing to the high prevalence of atherosclerosis (hardening of the arteries). In well-designed studies, GBE has displayed a statistically significant regression of the major symptoms of cerebral vascular insufficiency and impaired mental performance. These symptoms include short-term memory loss, vertigo, headache, ringing in the ears, and depression. The quality of research on GBE for cerebral vascular insufficiency is comparable to FDA-approved drugs. GBE works by a combination of effects, including an ability to improve blood supply to the brain and enhance energy production within the brain even if the oxygen supply is diminished.

Dementia and Alzheimer's disease

Ginkgo biloba extract has been shown to produce positive effects on mental function in many cases of dementia (senility), including Alzheimer's disease. In addition to GBE's ability to increase the functional capacity of the brain, it has also been shown to address many of the other major elements of Alzheimer's disease. Although double-blind studies in established Alzheimer's patients demonstrate that GBE produces some beneficial effects in improving mental function, memory, and mood, at this time it appears that GBE is most effective in delaying mental deterioration in the early stages of Alzheimer's disease. If the dementia is due to cerebral vascular insufficiency or depression and not Alzheimer's disease, GBE is usually effective in improving the deficit.

Depression

GBE was first shown to improve mood in double-blind studies in patients suffering from cerebral vascular insufficiency. Additional double-blind studies have confirmed the antidepressant effects of GBE. In one double-blind study, forty subjects (age fifty-one to seventy-eight) who had been diagnosed with depression and who had not benefited fully from standard antidepressant drugs were given either 80 mg of GBE three times daily or a placebo. By the end of the eight-week study, the average total score on the Hamilton Depression Scale fell from 14 to 4.5 in the GBE group. In comparison, the score in the placebo group dropped from 14 to only 13. The results of this study can be interpreted as suggesting that GBE may offer significant benefit as an antidepressant on its own or in combination with standard drug therapy (tricyclics and tetracyclics were used in the study).

Impotence

In cases of impotence (erectile dysfunction) due to impaired blood flow to erectile tissue, GBE may offer help, according to the results from preliminary and double-blind studies. In one of these studies, sixty patients with proven erectile dysfunction that had not responded to papaverine injections of up to 50 mg were treated with GBE at a dose of 60 mg per day for twelve to eighteen months. Penile blood flow was reevaluated by ultrasound every four weeks. The first signs of improved blood supply were seen after six to eight weeks. After six months of therapy, 50 percent of the patients had regained potency; in 20 percent a new trial of papaverine injection was successful; 25 percent of the patients showed improved blood flow, but papaverine was still not successful; 5 percent remained unchanged.

It should be noted that ginkgo's effects are more apparent with long-term therapy, and better results may be obtained with a dosage of 120 to 240 mg rather than the 60 mg per day used in this study.

Inner ear dysfunction (vertigo, tinnitus)

GBE has been shown to improve vertigo due to cerebral vascular insufficiency. In tinnitus (ringing in the ears) the results with GBE in double-blind studies are contradictory. The explanation for these differing results lies in the fact that people with recent-onset tinnitus are more likely to respond to GBE than those who have had tinnitus for at least three years.

Peripheral vascular insufficiency (intermittent claudication, Raynaud's phenomenon)

Peripheral arterial disease is caused by the same cholesterol-containing plaque that is responsible for other conditions associated with atherosclerosis, such as coronary artery disease and cerebral vascular insufficiency. In over a dozen double-blind studies, GBE has been shown to be quite active and superior to placebo and equal to the drug Trental (pentoxifylline). In the treatment of intermittent claudication (a peripheral vascular disease characterized by pain in the calf upon walking), not only did pain-free walking distance and maximum walking distance dramatically increase, but ultrasound measurements demonstrated increased blood flow through the affected limb. This indicates that GBE may be superior to pentoxifylline and standard medical therapy in the treatment of peripheral arterial insufficiency.

Premenstrual syndrome

Premenstrual syndrome (PMS) is often characterized by fluid retention, vascular congestion, increased capillary permeability, and breast tenderness during the later phase of the menstrual cycle. In one double-blind study, 165 women between the ages of eighteen and forty-five who had suffered from these congestive symptoms for at least three cycles were assigned to receive either the ginkgo extract (80 mg twice daily) or placebo from day sixteen of one menstrual period to day five of the next. Researchers concluded, on the basis of extensive symptom evaluation by the patients and physicians, that the ginkgo extract was effective against the congestive symptoms of PMS, particularly breast pain or tenderness. Patients taking the ginkgo extract also noted improvements in neuropsychological assessments. These results indicate that *Ginkgo biloba* extract may hold some promise in the treatment of PMS, but further studies are required to judge its true effectiveness.

Retinopathy (macular degeneration, diabetic retinopathy)

Ginkgo biloba extract appears to address quite effectively the underlying factors in several retinal disorders, including diabetic retinopathy and age-related macular degeneration (the latter is the most common cause of blindness in adults). In double-blind studies, GBE demonstrated a statistically significant improvement in long-distance visual acuity in both macular degeneration and diabetic retinopathy patients. *Ginkgo biloba* extract has demonstrated impressive protective effects against free-radical damage to the retina in experimental studies.

Available Forms

GBE is available as a fluid extract, capsules, and tablets. Whatever form of GBE is used, it appears to be essential that it be standardized for active ingredient content. Brands available include Ginkai, Ginkgold, and Ginkoba.

Cautions and Warnings

Crude ginkgo leaves contain a potential neurotoxin and should not be used, even as a tea.

GBE may potentiate the effects of the blood-thinning drug warfarin (Coumadin) as well as enhance the antiplatelet effects of drugs such as aspirin and ticlopidine (Ticlid), although this is quite rare.

Ginkgo use should be discontinued at least three days before any surgery, as it may increase bleeding tendency.

Possible Side Effects

Ginkgo biloba extract is extremely safe, and side effects are uncommon. In forty-four double-blind studies involving 9,772 patients taking GBE, the number of side effects reported was extremely small. The most common side effect, gastrointestinal discomfort, occurred in only twenty-one cases, followed by headache (seven cases) and dizziness (six cases).

In contrast to the lack of side effects of GBE, contact with the fruit pulp causes an allergic reaction similar to that caused by the poison ivy-oak-sumac group, while ingestion of as little as two pieces of fruit pulp has been reported to cause severe gastrointestinal irritation from the mouth to the anus.

Drug Interactions

GBE may potentiate the effects of the blood-thinning drug warfarin (Coumadin) as well as enhance the antiplatelet effects of drugs such as aspirin and ticlopidine (Ticlid), although this is quite rare. GBE in combination with these drugs has been associated with two cases of spontaneous bleeding, although GBE was not definitively shown to be the cause of the problem.

Antidepressant drugs such as fluoxetine (Prozac), paroxetine (Paxil), sertraline (Zoloft), and others are associated with reducing libido. In one preliminary study, GBE was shown to prevent loss of libido associated with these drugs.

Food and Nutrient Interactions

None known.

Usual Dosage

The typical dosage of GBE standardized to contain 24 percent ginkgo flavone glycosides has been 40 to 80 mg three times a day. It is difficult to devise a dosage schedule using other forms of ginkgo, owing to the extreme variation in the content of active compounds in dried leaf and crude extracts.

Overdosage

None known.

Special Populations

Pregnant/breast-feeding women
As the effects of GBE during pregnancy and lactation have not been sufficiently evaluated, it should not be used during these times.

Children
There does not appear to be an appropriate use of GBE in children at this time.

Seniors
No special precautions are known.

Ginkgold *(see Ginkgo biloba)*

General Information

Ginkgold is an extract from the leaves of *Ginkgo biloba* (EGB-761) developed by the Dr. Willmar Schwabe Company of Germany that has emerged as the premier ginkgo product in the world. EGB-761 has been the subject of over four hundred scientific studies and is the most clinically tested form of *Ginkgo biloba* extract. Each 40 mg enteric-coated tablet is standardized to contain 24 percent ginkgo flavone glycosides and 6 percent terpene lactones as well as over twenty other active and coactive constituents.

Ginsana (*see* Ginseng)

General Information

Ginsana is the most well researched and commercially successful Chinese or Korean ginseng *(Panax ginseng)* product. Each soft gelatin capsule provides 100 mg of *Panax ginseng* extract (G-115) standardized to contain 5 percent ginsenosides.

Ginseng *(Panax ginseng, Panax quinquefolius)*

Used For

Antifatigue effects
Effectiveness: B   Safety: C

Cancer prevention
Effectiveness: B   Safety: C

Cholesterol reduction
Effectiveness: B   Safety: C

Diabetes
Effectiveness: B   Safety: C

Enhancement of athletic and physical performance
Effectiveness: B–   Safety: C

Low immunity and immune support
Effectiveness: B   Safety: C

Menopause
Effectiveness: C   Safety: C

Reproductive effects
Effectiveness: C   Safety: C

Stress
Effectiveness: B   Safety: C

General Information

There are three major types of ginseng: Chinese or Korean *(Panax ginseng)*, American *(Panax quinquefolius)*, and Siberian *(Eleutherococcus senticosus)*. *Panax ginseng* is the most widely used and most extensively studied ginseng. Because American ginseng contains slightly different ratios of key compounds known as ginsenosides compared to *Panax ginseng*, it is generally regarded as providing similar effects for most indications but with less of a stimulatory effect (discussed in "Available Forms," below). Although **Siberian ginseng** *(Eleutherococcus senticosus)* also has many of the same effects as *Panax ginseng*, it is generally regarded as being milder in action.

Initial scientific research on ginseng focused on its adaptogenic qualities. An adaptogen is defined as a substance that (1) must be innocuous and cause minimal disorders in the physiological functions of an organism, (2) must have a nonspecific action (i.e., it should increase resistance to adverse influences by a wide range of physical, chemical, and biochemical factors), and (3) usually has a normalizing action on body functions. Tradition and scientific evidence suggest that ginseng exerts adaptogenic effects.

Antifatigue effects

Much of the early research on ginseng was performed during the late 1950s and early 1960s in Russia. In experiments in humans, subjects taking ginseng demonstrated improvement in both physical and mental performance. Experimental animal studies indicated that much of the antifatigue action of ginseng was due to its stimulant effect on the central nervous system. Ginseng also was shown to improve energy metabolism during prolonged exercise. In addition to the Russian studies, other studies showing the antifatigue and antistress effects of ginseng have been published. For example, in one double-blind study nurses who had switched from day to night duty demonstrated higher scores in competence, mood, and mental and physical performance when given ginseng compared with those receiving a placebo. In another double-blind study of university students in Italy, a standardized ginseng extract (Ginsana) produced positive effects on attention, mental arithmetic, logical thinking, and reaction time to sounds.

Cancer prevention

Regular ginseng consumption may protect against cancer. In one large population study, the risk of developing cancer was significantly lower among people who consumed ginseng on a regular basis. Ginseng extract and powder were shown to be more effective than fresh sliced ginseng, ginseng juice, or ginseng tea in reducing the cancer risk. A statistically highly significant dose-response relationship between ginseng intake and cancer risk was observed—that is, the higher the intake of ginseng, the lower the risk of cancer. These results support the preventive effects of ginseng suggested by earlier animal studies, but more research is required in this area.

Cholesterol reduction

In preliminary studies, ginseng administered to human subjects with elevated cholesterol and triglyceride levels was shown to produce modest reductions in total blood cholesterol, triglyceride, and fatty acid levels, while raising HDL cholesterol levels.

Diabetes

Ginseng, either alone or in combination with other herbs, has long been used in the treatment of diabetes. Ginseng has confirmed hypoglycemic (blood-sugar-lowering) activity in both animal and human experiments. In one double-blind study, ginseng was shown to improve glucose control and increase energy levels in patients with non-insulin-dependent diabetes mellitus (type 2 diabetes).

Enhancement of athletic and physical performance

The benefits of ginseng for athletic performance are not clear. Most recent double-blind studies have been negative. For example, in one study thirty-six healthy men received a standardized ginseng extract (Ginsana) at a dosage level of either 200 or 400 mg per day, but it appeared to have no effect on any exercise-related parameter (e.g., blood lactic acid concentration, heart rate, perceived exertion). Results to date do not offer support for claims that ginseng improves athletic performance.

Low immunity and immune support

Ginseng has been shown to enhance many immune functions in animal and double-blind human

studies. The research suggests that regular ingestion of ginseng by individuals with mild immune deficiency (i.e., those who get frequent colds) may
reduce the risk of viral infection. Use in this manner
is consistent with the historical use of ginseng.

Menopause

Ginseng components have shown estrogenlike
activity, and ginseng has historically been used to
address menopausal symptoms. However, there are
no double-blind studies to support or refute this use.

Reproductive effects

Although ginseng is claimed to be a "sexual rejuvenator," there are no human studies supporting
this belief. Ginseng has, however, been shown to
enhance reproductive function in animal studies and
may produce similar effects in humans. Effects
noted in animals include increased sperm count in
males, increased reproductive activity in both sexes,
and alleviating organic causes of female infertility.

Stress

Human and animal studies indicate that ginseng
enhances the ability to cope with various stressors,
both physical and mental. These antistress effects
are due largely to ginseng's effect on the adrenal
glands. Researchers have demonstrated that ginseng acts predominantly on the hypothalamus or pituitary to promote secretion of adrenocorticotropic
hormone (ACTH), which in turn promotes the manufacture and secretion of adrenal hormones. It appears that ginseng exerts a balancing effect on the
metabolic and functional systems governing hormonal control of the stress reaction.

Available Forms

There are many types and grades of ginseng and ginseng extracts that vary by the source, age, and parts of the root used, and by the methods of preparation. Old, wild, well-formed roots are the most valued, while rootlets of cultivated plants are considered the lowest grade. Ginseng is often processed in two forms, white and red. White ginseng is the dried root, whose skin is frequently peeled off. Red ginseng is the steamed root, which shows a caramel-like color. High-quality preparations consist of the main root of plants between four and six years of age, or extracts that have been standardized for ginsenoside content and ratio (see "Usual Dosage").

Brands available include Ginsana.

Cautions and Warnings

Do not use large dosages of ginseng during an acute infection. At higher dosages ginseng may inhibit some immune functions.

Individuals with diabetes need to be aware that taking ginseng may alter insulin or drug requirements. Consult a physician to discuss proper monitoring of blood sugar levels before taking ginseng.

Ginseng should not be used in patients taking warfarin (Coumadin) unless closely monitored by a physician.

Possible Side Effects

The problem of quality control in the marketplace has made the assessment of ginseng's side effects difficult to determine. Clinical studies performed with standardized ginseng extracts have demonstrated the absence of side effects. Nonetheless, possible side effects include a general stimulatory effect, including irritability and insomnia. Women taking *Panax ginseng* may experience breast tenderness and menstrual disturbances.

Drug Interactions

Taking ginseng preparations may increase the effectiveness of insulin and drugs that lower blood sugar levels, such as glyburide (Diabeta, Micronase). Consult a physician to discuss proper monitoring of blood sugar levels before taking ginseng.

Ginseng may interfere with the anticoagulant drug warfarin (Coumadin). People taking warfarin should not take ginseng unless they are being closely monitored by a physician.

Food and Nutrient Interactions

None known.

Usual Dosage

The appropriate dose of ginseng depends on the ginsenoside content. The standard dose for high-quality ginseng root is in the range of 4 to 6 g daily. For ginseng root extract containing 5 percent ginsenosides, the dose is typically 200 to 400 mg daily. As each individual's response to ginseng is unique, it is generally recommend to begin at lower dosages and increase gradually.

Overdosage

Excessive use or dosages of ginseng may produce a greater stimulatory effect.

Special Populations

Pregnant/breast-feeding women
As the effects of ginseng during pregnancy and lactation have not been sufficiently evaluated, it should not be used during these times.

Children
Ginseng is not usually recommended for use in children.

Seniors
No special precautions are known.

Goldenseal *(Hydrastis canadensis)*

General Information

Goldenseal is native to eastern North America. It is a perennial herb with a knotty yellow root that is used for medicinal purposes. Goldenseal shares similar indications and effects with other **berberine-containing plants** such as barberry and Oregon grape root. Due to environmental concerns about overharvesting, many herbalists recommend alternatives to goldenseal, such as Oregon grape root, barberry, or coptis.

Gotu Kola *(Centella asiatica)*

Used For

Burns
Effectiveness: B+   Safety: A

Cellulite
Effectiveness: B+   Safety: A

Cirrhosis of the liver
Effectiveness: B+   Safety: A

Keloids
Effectiveness: A   Safety: A

Leprosy
Effectiveness: B+   Safety: A

Scleroderma
Effectiveness: B+   Safety: A

Varicose veins
Effectiveness: A   Safety: A

Wound healing
Effectiveness: A   Safety: A

General Information

Gotu kola is a perennial plant native to India, China, Indonesia, Australia, the South Pacific, Madagascar, and southern and central Africa. Historically, the entire plant is used medicinally, with use centering on its ability to relieve leprosy and heal wounds. Both applications have been verified by modern science. In regard to its ability to promote wound healing, extracts of gotu kola have been shown to:

- Stimulate hair and nail growth
- Increase the development and maintenance of blood vessels in the support structures of skin
- Improve the structural framework of skin
- Promote proper collagen manufacture

The active compounds of gotu kola are known as triterpenoids. *Note:* Many people confuse gotu kola with cola nut and assume gotu kola produces a stimulant effect due to caffeine. However, gotu kola is not related to the cola nut *(Cola nitida)* nor does it contain any caffeine.

Burns

The triterpenic acid extract from gotu kola has been effectively used in the treatment of patients with second- and third-degree burns caused by boiling water, electrical current, or gas explosion. The extract prevented or limited the shrinking and swelling of the skin caused by skin infection, and it inhibited scar formation and improved healing time.

Cellulite

The triterpenic acid extract from gotu kola has demonstrated good results in the treatment of cellulite in several clinical studies. In one study over a period of three months, very good results were produced in 58 percent and satisfactory results in 20 percent of sixty-five women with cellulite. Other investigations have shown a similar success rate. The effect of gotu kola in the treatment of cellulite appears to be related to its ability to enhance the barrier of connective tissue that separates the outer skin from the underlying fat chambers.

Cirrhosis of the liver

Case reports have shown that the triterpenic acid extract from gotu kola was helpful in patients with alcohol-induced cirrhosis and cirrhosis of unknown cause. Improvements in symptoms and laboratory values were confirmed by liver biopsy. No effect was observed in patients with cirrhosis due to chronic hepatitis.

Keloids

There are basically two stages of scar formation, the inflammatory stage and the maturation phase. When the inflammatory stage is prolonged (months or even years), it can lead to the formation of a keloid—a large collection of scar tissue. The triterpenic acid extract from gotu kola has demonstrated impressive clinical results in the treatment of keloids. Its mechanism of action appears to be multifaceted, but it is basically due to reducing the inflammatory phase of scar formation while simultaneously enhancing the maturation phase of scar formation. In clinical trials, over 80 percent of subjects experienced relief of symptoms or complete maturation of the scar. In people who required surgical resection of the keloid, if a positive response is observed with gotu kola extract after two to three weeks of use, roughly 80 percent of subjects will have successful surgery.

Leprosy

In the United States today, leprosy is virtually unknown, but it still exists in other parts of the world, and gotu kola may offer successful treatment. The therapeutic response to gotu kola extract noted in clinical trials is comparable to that of dapsone, the standard drug used in the treatment of leprosy. In addition to its wound-healing activity, it appears that gotu kola extract may also inhibit *Mycobacterium leprae,* the causative organism involved with leprosy.

Scleroderma

Scleroderma is an autoimmune disease characterized by hardening of the skin, arthritis, and decreased blood flow to the hands and feet. The triterpenic acid extract of gotu kola was shown to produce significant benefit in relieving symptoms in several trials in subjects with scleroderma. Unfortunately, it has been more than twenty years since this study and others were performed. Given the positive results attained, it is unfortunate that more research has not been done.

Varicose veins

Numerous double-blind studies have demonstrated that the triterpenic acid extract of gotu kola is effective in the treatment of varicose veins. Again, this effect appears to be due to the ability of these compounds to enhance connective tissue structures—in this case, the connective tissue sheath that surrounds the vein, thus reducing hardening of the vein and improving venous blood flow. These effects produced significant improvement in symptoms such as feelings of heaviness in the lower legs, numbness and tingling sensations, and night cramps.

Wound healing

The triterpenic acid extract of gotu kola has been shown in a large number of clinical studies to greatly aid wound repair. The types of wounds healed include surgical wounds such as episiotomies or ear-nose-throat surgeries, skin ulcers due to arterial or venous insufficiency, traumatic injuries to the skin, gangrene, and skin grafts.

Available Forms

The majority of clinical studies used a triterpenic extract of gotu kola containing asiaticoside (40 percent), asiatic acid (29 to 30 percent), madecassic acid (29 to 30 percent), and madecassoside (1 to 2 percent); this solid extract is available in capsules and tablets. Gotu kola is also available in crude form (in bulk or in capsules, tablets, or tea bags), tinctures, and fluid extracts.

Cautions and Warnings

None known.

Possible Side Effects

Minor gastric irritation.

Drug Interactions

None known.

Food and Nutrient Interactions

None known.

Usual Dosage

The usual dosage of the triterpenic acid extract is 30 to 60 mg twice daily. Since the concentration of triterpenes in gotu kola can vary between 1.1 and 8 percent, it is best to use extracts standardized for triterpenic acids. Here are the approximate dosages for other forms:

Crude dried plant leaves: 1–2 g twice daily
Tincture (1:5): 5–10 ml twice daily
Fluid extract (1:1): 1–2 ml twice daily

Overdosage

None known.

Special Populations

Pregnant/breast-feeding women
Although studies to determine if gotu kola extracts are toxic to fetal development in rabbits proved negative, the effects of gotu kola during pregnancy and lactation in humans have not been sufficiently evaluated, so it cannot be considered safe during pregnancy and lactation at this time.

Children
Suitable for children at the adult dosage, but only under medical supervision.

Seniors
No special precautions are known.

Grape Seed Extract (*see* Procyanidolic Oligomers)

General Information

Extracts from skin surrounding the seeds of red grapes *(Vitex vinifera)* contain proanthocyanidins (also referred to as procyanidins), one of the most beneficial groups of plant flavonoids. Powerful antioxidants, the most active proanthocyanidins are those bound to other proanthocyanidins. Collectively, mixtures of proanthocyanidin dimers, trimers, tetramers, and larger molecules are referred to as procyanidolic oligomers (PCOs). Although PCOs exist in many plants, commercially available sources of PCOs include grape seed extracts and extracts from the bark of the maritime pine **(Pycnogenol).**

Grapefruit Seed Extract

Used For

Irritable bowel syndrome
Effectiveness: B   Safety: C

General Information

Grapefruit seed extract exerts significant antibiotic effects. Its internal use has not been sufficiently studied. In the only available published study, twenty-five patients with symptoms associated with irritable bowel syndrome such as intermittent diarrhea, constipation, flatulence, bloating, and abdominal discomfort (particularly after carbohydrate-rich meals) were treated with either two drops of a 0.5 percent oral solution of grapefruit seed extract twice daily or capsules containing 50 mg of grapefruit seed extract at a dosage of three capsules three times daily. After one month, gastrointestinal symptoms in two of ten patients on the liquid improved, while all fifteen of the patients on the capsules (which contained a higher dosage of the extract) noted definite improvement of constipation, flatulence, abdominal discomfort, and night rest. These results need confirmation in double-blind studies.

Available Forms

Grapefruit seed extract is available in liquid concentrate and in capsules and tablets. Brand names available include NutriBiotic.

Cautions and Warnings

The toxicity of grapefruit seed extract has not yet been determined.

Possible Side Effects

None known.

Drug Interactions

None known.

Food and Nutrient Interactions

None known.

Usual Dosage

The typical recommendation for the liquid concentrate is 10–12 drops in 200 ml of water one to three times daily. For capsules and tablets containing dried grapefruit seed extract, the usual recommendation is 100–200 mg one to three times daily.

Overdosage

Not yet determined.

Special Populations

Pregnant/breast-feeding women

As the effects of grapefruit seed extract during pregnancy and lactation have not been sufficiently evaluated, it should not be used during these times.

Children

Suitable for children over the age of six years at one-half the adult dosage. Consult a physician immediately when diarrhea or other gastrointestinal disturbance occurs in a child under six years of age.

Seniors

No special precautions are known.

Green Tea *(Camellia sinensis)*

Used For

Antioxidant supplementation
Effectiveness: B+   Safety: C

Cancer prevention
Effectiveness: B+   Safety: C

General Information

Both green tea and black tea are derived from the same plant, *Camellia sinensis.* Green tea is produced by lightly steaming the freshly cut leaves, while to produce black tea the leaves are allowed to oxidize. Oolong tea is partially oxidized. During oxidation, enzymes present in the tea convert polyphenols, which possess outstanding therapeutic action, to compounds with much less activity. With green tea, oxidation is not allowed to take place because the steaming process inactivates these enzymes. Green tea is very high in polyphenols with potent antioxidant and anticancer properties.

The major polyphenols in green tea are flavonoids (e.g., catechin, epicatechin, epicatechin gallate, epigallocatechin gallate, and proanthocyanidins). Epigallocatechin gallate is viewed as the most significant active component. Green tea also contains **caffeine** at about 30 to 50 mg per cup.

Antioxidant supplementation

Green tea polyphenols are potent antioxidant compounds that have demonstrated greater antioxidant protection than vitamins C and E in most but not all experimental studies. In addition to exerting antioxidant activity on its own, green tea may increase the activity of antioxidant enzymes in the small intestine, liver, and lungs. The ability of green tea extract to protect against oxidative damage to LDL cholesterol indicates that it may protect against atherosclerosis and heart disease.

Cancer prevention

Population studies have demonstrated that green tea consumption may be one of the major reasons why the cancer rate is lower in Japan. A number of experiments conducted in test tube and animal cancer models have shown that green tea polyphenols inhibit cancer by blocking the formation of cancer-causing compounds such as nitrosamines, suppressing the activation of carcinogens, and detoxifying or trapping cancer-causing agents. The forms of cancer that appear to be best prevented by green tea are cancers of the gastrointestinal tract, including cancers of the stomach, small intestine, pancreas, and colon; lung cancer; and estrogen-related cancers, including most breast cancers. These preliminary results need confirmation in double-blind studies in humans.

Available Forms

Green tea is most often consumed as a beverage from either loose green tea leaves or tea bags. Green tea extracts concentrated for polyphenol content (e.g., 70–80 percent) are available, including decaffeinated versions.

Cautions and Warnings

Do not exceed the recommended dosage of caffeine or caffeine-containing herb, especially if combined with other plant stimulants such as ephedrine.

Caffeine may have the potential to cause cardiac arrhythmia (irregular heartbeat). As a precaution, it is recommended that caffeine be avoided by individuals with a history of cardiac arrhythmia and/or palpitations and during the first month after suffering a heart attack.

Chronic caffeine consumption can lead to physical and psychological dependence. If caffeine intake is stopped abruptly, physical signs of withdrawal may occur. The most common symptoms of caffeine withdrawal are fatigue and headache. These symptoms usually begin twelve to twenty-four hours after caffeine intake is stopped and may last as long as a week.

Possible Side Effects

As with any caffeine-containing beverage, overconsumption of green tea or caffeine-containing green tea extract may produce a stimulant effect (nervousness, anxiety, insomnia, irritability). Other possible side effects include light-headedness, headache, nausea, gastric irritation, and vomiting.

Drug Interactions

The breakdown of caffeine is inhibited by the following drugs: birth control pills, estrogen (e.g., Premarin), mexiletine, cimetidine (Tagamet), and various antibiotics (e.g., norfloxacin, enoxacin, and ciprofloxacin). Tricyclic antidepressant drugs, ephedrine, and theophylline (used in asthma) all potentiate the effects of caffeine.

Food and Nutrient Interactions

Alcohol inhibits the breakdown of caffeine.

To avoid the potential danger of caffeine overdose, be aware of your consumption of caffeine-containing foods and beverages.

Usual Dosage

The average amount of green tea consumed by the Japanese and other green-tea-drinking cultures is about three cups daily, providing about 3 g of soluble components, and a daily dosage of roughly 240 to 320 mg of polyphenols (and roughly 90 to 150 mg of caffeine). To achieve the same degree of protection with a green tea extract standardized for 80 percent total polyphenols and 55 percent epigallocatechin gallate content, this would mean a daily dose of 300 to 400 mg.

Note: The caffeine content of green tea is roughly 30 to 50 mg per cup.

Overdosage

Doses of caffeine over 250 mg can produce definite signs of toxicity, such as stomach pain, nervousness, increased heart rate, elevation in blood pressure, frequent urination, and disordered thought and speech. More serious symptoms include arrhythmia (irregular heartbeat) and seizures.

Even if the victim is not displaying any of the symptoms above, do the following in case of accidental overdose: If the victim is unconscious or having convulsions, call for an ambulance immediately. If you take the victim to an emergency room, be sure to bring the bottle or container with you. If the victim is conscious, call your local poison control center or a health care professional. The poison control center may suggest inducing vomiting with ipecac syrup (available without a prescription at any pharmacy). *Do not* induce vomiting unless specifically instructed to do so.

Special Populations

Pregnant/breast-feeding women
Caffeine consumption, even from green tea, is best avoided during pregnancy and lactation. Caffeine has long been suspected of causing malformations in the fetus, although this is controversial. The dosage required for this effect is probably quite large, but the data are scant, as experimentation on humans is not feasible. Caffeine has been shown to cause malformations in rats when ingested at rates comparable to seventy cups a day for humans. In humans, daily doses of 300 mg per day or more in pregnant women have been linked to slowed growth and low birth weight of the infant.

Caffeine passes into breast milk and may cause wakefulness and irritability in nursing infants.

Children
There does not appear to be any appropriate use of caffeine or caffeine-containing beverages in children. The adverse effects of caffeine are usually more severe in children because their breakdown of caffeine is slower than that of adults.

Seniors
Seniors are often more sensitive to caffeine's stimulant effects and may be more likely to experience nervousness, anxiety, and insomnia. Seniors are also more likely to be taking drugs that interact with caffeine.

Guarana *(Paullinia cupana)*

General Information

Guarana is a caffeine-containing plant from the lower Amazon region of South America. Like other caffeine-containing plants, guarana has historically been used to sustain people during long journeys or long hours of work. The portion of the plant used is the seed from the small bright red fruit. Historically it is prepared by crushing the seeds to make a paste that is rolled into sticks and smoked. The form found in most commercial products is the powdered seed in tablets and capsules. Like **cola nut,** guarana extract is also used as a flavoring agent in cola beverages. The caffeine content of guarana ranges from 2.6–7.0 percent (see **caffeine**).

Guggul
(from *Commiphora mukul*)

Used For

Lowering cholesterol and triglyceride levels
Effectiveness: A   Safety: B

General Information

Guggul is a resinous material derived from the mukul myrrh tree *(Commiphora mukul),* native to Arabia and India. Upon injury, the tree exudes guggul—a yellowish gum resin that has a balsamic odor. The crude guggul must be purified to remove a toxin. For medicinal purposes, purified extracts standardized for guggulsterone content are recommended. Gugulipid is the most well studied guggul extract.

Numerous studies in humans and animals have shown that Gugulipid and other guggul preparations exert effective lipid-lowering activity, reducing LDL cholesterol while simultaneously elevating HDL cholesterol. In double-blind trials using Gugulipid, cholesterol levels typically dropped 14–27 percent in a four-to-twelve-week period, while triglyceride levels dropped 22–30 percent.

The primary mechanism of action responsible for the cholesterol-lowering effect is the stimulation of liver metabolism of LDL cholesterol. Specifically, the guggulsterones increase the uptake of LDL cholesterol from the blood by the liver.

In addition to lowering cholesterol levels, guggul preparations have been shown to prevent the formation of atherosclerosis, prevent the heart from being damaged by free radicals, improve the metabolism of the heart, prevent against clot formation, and exert mild anti-inflammatory effects.

Available Forms

Guggul is available as the crude resin and purified extract in tablets and capsules. Because of a potentially toxic component in crude preparations, purified extracts are recommended. Brands available include Gugulipid.

Cautions and Warnings

Allergic reactions have been reported with crude guggul preparations, but not with purified extracts such as Gugulipid.

Possible Side Effects

Crude guggul preparations are associated with gastrointestinal irritation, headache, mild nausea, and allergic skin reactions. These side effects have not been reported with purified extracts. In clinical studies, Gugulipid has not displayed any negative side effects.

Drug Interactions

Guggul preparations may decrease the absorption of propanolol (Inderal) and diltiazem (Cardizem).

There is some evidence that guggulsterones may stimulate thyroid function. People taking thyroid medication will need to monitor their blood thyroid hormones through their doctor if they elect to use guggul preparations.

Food and Nutrient Interactions

None known.

Usual Dosage

The dosage of guggul preparations is based on their guggulsterone content. Double-blind studies have demonstrated that 25 mg of guggulsterone three times per day is an effective treatment for elevated cholesterol levels, elevated triglyceride levels, or both. For a guggul extract containing 5 percent guggulsterones, this translates to a dose of 500 mg three times per day.

Overdosage

None known.

Special Populations

Pregnant/breast-feeding women

Although animal studies have shown that Gugulipid does not have any toxic effects on the fetus, the effects of guggul preparations during pregnancy and lactation in humans have not been sufficiently evaluated, and so they should not be used during these times.

Children

Suitable for children at one-half the adult dosage.

Seniors

No special precautions are known.

Gymnema Sylvestre

Used For

Diabetes
Effectiveness: B+   Safety: B

General Information

Gymnema sylvestre, a plant native to the tropical forests of India, has long been used as a treatment for diabetes. Recent scientific investigation has upheld its effectiveness in both type 1 and type 2 diabetes. Because *Gymnema sylvestre* has no apparent effect in animals that have had their pancreas removed, it is thought to enhance the production of insulin. There is also some evidence in animal studies that it can stimulate regeneration of the insulin-producing beta cells in the pancreas. *Gymnema sylvestre* extract has shown positive clinical results in both type 1 and type 2 diabetes. An extract of the leaves of *Gymnema sylvestre* given to twenty-seven patients with type 1 diabetes on insulin therapy was shown to reduce insulin requirements and fasting blood sugar levels and improve blood sugar control. In type 1 diabetes, it appears to enhance the action of insulin. In a study of type 2 diabetics, twenty-two were given *Gymnema sylvestre* extract along with their oral hypoglycemic drugs. All patients demonstrated improved blood sugar control; twenty-one of the twenty-two were able to reduce their drug dosage considerably, and five subjects were able to discontinue their medication and maintain blood sugar control with the extract alone. *Gymnema sylvestre* extract given to healthy volunteers does not produce any blood-sugar-lowering or hypoglycemic effects.

Animal studies also indicate the extract may lower blood cholesterol and triglyceride levels.

Available Forms

The portion of the plant used for medicinal purposes is the leaf. Extracts made from the leaves of *Gymnema sylvestre* are often standardized for gymnemic acid content.

Cautions and Warnings

Individuals with diabetes need to be aware that taking this herb may alter insulin or drug requirements. Consult a physician to discuss proper monitoring of blood sugar levels before taking gymnema extract.

Possible Side Effects

None known.

Drug Interactions

Taking *Gymnema sylvestre* preparations may increase the effectiveness of insulin and drugs that lower blood sugar levels. Consult a physician to discuss proper monitoring of blood sugar levels before taking gymnema extract.

Food and Nutrient Interactions

None known.

Usual Dosage

For *Gymnema sylvestre* extracts standardized to contain 24 percent gymnemic acids, the typical dosage recommendation is 200 mg twice daily.

Overdosage

None known.

Special Populations

Pregnant/breast-feeding women
As the effects of *Gymnema sylvestre* during pregnancy and lactation have not been sufficiently evaluated, it should not be used during these times.

Children
Suitable for children at one-half the adult dosage.

Seniors
No special precautions are known.

Hawthorn (*Crataegus* spp.)

Used For

Angina
Effectiveness: B+   Safety: A

Congestive heart failure (mild to moderate)
Effectiveness: A   Safety: A

High blood pressure
Effectiveness: B+   Safety: A

General Information

Hawthorn (*Crataegus* spp.) is a spiny tree or shrub that is native to Europe. Hawthorn leaves, berries, and blossoms contain many biologically active flavonoid compounds. These flavonoids are responsible for the red to blue colors not only of hawthorn berries, but also of blackberries, cherries, blueberries, grapes, and many flowers. These compounds are highly concentrated in hawthorn berry and flower extracts.

Hawthorn extracts are used primarily in cardiovascular disorders. Experimental studies indicate that the beneficial effects are the result of improvement of the blood supply to the heart along with improvement in the metabolic processes in the heart that results in an increase in the force of contraction of the heart muscle.

Angina

Hawthorn extracts exhibit a combination of effects that are of great value to patients with angina and other heart problems. Double-blind studies have shown that hawthorn extracts are effective in reducing angina attacks as well as in lowering blood pressure and serum cholesterol levels.

Congestive heart failure

Hawthorn has a long history of use in the treatment of congestive heart failure (CHF)—a condition of the heart characterized by an inability of the heart to effectively pump enough blood. CHF is most often due to long-term effects of high blood pressure, previous myocardial infarction, disorder of a heart valve or the heart muscle, or chronic lung disease such as asthma or emphysema. Several double-blind studies have shown that in mild to moderate cases of CHF, hawthorn extract alone may be sufficient, but for moderate to severe CHF, it is not strong enough and must be used in combination with prescription medications. In the double-blind studies in mild to moderate CHF, not only were resting heart measurements improved (e.g., reductions in blood pressure and heart rate), but subjects taking hawthorn extract also noted improved exercise performance.

High blood pressure

Hawthorn exerts a mild blood-pressure-lowering effect, according to results from experimental and clinical studies. Its action in lowering blood pressure is quite unique, in that it does so through a number of diverse pharmacological effects. The blood-pressure-lowering effect of hawthorn generally requires prolonged administration, and in many instances it may take up to two to four weeks before this mild effect is noted.

Available Forms

The dried berries and flowering tops (flowers and leaves in the blooming stage) are the portions of the plant used for medicinal purposes. The crude plant is available in bulk and in capsules and tablets; also available are tinctures, fluid extracts, and solid extracts in tablets and capsules. Extracts standardized for procyanidins (usually 10 percent) or vitexin-rhamnoside (usually 1.8 percent) are viewed by many experts as the most beneficial.

Brands available include HeartCare.

Cautions and Warnings

Theoretically, hawthorn may potentiate or interfere with the effects of drugs used for angina, arrhythmia, high blood pressure, and congestive heart failure such as digoxin, beta-blockers such as propanolol (Inderal), and calcium channel blockers such as diltiazem (Cardizem) and nifedipine (Procardia).

Possible Side Effects

Generally hawthorn is well tolerated and without side effects.

Drug Interactions

See "Cautions and Warnings."

Food and Nutrient Interactions

None known.

Usual Dosage

The dosage depends on the type of preparation and source material. The doses listed for the various hawthorn preparations are for use three times a day.

Berries or flowers (dried): 3–5 g or as an infusion
Tincture (1:5): 4–5 ml (alcohol may elicit an increase in blood pressure in some individuals)
Fluid extract (1:1): 1–2 ml
Freeze-dried berries: 1–1.5 g
Flower extract (standardized to contain 1.8 percent vitexin-rhamnoside or 10 percent procyanidins): 100–250 mg

Overdosage

None known.

Special Populations

Pregnant/breast-feeding women
As hawthorn's effects have not been sufficiently evaluated in pregnant and lactating women, it should not be used during these times unless directed to do so by a health care professional.

Children
Suitable for children at one-half the adult dosage.

Seniors
No special precautions are known.

Horse Chestnut
(Aesculus hippocastanum)

Used For

Hemorrhoids
Effectiveness: B+   Safety: C

Varicose veins
Effectiveness: A   Safety: C

General Information

Horse chestnut is a tree is native to Asia and northern Greece, but it is now cultivated in many areas of Europe and North America. The tree produces fruits that are made up of a spiny capsule containing one to three large seeds, known as horse chestnuts.

Double-blind human studies have shown that horse chestnut seed extracts are quite helpful in relieving symptoms of varicose veins and hemorrhoids. In fact, in the treatment of varicose veins, horse chestnut seed extract appears to be as effective as compression stockings in relieving symptoms such as heaviness of the legs, itching, and pins-and-needles sensation (paresthesia).

The key compound in horse chestnut is escin. Horse chestnut seed extracts standardized for escin exert anti-edema and anti-inflammatory properties and decrease capillary permeability by reducing the number and size of the small pores in the capillary walls. Investigators have also demonstrated that escin has venotonic activity. A venotonic is a substance that improves venous tone by increasing the contractile potential of the elastic fibers in the vein wall. Relaxation of the venous wall contributes greatly to the development of varicose veins and hemorrhoids.

Available Forms

Horse chestnut seed preparations are available in crude form in bulk, tea bags, capsules, and tablets. It is also available as a tincture, fluid extract, and solid extract in capsules and tablets. The best form appears to be solid extracts standardized for escin content; brand names available include Venastat. Crude preparations can contain a toxic compound (aesculin), which is removed during the extraction process.

Cautions and Warnings

Crude horse chestnut seed preparations as well as horse chestnut leaf and bark preparations should not be used. They definitely must be avoided by anyone with liver or kidney disease. Serious toxicity reactions have occurred after ingestion of crude preparations.

Possible Side Effects

Internal use of recommended amounts of horse chestnut extracts standardized for escin is generally safe. However, in rare cases oral intake of horse chestnut seed extract may cause nausea, upset stomach, and itching of the skin.

Drug Interactions

None known.

Food and Nutrient Interactions

None known.

Usual Dosage

Historically the dosage recommendation has been 0.2–1.0 g of the dried seeds per day. But given the toxicity of the crude seeds and the availability of safer horse chestnut seed extracts standardized for escin content (16–21 percent) or isolated escin preparations, the refined forms are often recommended in an amount that provides 50–75 mg of escin twice per day.

Overdosage

Overdosage of crude preparations of horse chestnut can be a medical emergency. Symptoms include shortness of breath, dizziness, vomiting, and severe trembling, possibly leading to loss of consciousness and death. The effects of an overdosage of horse chestnut seed extract standardized for escin are unknown. Do the following in case of accidental overdose: If the victim is unconscious or having convulsions, call for an ambulance immediately. If you take the victim to an emergency room, be sure to bring the bottle or container with you. If the victim is conscious, call your local poison control center or a health care professional. The poison control center may suggest inducing vomiting with ipecac syrup (available without a prescription at any pharmacy). *Do not* induce vomiting unless specifically instructed to do so.

Special Populations

Pregnant/breast-feeding women
Horse chestnut preparations have not been evaluated for use during pregnancy and lactation and should not be used by pregnant or lactating women.

Children
Horse chestnut seed preparations are not recommended for children under the age of twelve years unless under the supervision of a physician. Children over the age of twelve can take the adult dosage for standardized horse chestnut seed extracts.

Seniors
No special precautions are known.

Huperzine A

Used For

Alzheimer's disease
Effectiveness: A   Safety: B

General Information

The moss *Huperzia serrata* has been used in China since the start of recorded history. It is traditionally used to treat fever and inflammation, but modern scientific investigation has found a new use for this plant. Specifically, huperzine A, an alkaloid isolated from the moss, has produced extremely encouraging results in the treatment of Alzheimer's disease, a degenerative brain disorder that manifests itself as a progressive deterioration of memory and mental function.

The symptoms of Alzheimer's are believed to be caused by a reduced level of acetylcholine—a key neurotransmitter in the brain that is especially important for memory. Huperzine A enhances memory by preventing the breakdown of acetylcholine as a result of inhibiting the enzyme (acetylcholinesterase) responsible for breaking down acetylcholine. As a result, acetylcholine levels increase dramatically within the brain cell, and memory improves.

Huperzine A appears to be significantly more selective and substantially less toxic than synthetic acetylcholinesterase inhibitors such as physostigmine, tacrine, and donepezil. Huperzine A has been used as a prescription drug in China since the early 1990s and has reportedly been used by over a hundred thousand people with no serious adverse effects. Clinical studies conducted in China have shown considerable benefit in improving memory, cognitive function, and behavioral factors in roughly 60 percent of Alzheimer's patients taking huperzine A.

Available Forms

Huperzine A is available in capsules and tablets.

Cautions and Warnings

Given the mechanism of action of huperzine A and the lack of sufficient safety data, at this time huperzine A should not be used in people with liver disease characterized by elevations of serum transaminases, or prior to exposure to anesthesia.

Possible Side Effects

Although no significant side effects occurred in the studies conducted in China, given the mechanism of action of huperzine A, possible side effects include nausea, dry mouth, fatigue, and diarrhea.

Drug Interactions

Huperzine A should not be used prior to anesthesia, as it may exaggerate the anesthetic's effect.

Food and Nutrient Interactions

None known.

Usual Dosage

200 mcg twice daily.

Overdosage

Because of the potential for serious side effects at high dosages, do the following in case of accidental overdose: If the victim is unconscious or having convulsions, call for an ambulance immediately. If you take the victim to an emergency room, be sure to bring the bottle or container with you. If the victim is conscious, call your local poison control center or a health care professional. The poison control center may suggest inducing vomiting with ipecac syrup (available without a prescription at any pharmacy). *Do not* induce vomiting unless specifically instructed to do so.

Special Populations

Pregnant/breast-feeding women
Huperzine A is not recommended during pregnancy and lactation.

Children
Huperzine A is not recommended for children.

Seniors
No special precautions are known.

Iberogast

Used For

Drug-induced dyspepsia
Effectiveness: A   Safety: A

Gastroesophageal reflux disease
Effectiveness: A   Safety: A

Nonulcer dyspepsia (indigestion and heartburn)
Effectiveness: A   Safety: A

General Information

Iberogast is an herbal formula that contains digestion-stimulating substances (glucosinolates and cucurbitacins, derived from clown's mustard *[Iberis amara]*) in a base of liquid extracts of angelica, chamomile, caraway, milk thistle, melissa, peppermint, celandine, and licorice. Iberogast has been a popular herbal product in Germany since 1968. Detailed, well-designed clinical trials have confirmed its effectiveness in improving functional causes of indigestion such as nonulcer dyspepsia (NUD), gastroesophageal reflux disease (GERD), irritable bowel syndrome (IBS), and drug-induced dyspepsia.

Symptoms of NUD include symptoms of GERD (heartburn and/or upper abdominal pain) as well as difficulty swallowing, feelings of pressure or heaviness after eating, sensations of bloating after eating, stomach or abdominal pains and cramps, as well as all of the symptoms of irritable bowel syndrome (IBS).

Irritable bowel syndrome (IBS) is another very

common condition. While NUD involves a functional disturbance of the upper gastrointestinal tract, in IBS the large intestine, or colon, fails to function properly. IBS's characteristic symptoms include a combination of any of the following: abdominal pain and distension; more frequent bowel movements with pain, or relief of pain with bowel movements; constipation; diarrhea; excessive production of mucus in the colon; symptoms of indigestion such as flatulence, nausea, or anorexia; and varying degrees of anxiety or depression. About three out of ten patients with NUD also meet the criteria for IBS, and vice versa.

Iberogast has been evaluated in over fifteen clinical studies. The results from all of the studies indicate a high response rate—more than 80 percent of people with NUD, IBS, GERD, and drug-induced dyspepsia will experience significant relief without side effects.

Iberogast works by a complex mechanism. The glucosinolates and cucurbitacins from clown's mustard are believed to be the most active components, but compounds provided by the other ingredients are thought to play a role also. Four main mechanisms have been identified.

1. Stimulation of digestive secretions through interactions with the bitter receptors on the taste buds of the tongue
2. Regulation of peristalsis (the rhythmic contraction of the intestines) by exerting either a relaxing or stimulating effect on the intestinal smooth muscle
3. Protecting the lining of the stomach and intestines by stimulating the production of mucus by mast cells (mucus-producing cells of the stomach and intestines) as well as preventing the formation of

inflammatory substances within the intestinal
tract
4. Prevention of excessive flatulence by reducing the
formation of intestinal gases

Available Forms

Liquid preparation.

Cautions and Warnings

None known.

Possible Side Effects

No side effects have been reported in over thirty
years of use.

Drug Interactions

There are no known drug interactions.

Food and Nutrient Interactions

Generally recommended to be taken before meals.

Usual Dosage

The standard dosage for adults is 20 drops three
times daily. It is recommended that this dosage be
taken before or at meals with some liquid (warm
water is recommended).

Overdosage

No special precautions are necessary.

Special Populations

Pregnant/breast-feeding women
Considered safe during pregnancy and lactation.

Children
Iberogast is suitable for children under twelve at one-half the adult dosage, that is, 10 drops three times daily. Children over twelve can take the adult dosage.

Seniors
No special precautions are known.

Ivy (Hedera helix)

Used For

Asthma and chronic obstructive pulmonary disease
Effectiveness: B+   Safety: C

General Information

Ivy leaf has a long history of use in asthma and chronic obstructive pulmonary disease (COPD). Recent clinical research has validated its ability to reduce bronchial spasm and sputum viscosity. Several double-blind studies have shown that ivy extract improves lung function and reduces asthma attacks. For example, in one double-blind study twenty-five children age ten to fifteen years with asthma demonstrated improvements in lung capacity after ten days of treatment with ivy extract. Results from this study and others indicate that ivy extract requires some time to work but can produce clinical improvement in bronchial asthma and COPD.

Available Forms

Ivy leaf is available primarily as a tincture, fluid extract, and solid extract in capsules and tablets.

Cautions and Warnings

An acute asthma attack can be a medical emergency. If you are suffering from an acute attack, consult your physician or go to an emergency room immediately.

Possible Side Effects

None known.

Drug Interactions

None known.

Food and Nutrient Interactions

None known.

Usual Dosage

The typical dosage for adults is 100 mg once or twice daily.

Overdosage
None known.

Special Populations

Pregnant/breast-feeding women
As the effects of ivy during pregnancy and lacta-tion have not been sufficiently evaluated, it should not be used during these times.

Children
Suitable for children at one-half the adult dosage (i.e., 50 to 100 mg daily).

Seniors
No special precautions are known.

Juniper *(Juniperus communis)*

Used For

Diuretic
Effectiveness: C   Safety: D

Urinary tract infections
Effectiveness: C   Safety: D

General Information
Juniper is a well-known evergreen tree or shrub. The berries are the medicinal portions of the plant. Unlike other pine cones, the juniper cones are fleshy

and soft. Perhaps the best-known use of juniper
berries is as the flavoring agent in gin, but historically juniper berries were used for a wide range of
health conditions including various urinary tract and
kidney diseases. There has been no scientific validation of this historical use.

Available Forms

Juniper berries are available dried in bulk and in tea
bags; also available are tinctures, fluid extracts, and
solid extracts in capsules and tablets.

Cautions and Warnings

Must not be used by individuals with any serious
kidney disease.

Due to potential damage to the kidneys, juniper
berries should never be taken for more than four
weeks continuously.

Must not be used by pregnant or lactating women.

Possible Side Effects

The major concern with the use of juniper berries
is kidney irritation resulting in kidney pain, protein
or blood in the urine, and excessive urination.
Discontinue use immediately if any of these side effects appears.

Drug Interactions

None known.

Food and Nutrient Interactions

None known.

Usual Dosage

The typical dosage recommendation is 2–10 g of the dried fruit daily. To make a tea, 250 ml (1 cup) of boiling water is added to 1 tsp (5 grams) of juniper berries and allowed to steep for twenty minutes. One cup can be drunk each morning and night. As a capsule or tablet, 1–2 g can be taken three times per day, or 1–2 ml of tincture or fluid extract can be taken three times per day. Due to potential damage to the kidneys, juniper berries should never be taken for more than four continuous weeks.

Overdosage

Do the following in case of accidental overdose: If the victim is unconscious or having convulsions, call for an ambulance immediately. If you take the victim to an emergency room, be sure to bring the bottle or container with you. If the victim is conscious, call your local poison control center or a health care professional. The poison control center may suggest inducing vomiting with ipecac syrup (available without a prescription at any pharmacy). *Do not* induce vomiting unless specifically instructed to do so.

Special Populations

Pregnant/breast-feeding women
   Juniper berries must not be used by pregnant or lactating women, as they may interfere with implantation of the embryo or cause uterine contractions.

Children

Juniper berries do not appear to be appropriate for use in children.

Seniors

No special precautions are known.

Kan Jang (see Andrographis paniculata)

General Information

Kan Jang is a standardized extract of the plant *Andrographis paniculata* that has proven to significantly shorten the duration of the common cold in several double-blind studies.

Kava (Piper methysticum)

Used For

Anxiety
Effectiveness: A   Safety: C

Insomnia
Effectiveness: B   Safety: C

General Information

Kava is a plant that is native to the South Pacific, where it was used in ceremonies and celebrations because of its calming effect and ability to promote sociability. Preparations of kava root are now gaining popularity in Europe and the United States as a mild sedative and an anxiety-relieving medicine. Several European countries have approved kava preparations as a medical treatment for anxiety, insomnia, and restlessness based on the results of detailed scientific investigations and favorable clinical studies.

Most studies have featured kava extracts standardized to contain a specific percentage of compounds known as kavalactones. Evidence suggests that the whole complex of kavalactones and other compounds naturally found in kava produce greater pharmacological activity than isolated pure kavalactones.

Based upon the results of several double-blind studies in people with mild anxiety, kava appears to be as effective as standard drugs, yet it is believed to be considerably safer and nonaddictive. The result of these double-blind studies demonstrated that individuals taking the kava extract experience a statistically significant reduction in symptoms of anxiety, including feelings of nervousness, heart palpitations, chest pains, headache, dizziness, and gastric irritation. Two additional studies have shown that, unlike benzodiazepines (diazepam [Valium], triazolam [Halcion], alprazolam [Xanax] etc.), alcohol, and other drugs, kava extract is not associated with depressed mental function or impairment in driving or the operation of heavy equipment when used at recommended dosages.

Available Forms

The crude herb is available in bulk, capsules, and tablets; other forms available are tinctures, fluid extracts, and solid extracts in tablets and capsules. Extracts stating the concentration of kavalactones are preferred by most experts. Brands available include Kavatrol.

Cautions and Warnings

If you are currently on a tranquilizer or antidepressant, you will need to work with a physician to get off the drug. Stopping the drug on your own can be dangerous; you absolutely must have proper medical supervision.

Do not use kava if you have Parkinson's disease.

Do not take kava in combination with alcohol.

Do not take kava in combination with benzodiazepines such as diazepam (Valium) and triazolam (Halcion) unless under medical supervision.

Do not take kava for prolonged periods (more than six months) without medical supervision to monitor for possible liver damage.

Possible Side Effects

Although no significant side effects have been reported using standardized kava extracts at recommended levels in clinical studies, several case reports suggest that kava may cause liver damage, interfere with dopamine, worsen Parkinson's disease, exert an additive effect when combined with benzodiazepines, and impair driving ability when consumed in very large dosages. Until these issues are cleared up, kava extract should not be used without checks for liver damage every six months. It should not be used by Parkinson's patients, should be used with extreme caution and under medical supervision in people taking benzodiazepines such as diazepam (Valium) and triazolam (Halcion), and should only be taken at recommended levels.

Drug Interactions

Kava may potentiate the effects of benzodiazepines (diazepam [Valium], triazolam [Halcion], alprazolam [Xanax], etc.), barbiturates, and prescription sedatives. There is also evidence that kava interferes with drugs used in the treatment of Parkinson's disease.

Food and Nutrient Interactions

None known.

Usual Dosage

The dosage of kava preparations is based on the level of kavalactones. Based on clinical studies, the recommendation for anxiety-relieving effects is 45 to 70 mg of kavalactones three times daily. For sedative effects, the same daily quantity (135 to 210 mg) can be taken as a single dose one hour before retiring.

Overdosage

High dosages of kava beverage consumed daily over a prolonged period (a few months to a year or more) are associated with kava dermopathy, a condition of the skin characterized by a peculiar generalized eruption known as kani. The skin becomes dry and covered with scales, especially the palms of the hand, soles of the feet, forearms, back, and shins.

Other adverse effects seen with extremely high doses of kava (e.g., greater than 310 g per week) for prolonged periods include low levels of serum albumin, protein, urea, and bilirubin; presence of blood in the urine; increased red blood cell volume; decreased platelet and lymphocyte counts; and shortness of breath.

Special Populations

Pregnant/breast-feeding women
As the effects of kava during pregnancy and lactation have not been sufficiently evaluated, it should not be used during these times.

Children
Generally regarded as suitable for children at one-half the adult dosage.

Seniors
No special precautions are known.

Kelp (*see* Iodine)

General Information

Kelp is a seaweed that is most often utilized as a source of natural iodine.

Kira (*see* St. John's Wort)

General Information

Kira contains the St. John's wort extract known as LI-160, the most thoroughly researched extract of the plant. LI-160 has been proven to exert antidepressant activity in over twenty-five double-blind studies and is regarded as the gold standard of St. John's wort products. Each tablet contains 300 mg of St. John's wort extract standardized to contain 0.3 percent hypericin.

Kudzu *(Pueraria lobata)*

Used For

Alcohol cravings
Effectiveness: C   Safety: C

General Information

Kudzu is a coarse, high-climbing vine that grows in China and the southeastern United States. Kudzu root has been used in traditional Chinese medicine for centuries. One of its primary uses has been in the treatment of alcoholism. Several animal studies showed that kudzu extract and its primary components, daidzein (a key isoflavonoid also found in soy) and puerarin, inhibit the desire for alcohol. This effect has not yet been proven in controlled clinical studies with humans, however.

Available Forms

Crude kudzu root is available in bulk, capsules, and tablets; also available are tinctures, fluid extracts, and solid extracts in tablets and capsules. Extracts stating the concentration of isoflavones are preferred by most experts. Depending on growing conditions, the total isoflavone content varies from 1.77 to 12 percent.

Cautions and Warnings

None known.

Possible Side Effects

None known.

Drug Interactions

None known.

Food and Nutrient Interactions

None known.

Usual Dosage

The recommended dosage for the crude root is 9–15 g per day. For kudzu extract the recommended dosage is one to two capsules (each 100 or 150 mg capsule supplying 1 mg daidzein) three times daily. Kudzu tincture can be used in the amount of 1–2 ml taken three to five times per day.

Overdosage

None known.

Special Populations

Pregnant/breast-feeding women
As the effects of kudzu during pregnancy and lactation have not been sufficiently evaluated, it should not be used during these times.

Children
There does not appear to be a suitable use of kudzu in children.

Seniors
No special precautions are known.

Kwai (*see* Garlic)

General Information

Kwai is a special garlic preparation that contains all the beneficial elements of raw garlic without the odor. Kwai is the world's most thoroughly researched garlic product, having been the subject of over thirty double-blind studies. Each 100 mg tablet is specially coated so that the garlic components are released only when it's well into the digestive system. The typical dosage is 2 tablets three times daily.

Kyolic

Used For

Cancer protection
Effectiveness: C   Safety: A

Heart disease (atherosclerosis) prevention and high blood pressure
Effectiveness: B   Safety: A

Low immunity and immune support
Effectiveness: C   Safety: A

General Information

Kyolic is a form of **garlic** produced by a unique aging process. During aging (up to twenty months), many of the highly odorous compounds in fresh garlic are converted into more stable, less odorous compounds. Various studies have suggested that supplementation with aged garlic extract may be as beneficial as eating garlic or using garlic products that deliver the odorous compound allicin.

Cancer protection

Like garlic, Kyolic has demonstrated anticancer effects in test tube and animal studies. Preliminary studies suggest that Kyolic may reduce side effects such as fatigue and anorexia in cancer patients undergoing radiation therapy or chemotherapy, and possibly reduce the toxicity to the heart of the anticancer drug doxorubicin.

Heart disease (atherosclerosis) prevention and high blood pressure

Clearly, the most popular use of garlic is in lowering cholesterol and blood pressure. While there are some studies showing that Kyolic may lower both cholesterol and blood pressure, the clinical relevance of the reduction has not been sufficiently demonstrated. For example, in the best-designed double-blind study in men with beginning cholesterol levels in the 220–290 mg/dl range receiving either Kyolic (7.2 g per day) or placebo, after six months of use there was only a minimal reduction of total cholesterol (7 percent) and LDL cholesterol (4 percent) but no change in HDL cholesterol or triglyceride levels. The systolic blood pressure dropped an average of 5 mm/Hg, but there was no change in diastolic blood pressure. These results call into question whether Kyolic can produce meaningful reductions at normally recommended dosages.

Kyolic may offer better protection against heart disease and atherosclerosis by mechanisms other than lowering cholesterol. For example, Kyolic has demonstrated antioxidant effects in protecting LDL cholesterol from being damaged, and in turn contributing to arterial damage. It has also been shown to inhibit the development of arterial plaque.

Low immunity and immune support

Preliminary studies have suggested Kyolic may enhance the immune system. Specifically, in test tube studies Kyolic has been shown to enhance the function of white blood cells, while in animal studies it was shown to enhance the preventative effect of an influenza vaccine and when used alone was as effective as the vaccine. These preliminary results have not yet been followed up by human research.

Available Forms

Kyolic is available in several different forms—capsules, tablets, and liquid—in several different strengths.

Cautions and Warnings

None known.

Possible Side Effects

Although the odorous compounds have largely been removed, some people still experience a garlicky odor on their breath or through their pores with Kyolic.

Drug Interactions

Kyolic may reduce the toxicity to the heart of the anticancer drug doxorubicin.

Food and Nutrient Interactions

None known.

Usual Dosage

The typical recommendation is 600 to 2,400 mg per day for the extract in tablets or capsules and ¼ to ½ tsp per day for the liquid extract.

Overdosage

None known.

Special Populations

Pregnant/breast-feeding women
Kyolic is generally regarded as being safe during pregnancy and lactation.

Children
Suitable for children at one-half the adult dosage.

Seniors
No special precautions are known.

Licorice *(Glycyrrhiza glabra)*

Used For

AIDS and HIV infection
Effectiveness: B+   Safety: C

Common cold
Effectiveness: C   Safety: C

Hepatitis
Effectiveness: B+   Safety: C

Inflammation
Effectiveness: C   Safety: C

Premenstrual syndrome
Effectiveness: C   Safety: C

General Information

Licorice root is one of the most popular herbal medicines around the globe. The major active compo-

nent of licorice root is a compound known as glycyrrhizin, usually found in concentrations ranging
from 6 to 10 percent. Once ingested, glycyrrhizin is
broken down into glycyrrhetinic acid before it is absorbed. These compounds have shown a multitude
of pharmacological effects, including estrogenic,
anti-inflammatory (cortisone-like action), and antiviral actions. Many other licorice components, such as
flavonoids, also have shown significant effects.

As glycyrrhizin is 50 to a hundred times sweeter
than sucrose, licorice preparations are often used as
a sweetening or flavoring agent to mask the bitter
taste of other medications.

AIDS and HIV infection

Glycyrrhizin-containing preparations are showing
promise in the treatment of human immunodeficiency virus (HIV) infection and AIDS. Although
much of the research has featured injectable preparations, this route of administration may not be necessary, as glycyrrhizin and glycyrrhetinic acid are
easily absorbed orally and well tolerated. Several
double-blind studies have demonstrated that the
clinical effectiveness of oral administration of glycyrrhizin is equal to the results achieved via injection. In one of the studies, sixteen patients with
evidence of HIV infection received daily doses of
150–225 mg glycyrrhizin for three to seven years.
Helper T cell and total T lymphocyte numbers, other
immune system parameters, and glycyrrhizin and
glycyrrhetinic acid levels in the blood were monitored. None of the patients given the glycyrrhizin
had progression of immune system abnormalities
or progression to AIDS. In contrast, the group not receiving glycyrrhizin showed decreases in helper T
cell and total T lymphocyte counts and antibody levels. Two of the sixteen patients in the control group

developed AIDS. The results of this study and others in HIV-positive and AIDS patients are encouraging.

Common cold

Licorice has long been used in treating the symptoms of the common cold. This historical use is justified by its immune-enhancing and antiviral effects, but there are no clinical trials to justify or refute this use.

Hepatitis

Licorice exerts many pharmacological actions beneficial in the treatment of acute and chronic hepatitis, including protecting against liver damage, boosting immune function, and improving liver function. Clinical studies with a glycyrrhizin-containing product in Japan have shown excellent results in the treatment of acute and chronic hepatitis. The product, Stronger Neominophagen C (SNMC), consists of 200 mg glycyrrhizin, 100 mg cysteine, and 2,000 mg glycine in 100 ml of physiological saline solution. In the studies it was administered intravenously (oral administration may be just as effective, as discussed below). SNMC has demonstrated impressive results in treating hepatitis B and C. With either form, approximately 40 percent of patients will have complete resolution—a statistic that compares quite favorably to the 40–50 percent clearance rate seen with alpha-interferon (the conventional medical approach). SNMC has also been shown to lead to similar dramatic reductions in the risk for liver cancer (hepatocellular carcinoma) in patients with hepatitis C.

Inflammation

Licorice components have demonstrated significant anti-inflammatory and antiallergy actions in test tube and animal studies. Licorice has also been shown to enhance the action of corticosteroid drugs such as prednisone and prednisolone, as well as the levels of the body's own corticosteroids.

Premenstrual syndrome

It is thought that licorice exerts a balancing effect on estrogen metabolism—that is, when estrogen levels are too high, it will inhibit estrogen's action, and when estrogens are too low, it will enhance estrogen's action. One of its popular uses is in the treatment of premenstrual syndrome, although effectiveness for this application has not been confirmed in clinical studies.

Available Forms

Licorice root is available in crude (bulk) form, as a fluid extract, and as a dry powdered extract. Since the optimal dosage of licorice root often depends on the content of glycyrrhetinic acid, preparations standardized for this compound may produce more dependable results. These preparations are usually available in tablets or capsules. *Note:* In treating peptic ulcer, **deglycyrrhizinated licorice (DGL)** is preferred, as it produces equally effective results compared to glycyrrhetinic acid but is free from any side effects.

Cautions and Warnings

Licorice is not to be used by individuals with high blood pressure or kidney failure or who are currently taking digitalis (Digoxin) unless directed to do so by a physician.

Possible Side Effects

Glycyrrhetinic acid can raise blood pressure by causing sodium retention. There is great individual variation in the susceptibility to this side effect. Elevations in blood pressure are rarely observed at levels below 3 g of licorice root or 100 mg of glycyrrhetinic acid per day, while they are almost certain at levels above 12 g of licorice root or 400 mg of glycyrrhetinic acid per day. Monitoring of blood pressure is recommended with any long-term use of licorice.

Drug Interactions

Theoretically, licorice root preparations may counteract the effectiveness of drugs used to treat high blood pressure.

Licorice root preparations may potentiate corticosteroid drugs such as prednisone.

Licorice root preparations may offset some of the negative effects that drugs such as cimetidine (Tagamet) and ranitidine (Zantac) produce on the gastrointestinal tract.

Licorice root preparations may potentiate the effects of alpha-interferon in the treatment of chronic hepatitis.

Food and Nutrient Interactions

A high-potassium, low-sodium diet is recommended to prevent the blood-pressure-elevating effect of licorice root preparations.

Usual Dosage

The following dosages are typically taken three times daily:

Powdered root: 1–2 g
Fluid extract (1:1): 2–4 ml
Solid extract (5 percent glycyrrhetinic acid content):
   250–500 mg

Overdosage

Acute toxicity from licorice preparations is extremely rare.

Special Populations

Pregnant/breast-feeding women
   As the effects of licorice during pregnancy and lactation have not been sufficiently evaluated, it should not be used during these times unless directed to do so by a physician.

Children
   Suitable for children at one-half the adult dosage.

Seniors
   No special precautions are known.

Ma Huang (*see* Ephedra
[Ephedra sinica])

General Information

The name *Ma huang* refers to the aboveground portion of the most famous species of ephedra. Ma huang has been used as a medicine in China since before 2800 B.C. It is used primarily in the treatment of the common cold, asthma, hay fever, bronchitis, edema, arthritis, fever, low blood pressure, and hives.

Maté *(Ilex paraguariensis)*

General Information

Maté is a caffeine-containing plant from South America. Like other caffeine-containing plants, maté has historically been used to sustain people during long journeys or long hours of work. It is usually consumed as a beverage made from the dried minced or cut leaves. In addition to caffeine (0.9–1.7 percent), maté contains polyphenols; like other polyphenol-containing beverages (e.g., green tea and red wine), maté has been shown to provide significant antioxidant protection. For information on the uses and side effects of maté, see **caffeine**.

Mexican Wild Yam
(Dioscorea villosa)

Used For

Menopause
Effectiveness: C   Safety: C

General Information

Wild yam plants are found across the midwestern and eastern United States, Latin America (especially Mexico), and Asia. Several different species exist, all possessing similar constituents and properties. Components in wild yam root, such as diosgenin, can be converted in a laboratory environment into cortisone, estrogens, and progesteronelike compounds. Wild yam and other plants with similar constituents continue to be the main source of these drugs. However, contrary to popular claims, wild yam roots do not contain and are not converted into true progesterone, dehydroepiandrosterone (DHEA), or other hormones in the body.

Diosgenin and other wild yam components may act in a way similar to soy isoflavones—as phytoestrogens in the relief of menopausal symptoms. However, this possible application has not been studied in human clinical trials.

Available Forms

Mexican wild yam root is available as the dried root in tablets and capsules, as well as a tincture, a fluid extract, and a solid extract in tablets and capsules.

Cautions and Warnings

None known.

Possible Side Effects

At higher dosages it may induce nausea and vomiting.

Drug Interactions

None known.

Food and Nutrient Interactions

None known.

Usual Dosage

The typical dosage is based upon a diosgenin intake of 50 to 100 mg daily. For an extract standardized to contain 10 percent diosgenin, this amount translates to 500 to 1,000 mg of the extract. The diosgenin content of crude Mexican yam is roughly 2 percent, so the dosage for crude preparations is roughly 2,500 to 5,000 mg daily.

Overdosage

May produce nausea and vomiting.

Special Populations

Pregnant/breast-feeding women
As the effects of Mexican yam during pregnancy and lactation have not been sufficiently evaluated, it should not be used during these times.

Children

As the effects of Mexican yam in children have not been sufficiently evaluated, it should not be used in children unless directed to do so by a physician.

Seniors

No special precautions are known.

Milk Thistle
(Silybum marianum)

Used For

Hepatitis and cirrhosis of the liver
Effectiveness: B+   Safety: A

Gallstone prevention and dissolution
Effectiveness: B   Safety: A

Psoriasis
Effectiveness: B   Safety: A

General Information

Milk thistle contains silymarin, a mixture of flavonoid components (silybin, silidianin, and silichristine) that exert significant antioxidant and liver-protecting effects. Silymarin is at least ten times more potent in antioxidant activity than vitamin E and also increases the liver's own antioxidant, glutathione, by over 35 percent.

Hepatitis and cirrhosis of the liver

Milk thistle extracts (usually standardized to contain 70–80 percent silymarin) have been shown to exert positive effects in treating several types of liver disease, including hepatitis and cirrhosis. The therapeutic effect of milk thistle extracts in these disorders has been confirmed by biopsy as well as by clinical and laboratory data.

Although milk thistle extract has shown benefits in treating acute and chronic viral hepatitis, the results with milk thistle extract are most impressive when looking at studies evaluating its effectiveness in alcohol- or toxic-chemical-induced hepatitis. For example, in one double-blind study in workers exposed to toxic toluene and/or xylene vapors for five to twenty years, milk thistle extract (Thisilyn) was shown to significantly lower levels of two liver enzymes (AST and ALT) associated with liver damage and to significantly improve other blood measurements, such as platelet count, white blood cell count, and percentage of lymphocytes compared to other white blood cells.

Even in cirrhosis of the liver (serious liver damage associated with severe scarring), milk thistle extract has shown some benefits. Although not all studies have shown significant effects, in one controlled study the four-year survival rate was 58 percent in the milk thistle extract group compared to 39 percent in the control group.

Gallstones

Theoretically, milk thistle extract may help prevent or treat gallstones via its ability to increase the solubility of the bile (gallstones form when bile components fall out of solution). However, there have been no studies examining this application.

Psoriasis

Milk thistle extract has been reported to be of value in the treatment of psoriasis. This may be due to its ability to inhibit the synthesis of inflammatory compounds that stimulate psoriatic plaque formation as well as its ability to improve liver function. The liver is responsible for filtering out of the blood various gut-derived toxins that are implicated in psoriasis.

Available Forms

Milk thistle is available in bulk as the dried seeds, as tea bags, as a tincture, as a fluid extract, and as a solid extract in capsules and tablets. Extracts standardized for silymarin content are preferred over crude preparations by most experts. Brands available include Thisilyn. Another brand-name product, Silybin Phytosome, binds silybin, the key ingredient in silymarin, with **phosphatidylcholine**. Preliminary evidence indicates Silybin Phytosome is better absorbed and produces better clinical results than regular milk thistle extract.

Cautions and Warnings

None known.

Possible Side Effects

Milk thistle extract may increase the output of bile and as a result produce a looser stool. If this side effect occurs, it is often recommended to use fiber compounds (e.g., guar gum, pectin, psyllium, and oat bran; see **fiber**) to bind the bile components, thus preventing irritation and loose stools.

Drug Interactions

Milk thistle extract may reduce the toxicity to the liver caused by many drugs, including thyroid hormone, acetaminophen, butyrophenones, phenothiazines, phenytoin, and alcohol.

Food and Nutrient Interactions

None known.

Usual Dosage

The standard dosage for a milk thistle preparation is based on its silymarin content, with a goal of 70–210 mg of silymarin three times daily. For this reason, standardized extracts are preferred. The best results are achieved at higher dosages, that is, 210 mg of silymarin three times daily. The typical dosage for Silybin Phytosome is 80 to 120 mg two to three times daily between meals. The dosage for dried milk thistle seeds is 12 to 15 g daily.

Overdosage

None known.

Special Populations

Pregnant/breast-feeding women

As the effects of milk thistle preparations during pregnancy and lactation have not been sufficiently evaluated, it should not be used during these times unless directed to do so by a physician.

Children
   Suitable for children at one-half the adult dosage.

Seniors
   No special precautions are known.

Noni Fruit *(Morinda citrifolia)*

Used For

Low immunity and immune support
Effectiveness: C   Safety: C

General Information

Native to Polynesia, the noni plant (also known as Indian mulberry) is a small tree that usually grows to a height of 10 feet. The four-inch fruit is the portion of the plant used for medicinal purposes.

   Traditional Polynesian healers have used noni for the treatment of a broad range of disorders, but the terrible bitter taste has limited its use in modern times. Commercial products are now available that have either altered the taste of noni juice or made it available as an extract in tablets or capsules to increase acceptability. In the early 1990s noni juice became heavily marketed in the United States, primarily through network marketing companies. However, despite tremendous claims and testimonials, there is little scientific documentation on noni. Animal and test tube studies have shown some anticancer and immune-enhancing activity, and an earlier animal study seemed to indicate that the fruit exerts a mild sedative effect. But whether noni produces any real effects in humans has not been demonstrated.

Available Forms

Noni is available as juice in bottles or as an extract in tablets and capsules.

Cautions and Warnings

None known.

Possible Side Effects

Nausea and gastrointestinal irritation.

Drug Interactions

None known, although it has been suggested that it not be taken with coffee, tobacco, or alcohol.

Food and Nutrient Interactions

Generally recommended to be taken on an empty stomach.

Usual Dosage

The usual recommendation is the equivalent of 4 fluid ounces of noni juice half an hour before breakfast (effectiveness is thought to be best on an empty stomach). Labels of noni products in tablet or capsule forms usually give equivalent to ounces of juice.

Overdosage

Not known.

Special Populations

Pregnant/breast-feeding women
The safety of noni juice during pregnancy and lactation has not been determined, so it should not be used during these times.

Children
Suitable for children at one-half the adult dosage.

Seniors
No special precautions are known.

Olive Leaf *(Olea europa)*

Used For

Common cold and other viral infections
Effectiveness: C   Safety: C

Diabetes
Effectiveness: C   Safety: C

Heart disease (atherosclerosis) prevention
Effectiveness: C   Safety: C

High blood pressure
Effectiveness: B   Safety: C

General Information

Olive leaf extract contains many active compounds, including oleuropein and flavonoids. Preliminary studies indicate that olive leaf extract can act as an antioxidant in protecting against damage to LDL cholesterol, thereby preventing the initiation of the process of hardening of the arteries (atherosclerosis). Other effects that are thought to offer protection against atherosclerosis include inhibition of platelet aggregation and lowering of cholesterol levels. However, there is little clinical validation of these effects. In one double-blind study, olive leaf extract was shown to produce a modest lowering of blood pressure. This effect may be the result of decreasing the force of contraction of the heart.

Animal studies have also shown an ability to lower blood sugar levels, supporting a historical use of olive leaves. Olive leaf extract has also demonstrated some antibacterial and antiviral effects. Again, there have been no human studies to support this application.

Available Forms

Olive leaf is available in crude (bulk) form, as well as in fluid extracts and solid extracts. Since the optimal dosage of olive leaf depends on the content of oleuropein, preparations standardized for this compound may produce more dependable results. These preparations are usually available in tablets or capsules.

Cautions and Warnings

None known.

Possible Side Effects

None known.

Drug Interactions

Theoretically, olive leaf preparations may interfere with or enhance the effects of drugs used in the treatment of high blood pressure. Close monitoring of blood pressure is required in people taking olive leaf with any blood-pressure-lowering drug. Discontinue use immediately in the event blood pressure readings increase.

Food and Nutrient Interactions

None known.

Usual Dosage

The standard dosage for olive leaf preparation is based on its oleuropein content, with a typical recommendation of 50 to 100 mg of oleuropein three times daily. For this reason, standardized extracts are preferred. For an olive leaf extract standardized at 17 to 23 percent oleuropein, the typical dosage recommendation is 250 to 500 mg three times daily.

Overdosage

None known.

Special Populations

Pregnant/breast-feeding women
As the effects of olive leaf during pregnancy and lactation have not been sufficiently evaluated, it should not be used during these times.

Children
Suitable for use in children at one-half the adult dosage.

Seniors
No special precautions are known.

Oregon Grape Root *(Berberis aquifolium)* (*see* Berberine-Containing Plants)

General Information

The Oregon grape is an evergreen spineless shrub, 3 to 6 feet in height, native to the Rocky Mountains from British Columbia to California. The part used is the root. Oregon grape root shares indications and effects with other berberine-containing plants such as goldenseal and barberry.

Panax Ginseng (Chinese or Korean Ginseng) (*see* Ginseng)

General Information

Panax ginseng (Korean or Chinese ginseng) is the most widely used and most extensively studied ginseng. *Panax ginseng* is perhaps the most famous medicinal plant of China, where historically it was used alone or in combination with other herbs as a tonic and for its revitalizing properties, especially after a long illness.

Papain

General Information

Papain is a mixture of protein-digesting enzymes derived from unripe papaya. Papain is used commercially in many meat tenderizers. Although there has been little scientific investigation of papain, what is available indicates that papain has effects similar to those of bromelain. See **bromelain** for more information.

Passionflower

Used For

Insomnia
Effectiveness: C   Safety: C

General Information

Passionflower is a plant native to Latin and South America that derives its name from Spanish explorers who believed the flowers symbolized both Christ's passion and Christ's approval of their exploration. It was widely used by the Aztecs as a sedative and analgesic (pain reliever). There are animal studies that support these effects, but there have been no human studies. The active constituents of passionflower include harmine. This compound was originally known as telepathine because of its ability to induce a contemplative state and mild euphoria. It was later used by the Germans in World War II as "truth serum." Harmine and related compounds can inhibit the breakdown of serotonin and therefore may have a sleep-promoting effect. In addition to harmine, recent studies indicate that the flavonoids in passionflower also contribute to its sedative effects.

Available Forms

The crude dried flowers are available in bulk, in capsules and tablets, and in tea bags; also available are tinctures, fluid extracts, and solid extracts in capsules and tablets. Most solid extracts are standardized to contain no less than 0.8 percent total flavonoids.

Passionflower is often combined with valerian, lemon balm, and other herbs with sedative properties.

Cautions and Warnings

If you are taking an antidepressant drug, please consult your physician before taking passionflower.

Possible Side Effects

None known.

Drug Interactions

Many herbalists caution against use of passionflower by anyone taking an antidepressant drug. Theoretically, passionflower may enhance the effects of monoamine oxidase inhibitors, selective serotonin reuptake inhibitors, and tricyclic antidepressants.

Food and Nutrient Interactions

None known.

Usual Dosage

The recommended dosage as a sedative forty-five minutes before retiring for the various forms of passionflower are as follows:

Dried herb (or as tea): 4–8 g
Tincture (1:5): 6–8 ml (1½ –2 teaspoons)
Fluid extract (1:1): 2–4 ml (½ –1 teaspoon)
Solid extract (2.6 percent flavonoids): 300–450 mg

Overdosage

None known.

Special Populations

Pregnant/breast-feeding women
As the effects of passionflower during pregnancy and lactation have not been sufficiently evaluated, it should not be used during these times.

Children
Suitable for use in children at one-half the adult dosage.

Seniors
No special precautions are known.

Pau D'arco *(Tabebuia avellanedae)*

Used For

Cancer
Effectiveness: C   Safety: C

Infections
Effectiveness: C   Safety: C

General Information

Pau d'arco (also known as lapacho and taheebo) is a tree native to South America. Historically the inner bark was used as a folk remedy for a wide variety of indications, including infections and cancer. Pau d'arco has demonstrated some antimicrobial properties and anticancer effects; its components have shown activity against many disease-causing bacteria, viruses, and yeast (including *Candida albicans*). However, whether these effects apply to oral use of pau d'arco preparations has not been sufficiently studied in humans.

After hearing about pau d'arco's tumor-reducing qualities, the National Cancer Institute (NCI) subjected it to extensive study. After initial positive results, it was determined that the component lapachol was the most active anticancer agent. Lapachol entered human clinical trials at the NCI in 1968. During these trials it was difficult to obtain therapeutic blood levels of lapachol without some mild toxic side effects such as nausea, vomiting, and anti–vitamin K activity leading to bleeding tendencies. Research was halted at the NCI in 1970. At this time, despite many anecdotal reports of remission of different forms of cancer following the use of pau d'arco, it does not appear to offer significant effects against cancer.

Available Forms

Crude pau d'arco bark is available in bulk, tea bags, and capsules and tablets; also available are tinctures, fluid extracts, and solid extracts in capsules and tablets.

Cautions and Warnings

Do not use pau d'arco during pregnancy or lactation.

Due to the lack of documented benefit in cancer treatment in humans, pau d'arco should not be used as a primary therapy in cancer, which is a potentially life-threatening disease that requires proper medical treatment.

Possible Side Effects

No significant side effects have been seen when using preparations of the whole bark. However, high amounts (several grams daily over several days) of the isolated component lapachol can cause nausea and vomiting as well as lead to bleeding disorders.

Drug Interactions

Theoretically, because pau d'arco's components antagonize vitamin K, it may enhance the anticoagulant effects of warfarin (Coumadin).

Food and Nutrient Interactions

None known.

Usual Dosage

The usual form of administration of pau d'arco is as a decoction (tea made by boiling the bark) with the standard dose being 1 cup of the decoction two to eight times per day. The decoction is made by boiling 1 teaspoon of pau d'arco in a cup of water for five to fifteen minutes. The dosage of the dried or powdered crude bark is usually 300 to 1,000 mg three times daily. The dosage of other forms (tincture, fluid extract, and solid extract) should be equivalent to this amount; follow label instructions on these products.

Overdosage

Although overdosage with pau d'arco preparations is extremely unlikely, exposure to high levels of the isolated component lapachol can lead to significant toxicity. Do the following in case of accidental overdose: If the victim is unconscious or having convulsions, call for an ambulance immediately. If you take the victim to an emergency room, be sure to bring the bottle or container with you. If the victim is conscious, call your local poison control center or a health care professional. The poison control center may suggest inducing vomiting with ipecac syrup (available without a prescription at any pharmacy). *Do not* induce vomiting unless specifically instructed to do so.

Special Populations

Pregnant/breast-feeding women
As the effects of pau d'arco during pregnancy and lactation have not been sufficiently evaluated, it should not be used during these times.

Children
As the effects of pau d'arco during childhood have not been sufficiently evaluated, it should not be used by children unless under the direction of a physician.

Seniors
No special precautions are known.

Peppermint *(Mentha piperita)*

Used For

Common cold
Effectiveness: C   Safety: A

Irritable bowel syndrome
Effectiveness: A   Safety: B

General Information

Although peppermint was not officially recognized until the seventeenth century, various species of mint have been used for their medicinal effects for thousands of years. For medicinal effects, the above-ground portion of the plant is the most widely used. The major medicinal component of peppermint is its volatile oil and its chief component, menthol.

The most popular medicinal uses of peppermint and peppermint oil are for the treatment of the common cold and irritable bowel syndrome. Peppermint oil is also used extensively in antacid products, irritant laxatives, and mouthwash both for its flavor and for its therapeutic effects.

Common cold
Menthol and peppermint oil are often components of cough and throat lozenges as well as ointments, salves, and inhalants. The benefit of these products has not been proven in clinical studies, but they are generally regarded as being effective. Their popularity appears to be based on their ability to ease breathing during the common cold.

Irritable bowel syndrome
Peppermint tea and peppermint oil have long been used to calm intestinal spasms and reduce excessive flatulence. There is evidence to support this historical use. Peppermint oil has been shown in several clinical studies to be quite helpful in the treatment of irritable bowel syndrome. This syndrome is characterized by a combination of any of the following symptoms: abdominal pain and dis-

tension; more frequent bowel movements with pain, or relief of pain with bowel movements; constipation or diarrhea; excessive production of mucus in the colon; symptoms of indigestion such as flatulence, nausea, or anorexia; and varying degrees of anxiety or depression.

In order to be most effective, peppermint oil capsules should be enteric-coated to prevent the oil from being released in the stomach. Without enteric coating, peppermint oil tends to produce heartburn. With the enteric coating, the peppermint oil travels to the small and large intestine, where it relaxes intestinal muscles as well as promotes the elimination of excess gas.

Available Forms

Peppermint is available as the crude herb (fresh or dried leaves) in bulk as well as in capsules and tablets. Peppermint oil is available in enteric-coated soft-gelatin capsules. Brand names include Mentharil and Peppermint Plus.

Cautions and Warnings

Keep peppermint oil preparations away from children. Accidental poisonings are possible. The fatal oral dose in humans is 1 g per kg (2.2 pounds) body weight.

Possible Side Effects

Peppermint is generally regarded as safe when used as a tea; however, allergic reactions have been reported. Side effects with enteric-coated peppermint oil capsules are rare but can include allergic reactions (skin rash), heartburn, bradycardia, and muscle tremors.

Drug Interactions

None known.

Food and Nutrient Interactions

Peppermint oil is generally recommended to be taken on an empty stomach.

Usual Dosage

Peppermint is most widely used as a tea (infusion). The infusion is usually prepared with 1 to 2 teaspoons (1.5 to 3.0 g) of the dried leaves per 8 fluid ounces of water. For the tincture (1:5, 45 percent ethanol), take 2–3 ml three times daily. The dosage of peppermint oil administered in an enteric-coated capsule for the treatment of irritable bowel syndrome is 1–2 capsules (0.2 ml/capsule) three times daily between meals.

Overdosage

Overdosage with peppermint tea has not been reported. However, it is possible to overdose with peppermint oil. Do the following in case of accidental overdose: If the victim is unconscious or having convulsions, call for an ambulance immediately. If you take the victim to an emergency room, be sure to bring the bottle or container with you. If the victim is conscious, call your local poison control center or a health care professional. The poison control center may suggest inducing vomiting with ipecac syrup (available without a prescription at any pharmacy). *Do not* induce vomiting unless specifically instructed to do so.

Special Populations

Pregnant/breast-feeding women

Peppermint tea is considered safe during pregnancy and lactation, but peppermint oil should not be used during these times.

Children

Peppermint tea is suitable for children at one-half the adult dosage. If children can swallow enteric-coated peppermint oil capsules, it is suitable for them at a dosage of one capsule twice daily between meals.

Seniors

No special precautions are known.

Perika (*see* St. John's Wort)

General Information

Perika was the first St. John's wort extract on the market that was standardized to contain an effective amount of hyperforin, one of the key active ingredients responsible for the mood-enhancing effects of the herb.

Phytodolor

Used For

Arthritis (both osteoarthritis and rheumatoid arthritis)
Effectiveness: B+   Safety: A

Trauma and athletic injury
Effectiveness: B+   Safety: A

General Information

Phytodolor is a mixture of standardized fluid extracts from three medicinal plants: aspen *(Populus tremula)*, ash *(Fraxinus excelsior)*, and goldenrod *(Solidago virgaurea)*. It has been used in Germany since 1963, and it has been studied in over thirty clinical trials involving 1,151 patients. There have been six double-blind studies showing that Phytodolor is superior to a placebo and seven double-blind studies showing that it compares quite well to the nonsteroidal anti-inflammatory drugs (NSAIDs) in the treatment of osteoarthritis, trauma, and athletic injury. In regard to rheumatoid arthritis, Phytodolor on its own is not strong enough to provide significant clinical benefit, but studies demonstrate that it can significantly reduce the dosage of NSAIDs and other analgesics required to relieve pain in these patients.

Phytodolor works by a complex interplay of its plant constituents, which inhibit both formation and release of inflammatory compounds at sites of inflammation and trauma. One of the interesting aspects of Phytodolor's mechanism of action is that the most important constituents are not activated until they are chemically transformed inside the body. This fact is one of the key reasons why Phytodolor does not cause any of the harsh effects on the stomach and intestines characteristic of anti-inflammatory drugs. Phytodolor exerts no effect on blood clotting, as do aspirin and some other NSAIDs.

Available Forms

Phytodolor is a standardized fluid extract available in dropper bottles.

Cautions and Warnings

None known.

Possible Side Effects

None known.

Drug Interactions

Phytodolor has been shown to reduce the dosage required for pain management of rheumatoid arthritis patients taking NSAIDs and other pain relievers.

Food and Nutrient Interactions

Generally recommended on an empty stomach.

Usual Dosage

The typical dosage recommendation is 30 drops in 2–4 fluid ounces of water three times daily.

Overdosage

None known.

Special Populations

Pregnant/breast-feeding women
As the effects of Phytodolor during pregnancy and lactation have not been sufficiently evaluated, it should not be used during these times unless directed to do so by a physician.

Children
Suitable for children at one-half the adult dosage.

Seniors
No special precautions are known.

Pine Bark Extract (*see* Procyanidolic Oligomers)

General Information

Extracts from the bark of the maritime pine *(Pinus maritima)* contain proanthocyanidins (also referred to as procyanidins), one of the most beneficial groups of plant flavonoids. Powerful antioxidants, the most active proanthocyanidins are those bound to other proanthocyanidins. Collectively, mixtures of proanthocyanidin dimers, trimers, tetramers, and larger molecules are referred to as procyanidolic oligomers (PCOs). Although PCOs exist in many plants, commercially available sources of PCOs include grape seed and pine bark extracts.

Policosanol

Used For

Lowering cholesterol and triglyceride levels
Effectiveness: A   Safety: A

General Information

Policosanol is a mixture of fatty substances isolated and purified from the wax of sugar cane *(Saccharum officinarum)*. Policosanol has exceptional clinical documentation demonstrating efficacy, safety, and tolerability in lowering cholesterol and triglyceride levels. The clinical studies have included comparative studies versus conventional cholesterol-lowering drugs (e.g., lovastatin, pravastatin, simvastatin, gemfibrozil, and probucol). In these studies, policosanol in dosages ranging from 5 to 20 mg per day has resulted in significant improvements in cholesterol and triglyceride levels, with effects typically noticeable within the first six to eight weeks of use. At a daily dosage of 10 mg of policosanol at night, LDL cholesterol levels typically dropped by 20 to 25 percent within the first six months of therapy. At a dosage of 20 mg, LDL levels typically dropped by 25 to 30 percent. HDL cholesterol levels typically increased by 15 to 25 percent after only two months of use. The combined LDL reduction and HDL increase produced dramatic improvements in the LDL-to-HDL ratio.

In addition to its effects on cholesterol levels, policosanol also exerts additional positive effects in the battle against atherosclerosis (hardening of the arteries). It prevents excessive platelet aggregation without affecting coagulation, prevents smooth muscle cell proliferation into the lining of the artery, and exerts good antioxidant effects in preventing LDL oxidation and subsequent arterial damage.

Available Forms

Policosanol is not yet available in the United States, as it is manufactured in Cuba. It is, however, available in Canada from Natural Factors.

Cautions and Warnings

None known.

Possible Side Effects

None known.

Drug Interactions

No adverse drug reactions have been observed in clinical trials and safety studies.

Food and Nutrient Interactions

None known.

Usual Dosage

The recommended dosage of policosanol is 5 to 20 mg at the evening meal. It is given at night because most cholesterol manufacture occurs at night. As with other cholesterol-lowering therapies, dosage can be adjusted based upon checking blood cholesterol levels every eight weeks or so.

Overdosage

None known.

Special Populations

Pregnant/breast-feeding women
As the effects of policosanol during pregnancy and lactation have not been sufficiently evaluated, it should not be used during these times.

Children
As the effects of policosanol in children have not been sufficiently evaluated, it should not be used in children unless directed to do so by a physician.

Seniors
No special precautions are known.

Procyanidolic Oligomers

Used For

Antioxidant effects
Effectiveness: B   Safety: A

Venous and capillary disorders
Effectiveness: A   Safety: A

General Information

The proanthocyanidins (also referred to as procyanidins) are one of the most beneficial groups of plant flavonoids. The most active proanthocyanidins are those bound to other proanthocyanidins. Collectively, mixtures of proanthocyanidin dimers, trimers, tetramers, and larger molecules are referred to as procyanidolic oligomers (PCOs) or oligomeric proanthocyanidin complexes (OPCs). Although PCOs exist in many plants as well as red wine, commercially available sources of PCOs include extracts from grape seed skin *(Vitex vinifera)* and the bark of the maritime pine.

Antioxidant activity

Extracts of PCOs have demonstrated a wide range of activity, including exceptional antioxidant and free-radical-activity. In experimental models, the antioxidant activity of PCOs is much greater (approximately fifty times) that of vitamin C and vitamin E. From a cellular perspective, one of the most advantageous features of PCOs' free-radical-scavenging activity is that, because of their chemical structure, they are incorporated into cell membranes. This physical characteristic, along with their ability to protect against both water- and fat-soluble free radicals, provides significant cellular protection against free radical damage. The antioxidant activity of PCOs are thought to offer protection against heart disease, cancer, accelerated aging, and other health conditions linked to oxidative damage.

Since PCOs have a greater antioxidant effect than vitamins C and E, it is only natural to speculate they could offer greater protective effects against heart disease. There is evidence to support this hypothesis, as several studies indicate that heart disease is less frequent in people who consume higher levels of dietary flavonoids. Whether supplementation with PCOs protects against heart disease has not been demonstrated. What has been demonstrated in animal studies is that PCOs protect against oxidative damage to LDL cholesterol and the lining of the arteries, lower blood cholesterol levels and shrink the size of cholesterol deposits in arteries, and inhibit plaque formation.

Venous and capillary disorders

The primary clinical applications of PCOs are in the treatment of venous and capillary disorders, including venous insufficiency, varicose veins, and capillary fragility characterized by easy bruising. Good clinical studies have shown positive results in the treatment of these conditions, presumably as a result of PCOs strengthening the structure of veins and small blood vessels (capillaries).

Available Forms

Products containing PCOs from grape seed extracts and pine bark extracts are primarily available in capsules and tablets. Brands available include Leucoselect and Pycnogenol.

Cautions and Warnings

None known.

Possible Side Effects

None known.

Drug Interactions

There is one case report in which Pycnogenol improved the response to dextroamphetamine in a child with attention deficit disorder.

Food and Nutrient Interactions

None known.

Usual Dosage

For antioxidant support, a daily dose of 50 mg of PCOs from either grape seed or pine bark extract is suitable. When being used for therapeutic purposes, the daily dosage should be increased to 150 to 300 mg.

Overdosage

None known.

Special Populations

Pregnant/breast-feeding women

As the effects of PCOs during pregnancy and lactation have not been sufficiently evaluated, they should not be used during these times unless directed to do so by a physician.

Children

Suitable for use in children at one-half the adult dosage.

Seniors

No special precautions are known.

Promensil (*see* Red Clover)

General Information

Promensil is a red clover *(Trifolium pratense)* extract that has shown beneficial effects in preliminary studies in women with menopausal symptoms. Red clover is very rich in phytoestrogens—plant compounds capable of binding to estrogen receptors to produce a mild estrogenic effect.

Pseudoephedrine

Used For

Nasal congestion
Effectiveness: A   Safety: D

General Information

Pseudoephedrine is a compound that occurs naturally in **Ephedra sinica** (ma huang). As an isolated compound, it is an FDA-approved over-the-counter nasal decongestant. Pseudoephedrine works by constricting the blood vessels in the nose. By reducing the blood supply, it limits swelling in the lining of the nasal passages. Pseudoephedrine provides symptomatic relief for nasal congestion caused by the common cold or allergies.

Available Forms

Pseudoephedrine is available in many forms, including liquids, caplets, tablets, and capsules. Although it is available as a single ingredient, often pseudoephedrine is combined with other herbs or other approved synthetic cold or allergy compounds.

Brand names available include Actifed, Efidac 24, and Sudafed.

Cautions and Warnings

Use with caution if you suffer from diabetes, prostate enlargement, hypertension, or any other cardiovascular disease.

Do not take pseudoephedrine for periods longer than seven days without consulting a physician.

Do not exceed the recommended daily dosage.

Possible Side Effects

Pseudoephedrine has a low incidence of side effects in people taking recommended doses. Most of the side effects seen are related to a stimulant effect. If you develop any of the following side effects, stop taking pseudoephedrine:

- Stimulant effects: nervousness, restlessness, excitability, insomnia, dizziness, and weakness.
- Cardiovascular effects: increased blood pressure, increased heart rate, irregular heartbeat, and palpitations.
- Headache and drowsiness.

Drug Interactions

Pseudoephedrine should not be used at the same time as monoamine oxidase inhibitor (MAOI) drugs or within the first fourteen days after stopping treatment with an MAOI such as phenelzine (Nardil) or tranylcypromine (Parnate).

Pseudoephedrine may increase the stimulant effects of caffeine and ephedrine.

Food and Nutrient Interactions

None known.

Usual Dosage

For adults and children over twelve years of age: 60 mg every four to six hours, with a maximum of 240 mg in twenty-four hours.

Overdosage

Do the following in case of accidental overdose: If the victim is unconscious or having convulsions, call for an ambulance immediately. If you take the victim to an emergency room, be sure to bring the bottle or container with you. If the victim is conscious, call your local poison control center or a health care professional. The poison control center may suggest inducing vomiting with ipecac syrup (available without a prescription at any pharmacy). *Do not* induce vomiting unless specifically instructed to do so.

Special Populations

Pregnant/breast-feeding women
As the effects of pseudoephedrine during pregnancy and lactation have not been sufficiently evaluated, it should not be used during these times unless directed to do so by a physician.

Children
Suitable for use in children from six to eleven years of age at one-half the adult dosage (30 mg every four to six hours, with a maximum of 120 mg in twenty-four hours). For children under six years of age, consult a physician.

Seniors
No special precautions are known.

Pumpkin Seed Oil or Extract *(Cucurbita pepo)* (*see* Beta-sitosterol)

General Information

Pumpkin seed oil or extract is most often utilized as a source of beta-sitosterol in the treatment of benign prostatic hyperplasia (BPH).

Pycnogenol (*see* Procyanidolic Oligomers)

General Information

Pycnogenol is the brand name of an extract of the bark of French maritime pine *(Pinus maritima)* rich in flavonoid compounds known as procyanidolic oligomers (PCOs) or, alternatively, oligomeric proanthocyanidins (OPCs).

Pygeum Africanum

Used For

Benign prostatic hyperplasia (prostate enlargement)
Effectiveness: A   Safety: A

Erectile dysfunction
Effectiveness: B   Safety: A

Male infertility and impotence
Effectiveness: B   Safety: A

General Information

Pygeum africanum is an evergreen tree native to Africa that can grow to a height of 120–150 feet. An extract made from the bark has been well studied in the treatment of benign prostatic hyperplasia (BPH). Over thirty clinical studies, including a dozen double-blind studies, have shown *Pygeum africanum* extract to be effective in improving the major symptoms of BPH (nighttime urinary frequency, difficulty in starting urination, and incomplete emptying of the bladder). One of the shortcomings of some of the clinical research on *Pygeum africanum* is the lack in many of the studies of objective measures such as urine flow rate (ml/sec), residual urine content, and prostate size. Studies that have used objective measurements have shown some good results. For example, in one study, thirty patients with BPH given 100 mg per day of *Pygeum africanum* extract for seventy-five days demonstrated significant improvements in objective parameters of bladder obstruction: maximum urine flow rate increased from 5.43 ml/sec to 8.20 ml/sec, and the residual urine volume dropped from 76 ml to 33 ml.

Erectile dysfunction
Pygeum africanum extract can improve the capacity to achieve an erection in patients with BPH or prostatitis. Presumably by improving the underlying condition, pygeum can improve sexual function.

Male infertility
Pygeum africanum extract may be effective in improving fertility in cases where diminished prostatic secretion plays a significant role. It has been shown to increase prostatic secretions and improve the composition of the seminal fluid in men with decreased prostatic secretion.

Available Forms

The *Pygeum africanum* extract that has been used in the clinical studies, Prunuselect, is a fat-soluble

extract standardized to contain 14 percent triterpenes. It is available in soft gelatin capsules.

Cautions and Warnings

None known.

Possible Side Effects

The most common side effect is gastrointestinal irritation, resulting in symptoms ranging from nausea
to stomach pain. However, rarely are these side effects severe enough to discontinue use.

Drug Interactions

None known.

Food and Nutrient Interactions

None known.

Usual Dosage

The recommended dosage for *Pygeum africanum*
extract standardized to contain 14 percent triterpenes (Prunuselect) is 100 to 200 mg per day.

Overdosage

None known.

Special Populations

Pregnant/breast-feeding women
As the effects of *Pygeum africanum* extract during pregnancy and lactation have not been sufficiently evaluated, it should not be used during these times.

Children
There does not appear to be any suitable use of *Pygeum africanum* extract in children at this time.

Seniors
No special precautions are known.

Red Clover (*Trifolium pratense*)

Used For

Menopause
Effectiveness: B   Safety: C

General Information

Red clover contains high amounts of phytoestrogens—naturally occurring plant compounds that bind to estrogen receptor sites in humans. The four principal phytoestrogens in red clover are the isoflavones: formononetin, daidzein, biochanin, and genistein. The phytoestrogen (isoflavone) content of red clover is typically up to ten times higher than that of soy. Like soy isoflavones, preliminary research with a red clover extract standardized for isoflavone content (Promensil) is showing benefits in relieving menopausal symptoms such as hot flashes. It is also showing benefits in reducing the loss of elasticity in large arteries in menopausal women, which may predispose them to high blood pressure.

Available Forms

Red clover is available as the crude dried herb (flowers) in bulk, tea bags, and capsules or tablets; other forms include tinctures, fluid extracts, and solid extracts in capsules and tablets. Preparations standardized for isoflavone content are preferred. Brand names available include Promensil.

Cautions and Warnings

None known.

Possible Side Effects

Short-term safety studies with Promensil did not show any side effects. However, the long-term safety profile of red clover preparations is not as well established. Because the dosage is consistent with dietary intake of these compounds, red clover preparations such as Promensil are probably safe at recommended levels. However, there is an area of concern. Although most of the studies with dietary phytoestrogens are positive and show protective effects against breast cancer and other hormone-sensitive cancers, these compounds work by binding to estrogen and progesterone receptors (they actually act as antagonists to progesterone). Because of these effects, there is concern that they may stimulate breast cancer cells and uterine cancer cells. Test tube studies show that red clover extract increased the proliferation and growth of cancerous breast cells whether they had estrogen receptors or not.

Drug Interactions

Because the red clover phytoestrogens occupy estrogen receptors and are capable of producing antiestrogenic effects, the use of red clover is not recommended in women taking birth control pills or other sources of estrogen (e.g., Premarin).

Fermented red clover contains warfarin (sold as a drug under the name Coumadin), a substance that acts to block blood clotting by interfering with vitamin K. However, nonfermented red clover preparations do not exert any anticoagulant effects.

Food and Nutrient Interactions

None known.

Usual Dosage

The recommended dosage of red clover for the relief of menopausal symptoms is based upon the level of isoflavones. The suggested dosage of isoflavones is 40 to 80 mg daily. Promensil contains 40 mg of isoflavones per tablet.

As a tea, the usual dosage is 2 to 3 teaspoons (10–15 g) of dried flowers per cup of water, to be consumed up to three times daily. The dosage for the dried flowers in capsule or tablet form is 2 to 4 g daily. For the tincture, the dosage is 2 to 4 ml three times per day.

Overdosage

None known.

Special Populations

Pregnant/breast-feeding women
As the effects of red clover extract during pregnancy and lactation have not been sufficiently evaluated, it should not be used during these times unless directed to do so by a physician.

Children
There does not appear to be any suitable use for red clover extract in children at this time.

Seniors
No special precautions are known.

Remifemin (*see* Black Cohosh)

General Information

Remifemin is a special extract of black cohosh *(Cimicifuga racemosa)* that is by far the most widely used and thoroughly studied natural alternative to hormone replacement therapy (HRT) in the treatment of menopausal symptoms. In fact, several head-to-head comparison studies have shown Remifemin to produce better results than conjugated estrogens (i.e., Premarin) in relieving common menopausal symptoms such as hot flashes, vaginal atrophy, depression, and anxiety.

St. John's Wort
(Hypericum perforatum)

Used For

Anxiety
Effectiveness: A   Safety: A

Depression
Effectiveness: A   Safety: A

HIV and AIDS
Effectiveness: D   Safety: C

Seasonal affective disorder
Effectiveness: A   Safety: A

General Information

St. John's wort is a shrubby perennial plant with numerous bright yellow flowers. *Wort* is an Old English term for "plant"; its naming after St. John was based on the claim that red spots, symbolic of the blood of St. John, appeared on the leaves of the plant on the anniversary of the saint's beheading. St. John's wort is cultivated worldwide but grows quite well in northern California and southern Oregon.

Depression

St. John's wort extracts have been shown to produce significant antidepressant effects in over thirty double-blind studies involving over two thousand patients with mild to moderate depression. The quality of this research, particularly the studies since 1989, has been judged as acceptable by even the strictest criteria. Most patients begin reporting effects within the first two weeks. Like most antidepressant agents, maximum benefits are typically seen after six to eight weeks of continued use. While St. John's wort extract appears to be as effective as (or possibly even more effective than) conventional antidepressant drugs in mild to moderate depression, it does not appear to be as effective in severe depression as conventional drugs.

Originally it was thought that the antidepressant action of St. John's wort extract was due to hypericin acting as an inhibitor of the enzyme monoamine oxidase (MAO), thereby resulting in the increase of central nervous system monoamines such as serotonin and dopamine. However, newer information indicates that St. John's wort does not significantly inhibit of MAO in humans. At least two other mechanisms have been proposed: modulation of the hypothalamus and pituitary, and inhibition of the reuptake of serotonin similar to drugs such as fluoxetine (Prozac), paroxetine (Paxil), and sertraline (Zoloft).

HIV and AIDS

In response to test tube and animal studies showing that the St. John's wort compound hypericin inhibited the human immunodeficiency virus, many AIDS patients began self-administering St. John's wort. Although most patients reported feeling better, with a more positive outlook, more energy, and less fatigue, it was not known to what degree this was due to a placebo effect. To better determine the benefits, a number of trials evaluated the efficacy of St. John's wort extracts standardized for hypericin in the treatment of HIV-infected individuals. Despite good preliminary results, the trials proved disappointing, as significant blood levels of hypericin could not be achieved using the extract either orally or intravenously.

Seasonal affective disorder

St. John's wort extract also seems to provide improvement in seasonal affective disorder (SAD), a subgroup of major depression with a regular occurrence of symptoms in autumn/winter and full remission in spring/summer. Light therapy has become the standard treatment for this type of depression. However, several double-blind studies show that St. John's wort extract is effective when used alone as well as in combination with light therapy in SAD.

Available Forms

St. John's wort is available as the crude herb in bulk, tea bags, and capsules and tablets; also available are tinctures, fluid extracts, and solid extracts in capsules and tablets. The overwhelming majority of the studies in depression have used St. John's wort extract standardized to contain 0.3 percent hypericin, and more recently 3–5 percent hyperforin as well.

Brand names available include Harmonex, Kira, Movana, Perika, and Stjohnselect.

Cautions and Warnings

At this time, St. John's wort is most appropriate for the treatment of mild to moderate depression. For severe depression, at this time the best recommendation is to consult a physician.

Do not use St. John's wort if you are taking the drug digoxin (Lanoxin) without consulting a physician first.

Do not use St. John's wort if you are taking a prescription antidepressant or antianxiety drug without consulting a physician first.

Possible Side Effects

No significant side effects have been reported in the numerous double-blind studies. In a large-scale safety study involving 3,250 patients conducted in Germany, undesirable side effects were reported in 79 patients (2.4 percent). The most frequently noted side effects were gastrointestinal irritation (0.5 percent), allergic reactions (0.5 percent), fatigue (0.4 percent), and restlessness (0.3 percent).

Because of the possibility of photosensitivity (skin reactions to the sun), it is often recommended that individuals, especially those with fair skin, avoid exposure to strong sunlight and other sources of ultraviolet light when using St. John's wort. This is sensible, but it must be pointed out that the typical dosage of 2.7 mg hypericin per day is estimated to be well below the level required to produce photosensitivity.

Drug Interactions

St. John's wort appears to affect the enzymes in the liver and gut that metabolize certain drugs, including cyclosporine, digoxin, indinavir, oral contraceptives, theophylline, tricyclic antidepressants such as amitriptyline, and anticoagulants such as warfarin (Coumadin). Do not use St. John's wort if you are taking any of these drugs without consulting a physician first.

St. John's wort extract may potentiate prescription antidepressant and antianxiety drugs. There is one case report of simultaneous use of St. John's wort and paroxetine (Paxil) producing nausea, fatigue, lethargy, and weakness. Do not use St. John's wort if you are taking a prescription antidepressant or antianxiety drug without consulting a physician first.

Food and Nutrient Interactions

Initially it was recommended that those taking St. John's wort should also avoid tyramine-containing foods (cheeses, beer, wine, pickled herring, yeast, etc.), which are known to negatively interact with MAO-inhibiting drugs. However, given recent information on the lack of any significant MAO inhibition with St. John's wort extract, such foods do not appear to pose a problem.

Usual Dosage

The dosage of St. John's wort preparations is based upon the hypericin and hyperforin content. For St. John's wort extract standardized to contain 0.3 percent hypericin and 3–5 percent hyperforin, the recommended dosage is 900 mg daily.

To achieve the benefits noted in the clinical trials, it is difficult to recommend any other forms beyond standardized extracts. Nonetheless, here are dosage recommendations for various forms of St. John's wort.

Dried flowers: 2–4 g three times daily
Tincture (1:5): 2–4 ml three times daily
Fluid extract (1:1): 1–2 ml three times daily

Overdosage

Photosensitivity (skin reactions to the sun) may occur with overdosage (see "Possible Side Effects").

Special Populations

Pregnant/breast-feeding women
As the effects of St. John's wort during pregnancy and lactation have not been sufficiently evaluated, it should not be used during these times.

Children
Generally regarded as suitable for children at one-half the adult dosage.

Seniors
No special precautions are known.

Sambucol (*see* Elderberry)

General Information
Sambucol is the original elderberry extract developed by virologist Dr. Madeleine Mumcuoglu. Sambucol is the world's best-selling and most extensively researched elderberry extract and is produced through a patented process that isolates the key active constituent of elderberries. Sambucol is available in liquid (syrup) form as well as in chewable tablets.

Sarsaparilla
(Smilax sarsaparilla)

Used For

General tonic
Effectiveness: C   Safety: C

Psoriasis
Effectiveness: B   Safety: C

Sexual rejuvenator and muscle mass stimulator
Effectiveness: D   Safety: C

General Information

Sarsaparilla root has a long history of medicinal use, but there is little scientific information about the plant. From the limited information available, it appears that sarsaparilla binds bacterial toxins in the gut, rendering them unabsorbable. This effect greatly reduces stress on the liver and other organs and is probably responsible for sarsaparilla's historical use as a tonic—a substance that increases the tone of the entire body. This ability to bind toxins is also the probable reason why sarsaparilla was shown to produce some benefit in psoriasis in one clinical study, as elevated levels of gut-derived bacterial toxins are known to contribute to psoriasis.

Sarsaparilla has been widely touted as a "sexual rejuvenator," with some commercial suppliers even claiming that it is a rich source of human testosterone. The confusion arises because the sarsaparilla saponin, sarsasapogenin, can be synthetically transformed into testosterone in the laboratory.

However, it is extremely unlikely that this reaction could take place in the human body. There is no published evidence to support the contention that it acts like testosterone to stimulate libido or increase muscle mass.

Available Forms

Sarsaparilla root is available as the crude root in bulk, tea bags, capsules, and tablets; also available are tinctures, fluid extracts, and solid extracts in capsules and tablets.

Cautions and Warnings

None known.

Possible Side Effects

None known.

Drug Interactions

None known.

Food and Nutrient Interactions

None known.

Usual Dosage

The following dosages are typically recommended three times daily:

Dried root: 1–4 g or by decoction
Liquid extract (1:1): 8–12 ml (2–3 teaspoons)
Solid extract (4:1): 250 mg

Overdosage

None known.

Special Populations

Pregnant/breast-feeding women

As the effects of sarsaparilla root ingestion during pregnancy and lactation have not been sufficiently evaluated, it should not be used during these times.

Children

Suitable for use in children at one-half the adult dosage.

Seniors

No special precautions are known.

Saventaro (*see* Cat's Claw)

General Information

Saventaro is the only cat's claw (*Uncaria tomentosa*) extract that has been extensively studied and patented. Saventaro is cultivated, harvested, and extracted in such a manner as to contain only the beneficial pentacyclic alkaloids.

Saw Palmetto
(Serenoa repens)

Used For

Benign prostatic hyperplasia (prostate enlargement)
Effectiveness: A   Safety: A

General Information

Saw palmetto is a palm tree native to Florida. Numerous double-blind studies have shown an extract of the berries to significantly improve the signs and symptoms of benign prostatic hyperplasia (BPH), a condition that affects approximately 5 to 10 percent of males at age thirty and increases in incidence to eventually affect more than 90 percent of men over eighty-five years of age. Roughly 90 percent of men with mild to moderate BPH experience some improvement in symptoms during the first four to six weeks of therapy with saw palmetto. All major symptoms of BPH are improved, especially increased nighttime urination (nocturia). The mechanism of action is related to improving the hormonal metabolism within the prostate gland.

Available Forms

Crude saw palmetto is available in bulk as the dried berries and in tea bags. Also available are the tincture and fluid extracts, and the fat-soluble extract in soft gelatin and hard gelatin capsules and tablets. The overwhelming majority of the studies have

utilized fat-soluble saw palmetto extracts standardized to contain 85–95 percent fatty acids and sterols.

Brand names available include One-A-Day Prostate
Health and Sabalselect.

Cautions and Warnings

A prostate disorder can only be diagnosed by a
physician. Do not self-diagnose if you are experiencing any symptoms associated with BPH. See
your physician immediately for proper diagnosis.

Possible Side Effects

Saw palmetto extract is completely safe, as no significant side effects have ever been reported in the
clinical trials of the extract or with saw palmetto
berry ingestion. Detailed toxicology studies on the
extract have been carried out on mice, rats, and
dogs and indicate that the extract has no toxic effects. Saw palmetto extract does not affect the levels of serum prostate-specific antigen (PSA), used as
a screening tool for prostate cancer.

Drug Interactions

None known.

Food and Nutrient Interactions

None known.

Usual Dosage

The dosage for the fat-soluble extract of saw palmetto berries (containing 85–95 percent fatty acids
and sterols) is 320 mg daily. A similar dose using

fluid extracts and tinctures would require extremely large quantities of alcohol and therefore cannot be recommended. The dosage for the crude berries is roughly 10 g twice daily.

Special Populations

Pregnant/breast-feeding women
There does not appear to be a suitable application for saw palmetto during pregnancy or lactation at this time.

Children
There does not appear to be a suitable application for saw palmetto in children at this time.

Seniors
No special precautions are known.

Schisandra (*Schisandra chinensis*)

Used For

Antioxidant
Effectiveness: C   Safety C

Fatigue
Effectiveness: C   Safety: C

Stress
Effectiveness: C   Safety: C

General Information

Schisandra is a woody vine with numerous clusters
of tiny bright red berries native to northern Asia. The
fully ripe, sun-dried fruit has been a classic component in Chinese medicine for centuries. Scientific investigations indicate that a number of schisandra's
chemical components exert pharmacological effects; however, there have been no human clinical
studies with schisandra, so the relevance of animal
and test tube studies is unknown. Some of the effects noted in test tube and animal studies include
antioxidant effects; an adaptogenic action, much like
that of ginseng, in helping to combat fatigue and
stress; and an ability to protect the liver.

Available Forms

Schisandra berries are available as the crude herb in
bulk, tea bags, and capsules and tablets; also available are tinctures, fluid extracts, and the solid extract in capsules and tablets.

Cautions and Warnings

None known.

Possible Side Effects

Side effects are uncommon but may include decreased appetite, stomach upset, and skin rash.

Drug Interactions

None known.

Food and Nutrient Interations

None known.

Usual Dosage

The typical recommendation for the dried schisandra fruit range from 1.5 to 15 g per day. Dosages of other preparations should be equivalent to this range.

Overdosage

None known.

Special Populations

Pregnant/breast-feeding women
As the effects of schisandra during pregnancy and lactation have not been sufficiently evaluated, it should not be used during these times.

Children
As the effects of schisandra during childhood have not been sufficiently evaluated, it should not be used by children unless directed to do so by a physician.

Seniors
No special precautions are known.

Senna *(Cassia senna)*

Used For

Constipation
Effectiveness: A   Safety: C

General Information

Senna is a stimulant laxative made from the leaf and fruit of *Cassia senna.* The laxative components are compounds known as sennosides. Senna promotes its laxative effect in relieving constipation by increasing the strength of contraction of the intestinal muscles. Like other stimulant laxatives, senna has its place in clinical medicine. It should be limited to occasional use, as tolerance can develop. Long-term use of senna can lead to dependence and may increase the risk for colon cancer.

Available Forms

Senna is available in fluid extract, syrup, tablet, chewable tablet, and capsule form. Brands available include Ex-Lax and Senokot.

Cautions and Warnings

Do not use senna for more than seven days unless directed by your doctor.

Stimulant laxatives should not be used in patients with abdominal pain, nausea or vomiting, intestinal obstruction, inflammatory bowel disease, or appendicitis. They should not be used during pregnancy or lactation.

Do not take more than the recommended amount. Excessive laxative use or inadequate fluid intake may lead to significant fluid and electrolyte imbalance.

Possible Side Effects

Stimulant laxatives such as senna are likely to cause abdominal cramping, nausea, and increased mucus secretion. Less common side effects (muscle spasms, weakness, and fatigue) are associated with chronic use and are usually related to loss of potassium and other electrolytes. Call your doctor right away if you have any of these side effects: a sudden change in bowel habits that persists over a period of two weeks, rectal bleeding, or failure to have a bowel movement after use.

A benign blackish-brown pigmentation of the colonic mucosa (pseudomelanosis coli) may occur with prolonged use (at least four months) of senna due to its anthraquinone content. This condition is generally reversible within four to fifteen months after discontinuing the substance.

Drug Interactions

Senna and other stimulant laxatives may decrease the absorption of other drugs that pass through the gastrointestinal tract. If you are currently taking an oral medication, talk to your pharmacist or doctor before self-medicating with senna.

Senna may potentiate the action of digoxin and other heart medications, due to potassium depletion. The use of senna with thiazide diuretics and corticosteroids may further decrease potassium levels.

Food and Nutrient Interactions

Generally, senna is recommended on an empty stomach. Drink six to eight glasses of liquid daily while taking this laxative.

Usual Dosage

Follow manufacturer's instructions on package label. The usual dosage recommendation is based upon sennoside content: 15–30 mg sennosides at bedtime.

Overdosage

Symptoms of overdosage include persistent diarrhea and dehydration. In severe cases of accidental overdose, do the following: If the victim is unconscious or having convulsions, call for an ambulance immediately. If you take the victim to an emergency room, be sure to bring the bottle or container with you. If the victim is conscious, call your local poison control center or a health care professional. The poison control center may suggest inducing vomiting with ipecac syrup (available without a prescription at any pharmacy). *Do not* induce vomiting unless specifically instructed to do so.

Special Populations

Pregnant/breast-feeding women

Senna and other stimulant laxative should be avoided during pregnancy. Only bulk-forming laxatives or stool softeners are recommended for pregnant women.

Check with your doctor before using senna if you

are breast-feeding. Sennosides pass into the breast milk, but the concentration is usually insufficient to affect the infant.

Children

In general, stimulant laxatives should be avoided in children younger than six years of age unless prescribed by a physician. Senna is suitable for children older than six years of age at one-half of the adult dosage.

Seniors

Seniors commonly experience constipation and are most susceptible to becoming dependent on laxatives. Seniors are most likely to experience the more serious side effects of long-term use because of the potassium-depleting effects of senna and other stimulant laxatives. Bulk-forming laxatives are usually preferred for seniors.

Siberian Ginseng
(Eleutherococcus senticosus)

Used For

Adaptogenic effects
Effectiveness: B+   Safety: C

Fatigue
Effectiveness: B   Safety: C

Low immunity and immune support
Effectiveness: B   Safety: C

Stress
Effectiveness: B   Safety: C

General Information

Siberian ginseng is a popular medicinal plant that grows abundantly in parts of the Russian Far East, Korea, China, and Japan. There are three major types of ginseng: Chinese or Korean *(Panax ginseng)*, American *(Panax quinquefolius)*, and Siberian *(Eleutherococcus senticosus).* (See also **ginseng**.) Although Siberian ginseng possesses many of the same effects as these ginsengs, it is generally regarded as being milder in action.

Initial scientific research on Siberian ginseng focused on its adaptogenic qualities. An adaptogen is defined as a substance that (1) must be innocuous and cause minimal disorder in the physiological functions of an organism, (2) must have a nonspecific action (i.e., it should increase resistance to adverse influences by a wide range of physical, chemical, and biochemical factors), and (3) usually has a normalizing action on body functions. According to these criteria, Siberian ginseng appears to possess adaptogenic effects.

Siberian ginseng extract has been administered to more than 2,100 healthy human subjects in clinical trials for the purpose of evaluating its adaptogenic effects. These studies indicated that Siberian ginseng (1) increased the ability of humans to withstand many adverse physical conditions (i.e., heat, noise, motion, workload increase, exercise, and decompression), (2) increased mental alertness and work output, and (3) improved the quality of work produced under stressful conditions as well as athletic performance.

One of the more popular uses of Siberian ginseng is in the treatment of fatigue, including chronic fatigue syndrome (CFS). Central to CFS is a disturbed immune system. Siberian ginseng appears to address the fatigue, decreased sense of well-being, and impaired immune function in people with CFS. In regard to improving immune function, in one double-blind study, thirty-six healthy subjects received either 10 ml of a Siberian ginseng fluid extract or a placebo daily for four weeks. The group receiving the Siberian ginseng demonstrated significant improvements in a variety of immune system parameters.

Available Forms

Siberian ginseng is available in bulk as the dried root; crude root in capsules and tablets; tea bags; tincture; fluid extract; and dried powdered extraction capsules or tablets.

Cautions and Warnings

Do not use Siberian ginseng if you are taking digoxin (Lanoxin) without consulting a physician first.

Possible Side Effects

Siberian ginseng is generally well tolerated, and side effects are infrequent. However, side effects, including insomnia, irritability, melancholy, and anxiety, are often reported at higher dosages. In individuals with rheumatic heart disease, symptoms such as pericardial pain, headaches, and elevations in blood pressure have been reported.

Drug Interactions

Siberian ginseng has been shown to increase blood levels of the drug digoxin (Lanoxin). Do not use Siberian ginseng if you are taking digoxin without consulting a physician first.

Food and Nutrient Interactions

None known.

Usual Dosage

Dosages to be administered one to three times a day are as follows:

Dried root: 2–4 g
Tincture (1:5): 10–20 ml
Fluid extract (1:1): 2–4 ml
Solid extract (20:1, containing more than 1 percent eleutheroside E): 100–200 mg

Note: If Siberian ginseng is to be used in the long term, generally the recommendation is to take it in sixty-day courses, with an interval of fourteen to twenty-one days between courses.

Overdosage

None known.

Special Populations

Pregnant/breast-feeding women
As the effects of Siberian ginseng during pregnancy and lactation have not been sufficiently evaluated, it should not be used during these times.

Children
Suitable for use in children at one-half the adult dosage.

Seniors
No special precautions are known.

Silybin Phytosome (*see* Milk Thistle)

General Information
Silybin Phytosome binds silybin (the key flavonoid of milk thistle [*Silybum marianum*]) to **phosphatidylcholine**. This new molecule results in better absorption of the silymarin and better clinical results compared to milk thistle extract. The typical dosage for Silybin Phytosome is 80 to 120 mg two to three times daily between meals.

Silymarin (from *Silybum marianum*) (*see* Milk Thistle)

General Information

Silymarin is a mixture of flavonoid components (e.g., silybin, silidianin, and silichristine) from milk thistle. The concentration of silymarin is highest in the fruit, but it is also found in the seeds and leaves. Milk thistle extracts concentrated for silymarin (usually 70–80 percent) are most often used in liver disorders and psoriasis.

Sinupret

Used For

Common cold
Effectiveness: A   Safety: B

Sinus infection
Effectiveness: A   Safety: B

General Information

Sinupret is one of the most popular herbal products in Germany. It is a combination herbal product that contains gentian root *(Gentian lutea)*, elder flowers *(Sambucus nigra)*, vervain *(Verbena officinalis)*, and sorrel *(Rumex acetosa)*. Its primary application is in the treatment of sinus infections, but it has also shown usefulness in treating the common cold.

Although effective on its own in the treatment of bacterial and viral sinusitis, Sinupret has also been shown to enhance the effectiveness of antibiotics and nasal decongestants in patients with acute sinusitis, according to X-ray findings and patient assessments in double-blind studies.

Available Forms

Sinupret is available in tablet form.

Cautions and Warnings

Sinusitis can have serious consequences. Seek medical care in the event that sinusitis lasts longer than three days, is associated with a fever, and does not appear to be improving.

Possible Side Effects

None known. May be taken continuously for up to six weeks.

Drug Interactions

Sinupret has been shown to enhance the effectiveness of antibiotics and decongestants used in the treatment of sinusitis.

Food and Nutrient Interactions

None known.

Usual Dosage

One tablet three times daily.

Overdosage

None known.

Special Populations

Pregnant/breast-feeding women

As the effects of Sinupret during pregnancy and lactation have not been sufficiently evaluated, it should not be used during these times.

Children

Suitable for use in children at one-half the adult dosage.

Seniors

No special precautions are known.

Slippery Elm *(Ulmus rubra)*

Used For

Soothing effects on the throat and gastrointestinal tract

Effectiveness: C   Safety: C

General Information

The slippery elm tree is native to North America. The inner bark of the tree is the source of a mucilage that historically has been used to soothe internal membranes irritated by the common cold, coughs, ulcers, or inflammatory bowel disease (Crohn's disease and ulcerative colitis). Unfortunately, there have been no clinical studies documenting its effect. However, even the FDA acknowledges that slippery elm is of value in soothing a sore throat, having approved this claim for slippery elm products.

Available Forms

Slippery elm is available in bulk, as a tea, in capsules and tablets (including chewable tablets), and as throat lozenges.

Cautions and Warnings

None known.

Possible Side Effects

None known.

Drug Interactions

Slippery elm may interfere with the absorption of drugs. Take any medication at least forty-five minutes before or after using slippery elm.

Food and Nutrient Interactions

None known.

Usual Dosage

Slippery elm tea is made by boiling 0.5–2 g of the powdered bark in 8 ounces of water for ten to fifteen minutes; three to four cups a day can be used. For powdered slippery elm bark in tablets or capsules, the typical dosage is 400 to 1,000 mg three to four times daily. Slippery elm is also an ingredient of some cough lozenges and cough syrups; follow label instructions for proper dosages of these preparations.

Overdosage

None known.

Special Populations

Pregnant/breast-feeding women

Regarded by many herbal experts as safe during pregnancy and lactation. However, since its effects have not been sufficiently evaluated during these times, slippery elm should not be used at higher dosages or for long periods of time.

Children

Suitable for use in children at one-half the adult dosage.

Seniors

No special precautions are known.

Stinging Nettle *(Urtica dioica)*

Used For

Allergy
Effectiveness: B   Safety: C

Benign prostatic hyperplasia (prostate enlargement)
Effectiveness: B+   Safety: C

Osteoarthritis
Effectiveness: B   Safety: C

General Information

Stinging nettle has been used as a medicinal plant since ancient times in many parts of the world. The modern use of stinging nettle has focused on benign prostatic hyperplasia (BPH). The portion of the plant used for this purpose is the root. The aerial (aboveground) portion of the plant is used in the treatment of allergic rhinitis, osteoarthritis, and rheumatoid arthritis, and as a mild diuretic.

Allergy

Modest effects were reported with a freeze-dried preparation of the aerial parts of stinging nettle in one small double-blind study in patients with hay fever (allergic rhinitis). In the group receiving stinging nettle, 58 percent noted moderate improvement, compared to only 37 percent in the placebo group.

Benign prostatic hyperplasia (BPH)

Several double-blind studies have shown stinging nettle root extract to exert significant benefits in improving BPH symptoms as well as objective measurements such as urinary outflow. Its mechanism of action in BPH appears to be the result of (1) its ability to modulate the male sex hormones' stimulant effect on prostate cells and (2) a mild anti-inflammatory effect.

Osteoarthritis

Preparations of the aerial portions of stinging net tle have shown anti-inflammatory effects, and i preliminary clinical studies in patients with os teoarthritis it has produced some improvements Further research is needed to gauge its effectivenes compared not only to conventional drugs but also t other natural approaches.

Available Forms

The crude herb is available in bulk as the drie leaves or root, as tea bags, as root or leaf powder i capsules and tablets, and as freeze-dried leaves Also available are the tincture, fluid extract, an solid extract in capsules and tablets. In allergy, th freeze-dried leaves are recommended, as once th leaves have been air-dried, they lose their antial lergy effects. For BPH, extracts from the root hav been used. For osteoarthritis, extracts from th leaves and stems have been used.

Cautions and Warnings

None known.

Possible Side Effects

Although allergic reactions to oral stinging nettle ar rare, fresh nettles can cause a rash if they come int contact with the skin. Stinging nettle in any oral form may cause mild gastrointestinal upset in some people

Drug Interactions

Stinging nettle may enhance the effects of non steroidal anti-inflammatory drugs (NSAIDs) in the treatment of osteoarthritis and rheumatoid arthritis. Use of stinging nettle leaves, because of the vitamin K content, should be avoided in people who are taking warfarin (Coumadin).

Food and Nutrient Interactions

None known.

Usual Dosage

For allergies, the typical dosage has been two or three 300 mg freeze-dried nettle leaf capsules taken three times per day. In the treatment of BPH, the typical daily dosage of the root extract is 600 to 1,200 mg daily. In the studies in osteoarthritis, the dosages used were stewed nettle leaf (50 g/day) or extracts (1,340 mg/day).

Overdosage

None known.

Special Populations

Pregnant/breast-feeding women

As the effects of stinging nettle during pregnancy and lactation have not been sufficiently evaluated, it should not be used during these times.

Children

Suitable for use in children at one-half the adult dosage.

Seniors

No special precautions are known.

Synephrine (*see* Bitter Orange [*Citrus aurantium*])

General Information

Synephrine is a compound in bitter orange that appears to act in some ways like **ephedrine**. However, since synephrine does not cross the blood-brain barrier, it does not produce the stimulatory effects of ephedrine. Synephrine is marketed as a replacement for ephedrine in thermogenic formulas (see **ephedrine-caffeine combinations**), but it is not known if synephrine produces the same sort of weight-loss effects as ephedrine.

Thisilyn (*see* Milk Thistle)

General Information

Thisilyn contains the most widely researched milk thistle extract, standardized to 80 percent silymarin. Thisilyn has been shown to be better absorbed and utilized compared to other milk thistle brands, and clinical studies have indicated that it supports and promotes normal liver function.

Turmeric *(Curcuma longa)* (*see* Curcumin)

General Information

Turmeric is a perennial herb of the ginger family that is extensively cultivated in India, China, Indonesia, and other tropical countries. The powdered rhizome of turmeric is the major ingredient of curry powder and is also used in prepared mustard. It is extensively used in foods for both its color and flavor. In addition, turmeric is used in both the Chinese and Indian (Ayurvedic) systems of medicine as an anti-inflammatory agent and in the treatment of numerous conditions, including flatulence, jaundice, menstrual difficulties, bloody urine, hemorrhage, toothache, bruises, chest pain, and colic. Turmeric poultices are often applied locally to relieve inflammation and pain. The most popular use of turmeric as an alternative medicine is in the form of curcumin, the yellow pigment of turmeric.

Uva Ursi (*Arctostaphylos uva-ursi*)

Used For

Urinary tract infections
Effectiveness: B+   Safety: D

General Information

Uva ursi or bearberry is a small evergreen shrub
found in the northern United States and in Europe.
The leaves are the portions of the plant used for medicinal purposes, as they contain the compound arbutin. Uva ursi is helpful in preventing bladder
infections. In one double-blind study using a standardized uva ursi extract on recurrent bladder infections, at the end of one year, five of the twenty-seven
women in the placebo group had had a recurrence,
while none of the thirty women receiving uva ursi
extract had had a recurrence. No side effects were
reported.

Available Forms

Uva ursi is available as the crude leaves in bulk, capsules, and tablets as well as tinctures, fluid extracts,
and solid extracts in tablets and capsules. Extracts
stating the concentration of arbutin (e.g., 10 percent)
are preferred by most experts.

Cautions and Warnings

Do not use more than recommended amounts.
   Must not be used by children under twelve years
of age.
   Must not be used during pregnancy or lactation.

Possible Side Effects

Uva ursi can cause nausea, gastrointestinal discomfort, and a greenish brown discoloration of the
urine.

Drug Interactions

None known.

Food and Nutrient Interactions

None known.

Usual Dosage

The following dosages are generally taken three times a day with a glass of water for maximum benefit:

Dried leaves or by infusion (tea): 1½–4 g
Tincture (1:5): 4–6 ml
Fluid extract (1:1): ½–2 ml
Solid extract (10 percent arbutin content):
   250–500 mg

Overdosage

Uva ursi has the potential to cause serious toxicity. At higher dosages (i.e., 30 to 100 g) it can cause nausea, vomiting, a sense of suffocation, shortness of breath, cyanosis, convulsions, delirium, and collapse. Do the following in case of accidental overdose: If the victim is unconscious or having convulsions, call for an ambulance immediately. If you take the victim to an emergency room, be sure to bring the bottle or container with you. If the victim is conscious, call your local poison control center or a health care professional. The poison control center may suggest inducing vomiting with ipecac syrup (available without a prescription at any pharmacy). *Do not* induce vomiting unless specifically instructed to do so.

Special Populations

Pregnant/breast-feeding women
Uva must not be used during pregnancy or lactation.

Children
Uva ursi is not indicated for use in children under the age of twelve years.

Seniors
No special precautions are known.

Valerian *(Valeriana officinalis)*

Used For

Anxiety
Effectiveness: B   Safety: B

Insomnia
Effectiveness: A   Safety: B

General Information

Valerian is a perennial plant native to North America and Europe. The root is the portion of the plant used for medicinal effects. Historically valerian's primary use was as a sedative for the relief of insomnia, anxiety, and conditions associated with pain. Several recent clinical studies have substantiated this historical use.

Early studies in subjects who did not have insomnia showed that valerian could improve sleep quality and shorten sleep latency (the time required to go to sleep) but left no "hangover" the next morning. The same effects were later demonstrated for individuals with insomnia. In fact, in studies in patients suffering from insomnia, performed under strict laboratory conditions, valerian was shown to be as effective as low doses of prescription sedatives (specifically, valerian was as effective as low doses of barbiturates or benzodiazepines). However, while these latter compounds also increase morning sleepiness, valerian usually reduces morning sleepiness.

Valerian's success in helping anxiety has also been demonstrated in a few clinical studies, but not to the same degree as its confirmed effects in insomnia.

The important active compounds of valerian are the valepotriates (iridoid molecules) and valerenic acids. Valerian appears to work by binding to or enhancing the effects of the same brain receptors as diazepam (Valium) and other benzodiazepine drugs. However, valerian appears to be better tolerated, as side effects such as impaired mental function, morning "hangover," and dependency, which are such a problem with benzodiazepines, have not been reported with valerian.

Available Forms

The medicinal part is the dried root. It is available in bulk, capsules, and tablets as well as in tinctures, fluid extracts, and solid extracts in tablets and capsules. As the level of active constituents in the crude herb can vary greatly, preparations standardized for valerenic acid are recommended by most authorities. Brand names available include Silent Night.

Cautions and Warnings

The valepotriates have been suspected as possibly being carcinogens as well as potential liver toxicants. Until there is better information, the best choice may be to use water-soluble extracts standardized for valerenic acid content.

Possible Side Effects

Valerian is generally regarded as safe and is approved for food use by the United States Food and Drug Administration. Side effects can include morning sleepiness, headache, and gastrointestinal discomfort.

Drug Interactions

Given that the mechanism of action of valerian involves the same sort of receptor sites as benzodiazepine drugs, valerian should not be used in combination with these drugs unless being supervised by a health care professional. Examples of benzodiazepine drugs include diazepam (Valium), flurazepam (Dalmane), triazolam (Halcion), and temazepam (Restoril). These drugs are commonly prescribed for insomnia and anxiety.

Food and Nutrient Interactions

None known.

Usual Dosage

As a mild sedative, valerian may be taken at the following dose thirty to forty-five minutes before retiring:

Dried root (or as tea): 2–3 g
Tincture (1:5): 4–6 ml (1–1½ teaspoons)
Fluid extract (1:1): 1–2 ml (½ –1 teaspoon)
Solid extract (0.8 percent valerenic acid): 150–300 mg

Note: For best results, it is important to eliminate dietary factors such as caffeine and alcohol, which disrupt sleep, when using valerian. If the above dosage results in increased morning sleepiness, cutting the dosage in half will eliminate the problem.

For anxiety, the above dosage can be taken two to three times daily.

Overdosage

One case of valerian overdose has been reported. The individual presented with mild symptoms after taking valerian at approximately twenty times the recommended therapeutic dose. All symptoms disappeared within twenty-four hours.

Special Populations

Pregnant/breast-feeding women
Valerian is not contraindicated during pregnancy and lactation, according to various published authoritative texts. However, as its safety during pregnancy and lactation has not been adequately evaluated, valerian should not be used during these times except under the instruction of a health care professional.

Children
Suitable for children at one-half the adult dosage.

Seniors
No special precautions are known.

White Willow *(Salix alba)*

Used For

Arthritis (both osteoarthritis and rheumatoid arthritis)
Effectiveness: B   Safety: C

Trauma and athletic injury
Effectiveness: B   Safety: C

General Information

White willow bark contains the compound salicin, often referred to as "natural aspirin." In fact, salicin served as the starting point in the development of aspirin (acetylsalicylic acid). Once inside the body, salicin is converted into salicylic acid. This compound exerts many of the same effects as aspirin, although it does not prevent platelet aggregation like aspirin. The salicin content of white willow bark is thought to be responsible for most of the substance's anti-inflammatory and pain-relieving actions. Most clinical studies of preparations containing white willow also contain other anti-inflammatory herbs, so it is difficult to ascertain the true effect of white willow alone. Nonetheless, based on existing evidence, it appears that it does possess some benefit in relieving pain and inflammation in osteoarthritis and injuries.

Available Forms

White willow is available in several different forms: as the crude herb in bulk, tea bags, and capsules and tablets; as a tincture; as a fluid extract; and as a solid extract in capsules and tablets. White willow extracts standardized for salicin content are preferred because of the tremendous variation in salicin content in various preparations.

Cautions and Warnings

White willow bark preparations are not recommended for people who are sensitive or allergic to aspirin.

Possible Side Effects

None has been reported. Theoretically, allergic reactions are possible. Most experts recommend that aspirin-sensitive people avoid using white willow bark.

Drug Interactions

None known.

Food and Nutrient Interactions

None known.

Usual Dosage

White willow extracts standardized for salicin content are preferred. The dosage is based upon providing a daily intake of salicin between 60 and 120 mg. An approximate dosage using white willow tea is 1 to 3 g of bark boiled in 8 ounces of water for ten minutes. Five or more cups of this tea can be drunk per day. Tinctures are also available, with a recommended dosage of 1 to 2 ml three times per day.

Overdosage

None known.

Special Populations

Pregnant/breast-feeding women
As the effects of white willow bark during pregnancy and lactation have not been sufficiently evaluated, it should not be used during these times.

Children
Suitable for use in children at one-half the adult dosage.

Seniors
No special precautions are known.

Yohimbe Bark
(Pausinystalia johimbe)

Used For

Erectile dysfunction
Effectiveness: A   Safety: D

General Information

Yohimbe bark is a source of the alkaloid yohimbine, a drug approved by the FDA for erectile dysfunction (impotence). When used alone, yohimbine is successful in 34 to 43 percent of cases of erectile dysfunction. Unfortunately, a 1995 analysis showed that while crude yohimbe bark typically contains 6 percent total alkaloids, most commercial products contained virtually no yohimbine—of the twenty-six samples, nine were found to contain absolutely zero yohimbine, seven contained only trace amounts, and the rest contained small amounts. These results and the problems with side effects call into question the use of over-the-counter yohimbe preparations and suggest that men wanting to use yohimbine should discuss it with their doctor and get the prescription form.

Available Forms

Yohimbe bark is available in crude (bulk) form, fluid extracts, and solid extracts. Since the optimum dosage of yohimbe depends on the content of yohimbine, preparations standardized for yohimbine may produce more dependable results. These preparations are usually available in tablets or capsules. Brand names available include Male Fuel.

Cautions and Warnings

May induce anxiety, panic attacks, and hallucinations in some individuals.

Must not be used by individuals with kidney disease or psychological disease.

Must not be used during pregnancy or lactation, or by children.

Possible Side Effects

Yohimbine can produce significant side effects, including anxiety, panic attacks, and hallucinations, but it is most often associated with feelings of nervousness, elevations in blood pressure and heart rate, dizziness, headache, and skin flushing.

Drug Interactions

If you are taking any prescription medication, please consult your physician or pharmacist before taking yohimbe products. Yohimbine theoretically may interact with many different types of medications. In particular, it is generally recommended that yohimbe preparations be avoided in people taking blood-pressure-lowering drugs, including beta-blockers such as propanolol (Inderal), tricyclic antidepressants (e.g., imipramine, desipramine), monoamine oxidase inhibitors (MAOIs), and various antipsychotic medications.

Food and Nutrient Interactions

None known.

Usual Dosage

The dosage of yohimbe bark is dependent upon its yohimbine content. The standard dose for yohimbine is 15 to 20 mg per day.

Overdosage

None known.

Special Populations

Pregnant/breast-feeding women
Yohimbine must not be used during pregnancy and lactation.

Children
Yohimbine must not be used by children.

Seniors
Seniors may be more sensitive to the effects and side effects of yohimbine.

PART V
Natural Ingredients Used in Topical Preparations

Natural compounds have long been used in cosmetics and skin care products. In addition to providing aesthetic and functional benefits to the skin, a number of natural compounds have demonstrated therapeutic benefits as well. In this section each of the entries is organized according to the following outline:

Name

The common name of the natural product is used for all entries (e.g., vitamin C instead of ascorbic acid).

Used For

A listing of the popular uses for each entry is given. In an effort to provide information on the effectiveness and safety of the entries, a rating system was developed based upon currently available information. The rating is based upon the level of scientific support for a particular application or its general acceptance in regard to effectiveness or safety.

Effectiveness
The following rating scale is used:
A = Excellent, with multiple double-blind studies or generally accepted as effective

B+ = Very good results in a small number of double-blind studies

B = Some clinical evidence of effectiveness

B– = Some clinical evidence of effectiveness but also some studies showing no effect

C = Strong historical use or scientific rationale but no clinical trials to show effectiveness in humans

D = No significant documentation of historical use or scientific rationale, or majority of clinical studies show no effect

F = Documentation that it is *not* effective

Safety

The following rating scale is used:

A = Excellent safety profile

B = Good safety profile

C = Generally regarded as safe at recommended levels

D = Generally regarded as safe at recommended levels but must be used with caution;

F = Potentially dangerous, should not be used.

General Information

Under this heading you will find a description of the product's effects and uses, including results from clinical trials in humans.

Brand names are given when a brand has a substantial amount of original scientific research behind it or has established its identity in the marketplace by an extensive marketing effort.

Cautions and Warnings

Although generally safe, some natural products carry warnings and cautions. This heading will alert you to any concerns.

Possible Side Effects

A description of possible side effects is presented to alert you to any problems that may occur when using a particular natural product.

Note: For information on dosage and method of application, please follow label instructions.

Allantoin

Used For

Skin moisturizer and protectant
Effectiveness: A   Safety: A

General Information

Allantoin is a compound originally isolated from comfrey *(Symphytum officinale)* that has a long history of use in various skin care products. Its effects on the skin are to soften, protect, and stimulate normal cell growth. These effects make allantoin useful in many skin complaints, especially those involving dry, scaly, or flaky skin, such as eczema and psoriasis. It is usually contained in products at a level of 0.5 to 2 percent.

Cautions and Warnings

None known.

Possible Side Effects

Allantoin is completely nontoxic, nonallergenic, and nonirritating.

Aloe Vera

Used For

Minor skin irritations
Effectiveness: A   Safety: A

Psoriasis
Effectiveness: B   Safety: A

Sunburn
Effectiveness: A   Safety: A

Wound healing
Effectiveness: A   Safety: A

General Information

The soothing and wound-healing effects of *Aloe vera* have been chronicled since ancient times—both Pliny (A.D. 23–79) and Dioscorides (first century A.D.) wrote of aloe's ability to treat wounds and heal infections of the skin. A major development in the modern use of aloe occurred in 1935 when a group of physicians successfully used the fresh juice to treat a patient suffering from facial burns.

The relief offered by aloe in the topical treatment of burns, minor irritations, skin ulcers, and other skin disorders is a major reason why companies supplying skin care and cosmetic products have incorporated aloe into many of their formulations. Yet despite this popularity, few human studies have been carried out. Most of the studies on *Aloe vera* have utilized different animals in various models of inflammation and wound healing. Virtually all of the studies support the topical use of *Aloe vera* gel, especially in minor burns or skin inflammation. Aloe gel may also be shown to be helpful in psoriasis, as one double-blind study found that a topical preparation containing 0.5 percent *Aloe vera* extract produced impressive results. By the end of the sixteen-week study, the *Aloe vera* extract cream had cured twenty-five of thirty patients (83.3 percent) compared to the placebo cure rate of only two of thirty (6.6 percent).

Cautions and Warnings

None known.

Possible Side Effects

None known.

Alpha-hydroxy Acids

Used For

Antiwrinkle and antiaging effects
Effectiveness: A   Safety: A

General Information

Alpha-hydroxy acids (AHAs) are naturally occurring acids found in fruits that are now incorporated into most antiwrinkle and antiaging products. They include glycolic, lactic, tartaric, malic, and citric acids. First used in 1974, AHAs were quickly adopted by the cosmetic and dermatology worlds. Besides improving wrinkles, AHA-containing preparations are used as moisturizers for dry skin and in the treatment of acne and age spots. They also help the skin look younger. Dermatologists use AHAs to perform chemical peels of the skin—a procedure where the AHAs literally dissolve or peel away layers of skin. The amount of free acid in the product determines whether it will moisturize, eliminate wrinkles, or act as a chemical peel. The higher the percentage of AHA, the greater the peeling effect. While dermatologists use products with 70 percent free acids, most over-the-counter AHA products contain only 4 percent—the minimum amount needed to produce skin cell renewal.

Cautions and Warnings

Only use AHA-containing products according to label recommendations.

Possible Side Effects

When using AHAs, be aware that your skin is now even more vulnerable to the negative effects of the sun. Use an effective sun block before exposing your skin to the sun.

Capsaicin

Used For

Arthritis (both osteoarthritis and rheumatoid arthritis)
Effectiveness: A   Safety: D

Diabetic neuropathy
Effectiveness: A   Safety: D

Pain disorders
Effectiveness: A   Safety: D

Psoriasis
Effectiveness: B+   Safety: D

General Information

Capsaicin is the active component of cayenne pepper (also known as chili or red pepper), the fruit of *Capsicum frutescens*. Capsaicin is the component responsible for the pungent and irritating effects of cayenne pepper. Typically, cayenne pepper contains about 1.5 percent capsaicin and related principles. Topical preparations containing 0.025 to 0.075 percent capsaicin are popular over-the-counter products for the relief of pain. A stronger concentration (0.25 percent) is available by prescription (Dolorac). When applied to the skin, capsaicin is known to first stimulate and then block small-diameter pain fibers by depleting them of the neurotransmitter substance P. Substance P is thought to be the principal chemical mediator of pain impulses from the peripheral nerves. In addition, substance P has been shown to activate inflammatory mediators into joint tissues in osteoarthritis and rheumatoid arthritis. In order to be effective, capsaicin-containing creams must be applied according to label or insert instructions. Usually results are most apparent after one week of continuous use.

Brands available include ArthriCare, Capzasin-HP, Capzasin-P, Dolorac (by prescription), and Zostrix.

Arthritis

Topically applied capsaicin can be effective in relieving the pain of either osteoarthritis or rheumatoid arthritis. In fact, capsaicin is so effective in relieving pain in most cases of arthritis that it is now the most widely used and recommended over-the-counter topical analgesic.

Diabetic neuropathy

Diabetic neuropathy refers to a painful nerve disorder caused by long-term diabetes. Topically applied capsaicin has been shown to be of considerable benefit in relieving the pain of diabetic neuropathy in numerous double-blind studies. For example, in one large double-blind eight-week study involving 277 subjects with painful diabetic neuropathy of the hands and feet, 69.5 percent of the group applying 0.075 percent capsaicin cream showed improvement, compared to 53.4 percent of the group applying simply the vehicle cream.

Pain disorders

The first studied and approved use for topically applied capsaicin was in relieving the pain associated with shingles (herpes zoster), a clinical condition known as postherpetic neuralgia. Numerous studies now document this FDA-approved application. Topically applied capsaicin is also effective in reducing the pain of trigeminal neuralgia (also known as tic douloureux), a painful disorder of the main nerve of the face characterized by severe, stabbing pain affecting the cheek, lips, gums, or chin on one side of the face; the pain after breast reconstruction or mastectomy; and postamputation (phantom) pain.

Psoriasis

Excessive substance P levels in the skin have been linked to psoriasis. This finding prompted researchers to study the effects of topically applied capsaicin. In one double-blind study, 197 patients applied 0.025 percent capsaicin cream or placebo cream four times a day for six weeks. Capsaicin-treated patients demonstrated significantly greater improvement.

Cautions and Warnings

For external use only. Avoid contact with the eyes and mucous membranes.

Wash hands with soap and water immediately after applying.

Do not use a heating pad or bandage on the area.

Possible Side Effects

A transient burning sensation is usually noticed, but this generally lessens or disappears after several days of use. If severe burning or blisters occur, discontinue use and apply vegetable oil to the skin to dilute.

Chamomile (topical)

Used For

Dry, flaky, irritated skin
Effectiveness: B   Safety: A

General Information

Chamomile preparations are widely used in cosmetics, including bath and hair preparations. They are also used in Europe for the treatment of a variety of common skin complaints, including dry, flaky, irritated skin. The flavonoid and essential oil components of chamomile possess significant anti-inflammatory and antiallergy activity. Chamomile preparations may prove useful in eczema, psoriasis, and other skin disorders that are often treated with topical corticosteroids.

   Brand names include CamoCare.

Cautions and Warnings

None known.

Possible Side Effects

None known.

Glycyrrhetinic Acid

Used For

Eczema
Effectiveness: B   Safety: A

Herpes
Effectiveness: B   Safety: A

Psoriasis
Effectiveness: B   Safety: A

General Information

Glycyrrhetinic acid is a compound from licorice (*Glycyrrhiza glabra*) that exerts an effect similar to that of topical hydrocortisone in the treatment of eczema, contact and allergic dermatitis, and psoriasis. In fact, in several studies, glycyrrhetinic acid was shown to be superior to topical cortisone, especially in chronic cases. For example, in one study in patients with eczema, 93 percent of the patients applying glycyrrhetinic acid demonstrated improvement compared to 83 percent using cortisone. Glycyrrhetinic acid can also be used to potentiate the effects of topically applied hydrocortisone.

In the treatment of lesions due to the herpes simplex virus (HSV-1 and HSV-2), topical glycyrrhetinic acid was shown to be quite helpful in reducing the healing time and pain associated with cold sores and genital herpes in preliminary clinical studies. In test tube studies, glycyrrhetinic acid permanently inactivates the herpes simplex type 1 virus and stimulates the synthesis and release of interferon—the body's own antiviral compound.

Cautions and Warnings

None known.

Possible Side Effects

None known.

Hydroquinone

Used For

Age-spot removal
Effectiveness: A   Safety: C

General Information

Hydroquinone is a naturally occurring compound used as an antioxidant and skin bleaching agent. In lighter-skinned people, large, frecklelike discolorations may appear on the skin with advancing years. These blemishes—commonly called age spots—result from the buildup of a dark substance known as lipofuscin that is mostly composed of cellular debris from molecules that have been damaged by free radicals. Creams containing hydroquinone can reduce the darkness of age spots by about 50 percent after three to four weeks of use. The effect lasts for about two to six months, with darker lesions repigmented more quickly than lighter lesions.

Cautions and Warnings

Due to the lack of safety data, hydroquinone is not recommended for children under twelve years of age or for pregnant or breast-feeding women.

Possible Side Effects

At recommended concentrations (1.5–2.0 percent), hydroquinone's side effects are very mild and include tingling or burning on application, some redness, and inflammation.

Lemon Balm
(Melissa officinalis)

Used For

Cold sores and genital herpes lesions
Effectiveness: B+   Safety: A

General Information

Lemon balm contains components that exert activity against the herpes simplex virus—the cause of cold sores and genital herpes. A cream containing a concentrated extract (70:1) of lemon balm has shown positive effects in clinical studies conducted in three German hospitals and a dermatology clinic. When the lemon balm cream was used, it produced a rapid interruption of the infection and promoted healing of the herpes blisters much more quickly than normal. The control group receiving other topical creams had a healing period of ten days, while the group receiving the lemon balm cream was completely healed within five days. Researchers also found that if subjects used the lemon cream regularly, they either stopped having recurrences or experienced a tremendous reduction in the frequency of recurrences (an average cold-sore-free period of greater than three and a half months).

The lemon balm cream should be applied to the lips two to four times a day during an active recurrence. It can be applied fairly thickly (1–2 mm). Detailed toxicology studies have demonstrated that lemon balm is extremely safe and suitable for long-term use.

Brand names include Herpilyn and Herpalieve.

Note: The antiviral effects of the lemon balm extract are due to direct action on the virus. In order to achieve this killing effect, a relatively high concentration of the extract's antiviral compounds must attach directly to the herpes virus. When applied topically, the concentration of active compounds is sufficient to inactivate the virus, but taking the extract internally would require huge amounts in order to achieve concentrations that would inhibit the virus. It is simply not feasible to get the necessary amounts of lemon balm into the body.

Cautions and Warnings

None known.

Possible Side Effects

None known.

Menthol

Used For

Headache
Effectiveness: A   Safety: A

Musculoskeletal pain relief
Effectiveness: A   Safety: A

General Information

Menthol is a volatile oil that is a component of peppermint oil and oils from other mint species. The external analgesic and counterirritant effects of menthol are well known. When applied to the skin, menthol stimulates nerves that perceive cold while simultaneously depressing those that perceive pain. The initial cooling effect is followed by a period of warmth. Menthol and related substances such as methylsalicylate are useful in the treatment of arthritis, muscle pains, tendonitis, and other inflammatory conditions involving the musculoskeletal system.

Topical application of menthol or other volatile oils is also of benefit in tension headaches, as they help to relax the temporal muscles. In one study, Tiger Balm (a proprietary preparation containing menthol, camphor, and peppermint oil) was shown to produce results on a par with oral headache medications. Tiger Balm was applied to the temple, then repeated at thirty minutes and one hour. Similar results were noted in studies with topical application of peppermint oil or eucalyptus oil to the forehead and temples.

Brand names include White Flower and Tiger Balm.

Cautions and Warnings

Allergic reactions to the skin have been reported. It is recommended that individuals apply the menthol product to a small area of skin before using it extensively for the first time, so as to avoid developing contact dermatitis (an allergic reaction of the skin) over a larger area.

Menthol preparations should not be used more than three or four times per day and should not be applied to an area larger than 8 inches by 8 inches.

Possible Side Effects

Generally, the application of menthol is without side effects. Allergic reactions, however, have been reported (see "Cautions and Warnings," above). The likelihood of developing such a reaction is increased when heating pads are used in conjunction with topically applied preparations containing menthol.

Tea Tree Oil (from *Melaleuca alternifolia*)

Used For

Acne
Effectiveness: B   Safety: A

Athlete's foot and other common foot problems
Effectiveness: B   Safety: A

Fungal nail infections
Effectiveness: B   Safety: A

Topical antiseptic
Effectiveness: B+   Safety: A

Vaginal infections
Effectiveness: B   Safety: A

General Information

Tea tree is a small tree native to only one area of the world—the northeast coastal region of New South Wales, Australia. The leaves are the source of tea tree oil. The medical world's first mention of tea tree appeared in the *Medical Journal of Australia* in 1930, where a surgeon in Sydney reported impressive results from a solution of tea tree oil for cleaning surgical wounds. Tea tree oil possesses significant antibiotic effects and is an ideal skin disinfectant, as it is active against a wide range of organisms, possesses good penetration, and is nonirritating to the skin.

A variety of tea tree oil products are on the market, including toothpastes, shampoos and conditioners, creams, hand and body lotions, soaps, gels, liniments, and nail polish removers.

Acne

Topical application of tea tree oil is a suitable alternative to benzoyl peroxide preparations. In one study, 124 patients with mild to moderate acne applied either a 5 percent gel of tea tree oil or 5 percent benzoyl peroxide lotion daily. After three months, both treatments produced a significant improvement in mean number of both noninflamed and inflamed lesions—only with noninflamed lesions was benzoyl peroxide found to be more effective. An important finding was that there were fewer reports of side effects (dryness, itchiness), stinging, burning, and skin redness) with tea tree oil (44 percent versus 79 percent).

Athlete's foot and other common foot problems

Tea tree oil, in emollient form (8 percent tea tree oil) or in solution (40 percent), can be massaged into the feet daily for the treatment of athlete's foot (*tinea pedis*), foot irritation, and bromhidrosis (severely foul-smelling feet).

Fungal nail infection

Fungal nail infections (onychomycosis) are the most frequent cause of nail disease, affecting between 2 and 13 percent of the population. Topical therapy with 100 percent tea tree oil, in conjunction with debridement (the clearing away of dead tissue), provides excellent improvement in nail appearance and symptoms. The degree of improvement is on a par with topically applied antifungal drugs (e.g., 1 percent clotrimazole solution).

Topical antiseptic

Tea tree oil is useful in a broad range of skin infections, not only because of its broad-spectrum antibiotic properties, but also because of its capacity to mix with sebaceous secretions and penetrate the epidermis. A clinical trial in patients with boils demonstrated that tea tree oil encouraged more rapid healing without scarring, compared to matched controls. Presumably the positive clinical effects were due to the oil's germicidal activity against *Staphylococcus aureus*. The method of application included cleaning the site and painting the surface of the boil freely with tea tree oil two or three times a day.

Vaginal infections

Tea tree oil has demonstrated activity against a number of organisms that can cause vaginal infections, including *Trichomonas vaginalis* and *Candida albicans.* For vaginal infections, daily vaginal douches with one quart of water containing 4 to 5 ml of tea tree oil is often recommended.

Cautions and Warnings

Allergic reactions are not uncommon. It is recommended that individuals apply the oil to a small area of skin before using tea tree oil extensively for the first time, so as to avoid developing contact dermatitis (an allergic reaction of the skin) over a larger area.

Possible Side Effects

Generally, the application of tea tree oil is without side effects. Allergic reactions, however, have been reported.

Vitamin A

Used For

Dry eye disorders
Effectiveness: A   Safety: A

General Information

Vitamin A eyedrops have shown impressive results in relieving dry eye disorders, a complex group of diseases that can be characterized by (1) a localized water deficiency in the tear ducts, (2) a mucin deficiency, or (3) a combination of the two. Despite the diversity of underlying causes, the changes in the lining of the eye (conjunctiva) are similar in all cases: loss of goblet cells (mucin-producing cells), abnormal enlargement of surface cells, and an increase of cellular layers and the depositing of keratin (a hard protein).

Considering vitamin A's vital role in epithelial tissue, the hypothesis that a localized vitamin A deficiency in the lining of the outer eye may be responsible for dry eye seems obvious. Clinical studies featuring a commercial formula (Viva-Drops) have yielded impressive clinical results in the treatment of dry eye. Unlike other dry-eye preparations, however, the underlying cellular changes causing the dry eye are reversed by topical vitamin A.

Brand names available include Viva-Drops.

Cautions and Warnings

Use only sterile vitamin A preparations for topical application in the eye.

Possible Side Effects

None known.

Vitamin C (topical)

Used For

Antiwrinkle and antiaging effects
Effectiveness: A   Safety: A

General Information

As vitamin C is an alpha-hydroxy acid, it has shown the same effect as the other **alpha-hydroxy acids (AHAs)** in helping the skin look younger.

Cautions and Warnings

Only use vitamin C and other AHA-containing products according to label recommendations.

Possible Side Effects

When using vitamin C and other AHAs, be aware that your skin is now even more vulnerable to the negative effects of the sun. Use an effective sun block before exposing your skin to the sun.

Vitamin E (topical)

Used For

Prevention of scar formation and wound healing
Effectiveness: F   Safety: A

Skin moisturizer and protectant
Effectiveness: A   Safety: A

General Information

Vitamin E is believed to exert a moisturizing effect on the skin. It is often recommended for application to wounds to reduce or soften scar formation. However, clinical studies have shown that this practice is without merit.

Cautions and Warnings

None known.

Possible Side Effects

None known.

Witch Hazel (Hamamelis virginiana)

Used For

Eczema and minor skin irritations
Effectiveness: B+   Safety: A

General Information

Witch hazel has a long history of use in treating minor skin irritations. In Germany, witch hazel distillates are viewed as safe and effective alternatives to topical corticosteroids. The anti-inflammatory effect

of witch hazel appears to be due primarily to reduced blood flow to the skin caused by the vaso-
constrictive effects of witch hazel tannins. Several
double-blind studies have shown witch hazel preparations to be helpful in the treatment of eczema
(atopic dermatitis) and other minor skin irritations.

Cautions and Warnings

None known.

Possible Side Effects

None known.

PART VI
Common Health Conditions

This section provides a quick guide to common health conditions. Each entry is organized as follows:

Health condition

Definition

A brief description of the condition.

Signs and Symptoms

What a person generally experiences if he or she has the condition.

Causes

A brief description of the primary or suspected causes of the condition.

Dietary Factors

A description of the key dietary factors to focus on in improving the condition.

Conventional Drugs

A complete listing of the current drugs in use for a particular condition. The generic name is given first, in lower case, and brand names are capitalized. If you are taking a prescription drug, please check with

your physician or pharmacist regarding any con-
traindications or drug interactions with natural products.

Natural Medicines

A listing of the natural products most often used for
the condition, complete with the effectiveness and
safety ratings given in the previous sections. The
safest and most effective natural medicines are
listed, but also others that enjoy wide popularity or
are often marketed for the condition. In this way,
you can assess the relative merits of remedies that
are likely to be suggested to you.

Commentary

Key points regarding the condition that you can use
to improve your health.

ACNE

Definition

Acne is a common skin disorder that occurs in two forms: superficial (acne vulgaris—affecting the hair follicles and oil-secreting glands of the skin and manifesting as blackheads, whiteheads, and inflammation) and cystic (acne conglobata—a more severe form, with deep cyst formation and subsequent scarring). In both forms, the lesions occur predominantly on the face and, to a lesser extent, on the back, chest, and shoulders. These areas of the skin have more sebaceous glands that produce sebum, a mixture of oils and waxes that lubricates the skin and prevents loss of water.

Signs and Symptoms

Acne is associated with the presence of blackheads, pimples, nodules (tender collections of pus deep in the skin that discharge to the skin's surface), and cysts (deep nodules that fail to discharge contents to the surface).

Causes

Acne is most common at puberty due to increased levels of the male sex hormone testosterone. Although men have higher levels of testosterone than women, during puberty there is an increase of testosterone in both sexes, making girls in this age group just as susceptible to acne. Testosterone causes the sebaceous glands to enlarge and produce more sebum. In addition, the cells that line the pores produce more keratin, a waxy protein. The combination of increased secretion of sebum and keratin can lead to blockage of the pore and formation of a blackhead. With the blockage of the pore, bacteria overgrow and release enzymes that break down sebum and promote inflammation. This forms what is known as a whitehead or pimple.

Dietary Factors

It is often recommended that all refined and/or concentrated simple sugars and foods containing transfatty acids (milk and milk products as well as margarine, shortening, and other synthetically hydrogenated vegetable oils) and oxidized fatty acids (fried foods) be avoided.

Conventional Drugs

- *Vitamin A derivatives:* isotretinoin (Accutane)
- *Oral antibiotics:* minocycline (Dynacin, Minocin, Vectrin); tetracycline; demeclocycline (Declomycin), doxycycline (Vibramycin Monodox)
- *Topical antibiotics:* azelaic acid (Azalex); clindamycin (Cleocin T, Clindets, Pledgets); erythromycin (A/T/S 2%, Emgel 2%, Erycette, T-Stat 2%, Theramycin Z); erythromycin/benzoyl peroxide (Benzamycin); benzoyl peroxide (Benzac, Benzashave, Brevoxyl, Desquam-EX, Triaz); hydrocortisone/benzoyl peroxide (Vanoxide-HC)
- *Topical vitamin A derivatives:* adapalene (Differin); tretinoin (Retin-A, Avita Cream)

Natural Medicines

Vitamin A
Effectiveness: B   Safety: D

Tea tree oil (topical)
Effectiveness: B   Safety: A

Zinc
Effectiveness: B   Safety: A

Commentary

Topical treatment with tea tree oil has produced results equal to benzoyl peroxide but with fewer side effects. To remove excess sebum and oil from the face, wash thoroughly twice daily (more if necessary). Also, avoid the use of greasy creams or cosmetics, and wash pillowcases regularly in chemical-free (no added colors or fragrances) detergents.

AIDS AND HIV INFECTION

Definition

Acquired immunodeficiency syndrome (AIDS) is characterized by a profound defect in immune function. The cause of AIDS is infection with the human immunodeficiency virus (HIV). Diagnosis of HIV is made by a positive blood test for HIV antigen and antibodies. Diagnosis of AIDS depends on meeting certain criteria, such as a positive HIV test plus a total helper T cell count (CD4 count) of less than 200 cells per mcl, or a ratio of helper cells to total lymphocytes (CD8 count) that is less than 14 percent.

Signs and Symptoms

The spectrum of HIV infection ranges from a person who tests positive for HIV but has no signs of immune deficiency to a person with full-blown AIDS. Onset of AIDS can be either sudden (with the development of fevers, sweats, malaise, fatigue, joint and muscle pain, headaches, sore throat, diarrhea, generalized swelling of lymph glands, and/or rash on the trunk) or more insidious (presenting as unexplained progressive fatigue, weight loss, fever, diarrhea, and/or generalized swelling of the lymph glands). Anyone experiencing symptoms suggestive of AIDS or HIV infection should consult a physician.

Causes

Primary risk factors for developing AIDS and HIV infection include sexual contact with an HIV-infected person, intravenous drug use involving needle sharing, or being born to a mother who has HIV.

Dietary Factors

The immune system requires a constant supply of nutrients to function properly. Unfortunately, the AIDS patient has many obstacles to overcome in order to supply the immune system with the nutrition it needs. Chief among these obstacles are gastrointestinal tract infection and the wasting (muscle breakdown) promoted by the progressing infection. It is easier to institute nutritional therapies early on than after full-blown AIDS has developed.

It is often recommended that the diet should be rich in whole, natural foods, such as fruits, vegetables, grains, beans, seeds, and nuts; be low in fats and refined sugars; and contain adequate but not excessive amounts of protein. For the person with AIDS, the protein requirement is at least 2 g per kg (2.2 pounds) of body weight. Supplementing the diet with whey protein (high in the amino acid glutamine) appears particularly useful in cases of AIDS, in terms of both its potential for addressing the wasting syndrome of AIDS and its ability to heal the gastrointestinal tract. High-quality whey protein (microfiltered, ion-exchanged) at a dosage of 1 g per kg of body weight is recommended for people who show signs of weight loss or the wasting syndrome (progressive weight loss and weakness, often associated with fever and diarrhea).

Conventional Drugs

- *Antibiotics:* clarithromycin (Biaxin); sulfamethoxazole /trimethoprim (Bactrim, bethaprim, Cotrim, Septra, Sulfaprim, Sulfatrim, Sultrex); daunorubicin citrate (DaunoXome); doxorubicin (Doxil)
- *Antifungal:* itraconazole (Sporanox)
- *Antimycobacterium:* rifabutin (Mycobutin)
- *Antivirals (HIV-specific):* abacavir sulfate (Ziagen); delavirdine mesylate (Rescriptor); didanosine (Videx); efavirenz (Sustiva); lamivudine (Epivir); nevirapine (Viramune); stavudine (Zerit); zalcitabine (Hivid); zidovudine (Retrovir); zidovudine/lamivudine (Combivir)
- *Protease inhibitors:* amprenavir/vitamin E (Agenerase); indinavir sulfate (Crixivan); nelfinavir mesylate (Viracept); ritonavir (Norvir); saquinavir (Fortovase; Invirase)
- *Growth hormone:* somatropin (Genotropin, Humatrope, Norditropin, Nutropin, Saizen, Serostim)

- *Hematinics:* epoetin-alfa (Epogen, Procrit)
- *Immunomodulators:* aldesleukin (Proleukin); in-terferon alfa-2a (Roferon-A, Intron A)

Natural Medicines

Aloe vera gel
Effectiveness: B   Safety: C

Cat's claw (Uncaria tomentosa)
Effectiveness: B   Safety: C

Licorice (Glycyrrhiza glabra)
Effectiveness: B+   Safety: C

Lipoic acid
Effectiveness: B   Safety: A

N-acetylcysteine
Effectiveness: D   Safety: C

St. John's wort (Hypericum perforatum)
Effectiveness: D   Safety: C

Thymus extract
Effectiveness: B   Safety: B

Vitamin A
Effectiveness: B   Safety: B

Vitamin B$_{12}$
Effectiveness: B+   Safety: C

Commentary

The obvious goal of treatment for HIV-positive indi-viduals is to slow the progression of HIV to AIDS. This goal is accomplished by utilizing appropriate drug therapy, optimizing nutritional status, follow-ing a health-promoting lifestyle, and employing measures to enhance immune function.

ALCOHOLISM

Definition

Alcoholism has been defined by the World Health Organization as "alcohol consumption by an individual that exceeds the limits accepted by the culture or injures health or social relationships." Current estimates indicate that over eighteen million people in the United States (roughly 10 percent of the adult population) are alcoholics, making alcoholism one of the most serious health problems today.

Signs and Symptoms

Psychological and social signs of excessive alcohol consumption include depression, loss of friends, arrest for driving while intoxicated, excessive drinking, drinking before breakfast, frequent accidents, and unexplained work absences. Physical signs of excessive alcohol consumption include alcohol odor on the breath, flushed face, tremor, and unexplained bruises.

Causes

Alcoholism represents a multifactorial condition with genetic, physiological, psychological, and social factors, all of equal importance.

Dietary Factors

While many of the nutritional problems of alcoholics relate directly to the effects of alcohol, a major contributing factor is that alcoholics tend not to eat; they substitute alcohol for food. As a result, the alcoholic has to deal not only with secondary nutritional deficiencies caused by excessive alcohol consumption, but also with primary nutritional deficiencies due to inadequate intake.

It is important for alcoholics to avoid refined sugars and caffeine, as these substances stress blood sugar control mechanisms, potentially increasing the craving for alcohol.

Conventional Drugs

- *Antialcoholic preparations:* disulfiram (Antabuse, Disulfiram)

Natural Medicines

Kudzu (Pueraria lobata)
Effectiveness: C   Safety: C

Commentary

A high-potency multiple vitamin and mineral formula (zinc is especially important) or a B vitamin complex is the best first-step nutritional supplement. B vitamins are extremely critical in the nutritional support for alcoholism. Alcoholics are almost always deficient in at least one of the B vitamins; a thiamin (vitamin B_1) deficiency is both the most common and the most serious of the B vitamin deficiencies in the alcoholic. In addition, recent evidence indicates that a thiamin deficiency results in greater intake of alcohol, suggesting that thiamin deficiency is a predisposing factor for alcoholism. A good dosage for thiamin is 50 to 100 mg daily.

ALZHEIMER'S DISEASE

Definition

Alzheimer's disease (AD) is a degenerative brain disorder that manifests as a progressive deterioration of memory and mental function, commonly referred to as dementia. In the United States, 5 percent of the population over sixty-five suffer from severe dementia, while another 10 percent suffer from mild to moderate dementia. With increasing age, there is a rise in frequency. For example, in people over eighty, the rate of dementia is more than 25 percent.

Signs and Symptoms

Progressive mental deterioration, loss of memory and cognitive functions, and inability to carry out activities of daily life are the characteristic symptoms of AD. These symptoms are related to a reduced level of acetylcholine, a key neurotransmitter in the brain that is especially important for memory.

Causes

Alzheimer's disease is characterized by distinctive changes in the brain. The primary feature is the formation of what are referred to as neurofibrillary tangles and plaques. Simplistically speaking, these neurofibrillary tangles and plaques are "scars," composed of deposits of various proteins and cellular debris. The result is massive loss of brain cells, especially in key areas of the brain that control mental function. Although genetic factors probably play a significant role in determining who is going to develop AD, environmental factors are important. Increased oxidative damage, traumatic injury to the head, chronic exposure to aluminum and/or silicon, and exposure to toxins from environmental sources have all been implicated as causative factors.

Considerable attention has been given to the aluminum concentration in the neurofibrillary tangle. Whether the aluminum concentration develops in response to AD or initiates the lesions has not yet been determined, but significant evidence shows that it contributes, possibly very significantly, to the disease. It certainly seems appropriate to avoid all known sources of aluminum: antacids and antiperspirants that contain aluminum; aluminum pots and pans; aluminum foil as food wrapping; and nondairy creamers.

Dietary Factors

In the elderly, studies have shown that mental function is directly related to nutritional status. High nutritional status equals higher mental function. Given the frequency of nutrient deficiency in the elderly population, it is likely that many cases of impaired mental function may have a nutritional cause. Also, since there is considerable evidence that oxidative damage plays a major role in the development and progression of AD and that diets high in antioxidants such as vitamins C and E prevent AD, it makes sense to eat a diet rich in green leafy vegetables; highly colored vegetables such as carrots, yams, and squash; and flavonoid-rich fruits such as citrus, berries, and cherries. Folic acid and vitamin B_{12} also appear to be important in preventing AD.

Conventional Drugs

- *Acetylcholinesterase inhibitors:* donepezil (Aricept); tacrine (Cognex)

Natural Medicines

Carnitine (L-acetylcarnitine)
Effectiveness: B+   Safety: B

DMAE (2-dimethylaminoethanol)
Effectiveness: B–   Safety: C

Ginkgo biloba *extract*
Effectiveness: A   Safety: A

Huperzine A
Effectiveness: A   Safety: B

NADH (niacinamide adenine dinucleotide)
Effectiveness: B   Safety: A

Phosphatidylcholine
Effectiveness: B–   Safety: A

Phosphatidylserine
Effectiveness: B+   Safety: A

Thiamin
Effectiveness: B+   Safety: A

Vitamin C (prevention)
Effectiveness: B   Safety: A

Vitamin E
Effectiveness: B+   Safety: A

Vitamin B_{12}
Effectiveness: B   Safety: A

Zinc
Effectiveness: B   Safety: A

Commentary

Significant improvements in mental function and mood in patients in the early stages of Alzheimer's disease have been reported with the natural medicines listed above. However, less noticeable improvements have been noted in patients with more advanced stages of Alzheimer's disease. Huperzine A is probably the most active in these patients.

ANEMIA

Definition

Anemia refers to a condition in which the blood is deficient in red blood cells or the hemoglobin (iron-containing) portion of red blood cells. The primary function of the red blood cell is to transport oxygen from the lungs to the tissues of the body in exchange for carbon dioxide. The symptoms of anemia, such as extreme fatigue, are caused by a lack of oxygen being delivered to tissues and a buildup of carbon dioxide.

Signs and Symptoms

Anemia can lead to pallor, weakness, and a tendency to become fatigued easily. Laboratory results may indicate a low volume of blood, low level of total red blood cells, or abnormal size or shape of red blood cells.

Causes

Anemia can be due to excessive blood loss, excessive red blood cell destruction due to abnormal red blood cell shape (as in sickle cell anemia), or, most commonly, inadequate red blood cell production as a result of nutritional deficiencies. Although deficiency of any of several vitamins and minerals can produce anemia, the most common causes are deficiencies of iron, vitamin B_{12}, or folic acid.

Dietary Factors

Calf liver is often recommended for anemia, as it is rich not only in iron but also in all B vitamins. Green leafy vegetables are also of great benefit to individuals with any kind of anemia. These vegetables contain not just iron and folic acid but also natural fat-soluble chlorophyll. The chlorophyll molecule is similar to the heme part of the hemoglobin molecule. Fat-soluble (but not water-soluble) chlorophyll is efficiently absorbed from the gastrointestinal tract.

Conventional Drugs/Natural Medicines

Conventional and natural treatments used in the treatment of nutrition-related anemias are identical—that is, supplementation with the nutrient to address the deficiency. For example, supplementing with iron is the treatment for anemia due to iron deficiency, and vitamin B_{12} is used in treating anemia due to vitamin B_{12} deficiency.

Commentary

It is important to work with your physician to identify the exact cause of the anemia; a comprehensive laboratory analysis of the blood will be performed.

ANGINA

Definition

Angina pectoris is caused by an insufficient supply of oxygen to the heart muscle, which produces a squeezing or pressurelike pain in the chest. Angina often serves as a harbinger of a future heart attack. Since physical exertion and stress increase the heart's need for oxygen, they are often the triggering factors.

Signs and Symptoms

The characteristic symptoms are a squeezing or pressurelike pain in the chest occurring immediately after exertion. Angina can also be triggered by emotional tension, cold weather, or large meals. The pain may radiate to the left shoulder blade, left arm, or jaw. The pain typically lasts for one to twenty minutes.

Causes

Angina is almost always due to atherosclerosis—the buildup of cholesterol-containing plaque that progressively narrows and ultimately blocks the blood vessels supplying the heart (the coronary arteries).

This blockage results in a decreased supply of blood and oxygen to the heart tissue. When the flow of oxygen to the heart muscle is substantially reduced, or when there is an increased need by the heart for oxygen, the result is angina.

Dietary Factors

See **atherosclerosis**.

Conventional Drugs

- *Alpha/beta-adrenergic blocking agents:* labetalol (Labetalol, Normodyne, Trandate)
- *Beta-adrenergic blocking agents:* acebutolol (Acebutolol, Sectral); atenolol (Atenolol, Senormin, Tenormin); bisoprolol fumarate (Zebeta); carteolol (Cartrol, Ocupress); metoprolol (Toprol-XL, Lopressor); nadolol (Corgard); penbutolol sulfate (Levatol); pindolol (Visken); propranolol (Betachron, Inderal, Pronol); timolol malteate (Blocadren)
- *Calcium channel blocking agents:* diltiazem (Cardizem CD, Cartia, Dilacor XR, Diltia XT, Tiazac); nifedipine (Adalat CC, Procardia XL); verapamil (Calan, Covera-HS, Isoptin, Verelan)
- *Nitrate coronary vasodilators:* isosorbide dinitrate (Dilatrate-SR, Isd, Isordil, Sorbitrate); isosorbide mononitrate (Imdur, Ismo, Isotrate ER, Monoket); nitroglycerin (Nitro-Bid, Nitro-Dur, Nitrolingual, NitroStat, Transderm-Nitro)

Natural Medicines

Arginine
Effectiveness: A   Safety: A

Carnitine
Effectiveness: B+   Safety: B

Coenzyme Q$_{10}$ (CoQ$_{10}$)
Effectiveness: B+   Safety: A

Fish oils (eicosapentaenoic acid and docosahexaenoic acid)
Effectiveness: B+   Safety: A

Hawthorn (Crataegus spp.)
Effectiveness: B+   Safety: A

Magnesium
Effectiveness: B+   Safety: A

Commentary

Angina is a serious condition that requires careful treatment and monitoring. In severe cases, as well as in the initial stages of mild to moderate angina, prescription medications may be necessary. Natural medicines should be reserved for minor cases and as supportive therapy for more severe cases.

ANXIETY

Definition

Anxiety is an unpleasant emotional state ranging from mild unease to intense fear. Anxiety differs from fear in that while fear is a rational response to a real danger, anxiety usually lacks a clear or realistic cause. Though some anxiety is normal and, in fact, healthy, higher levels of anxiety not only are uncomfortable, but can lead to significant problems.

Signs and Symptoms

Anxiety is often accompanied by a variety of symptoms. The most common symptoms relate to the chest, such as heart palpitations (awareness of a more forceful or faster heartbeat), throbbing or stabbing pains, a feeling of tightness and inability to take in enough air, and a tendency to sigh or hyperventilate. Tension in the back and neck muscles often leads to headaches, back pains, and muscle spasms. Other symptoms can include excessive sweating, dry mouth, dizziness, digestive disturbances, and an unusually frequent need to urinate or defecate.

The anxious individual usually has a constant feeling that something bad is going to happen. Such a person may fear that he or she has a chronic or dangerous illness—a belief that is reinforced by the symptoms of anxiety. Inability to relax may lead to difficulty in getting to sleep and to constant waking through the night.

Causes

Anxiety can be the result of both physical and psychological factors. For example, extreme stress can definitely trigger anxiety, and so can certain stimulants such as caffeine. Anxiety can also be triggered by elevations in blood lactic acid level. Lactic acid is the final product in the breakdown of blood sugar (glucose) when there is a lack of oxygen.

Dietary Factors

There are at least seven nutritional factors that may be responsible for triggering anxiety by raising blood lactic acid levels: caffeine, sugar, deficiency of B vitamins, deficiency of calcium, deficiency of magnesium, food allergies, and alcohol. Simply avoiding caffeine, sugar, alcohol, and food allergens along with boosting B vitamins, calcium, and magnesium can go a long way in relieving anxiety. Cutting out caffeine alone often results in complete elimination of symptoms.

Conventional Drugs

- *Benzodiazepine and other antianxiety drugs:* alprazolam (Xanax); buspirone (BuSpar); chlordiazepoxide (Librium); clorazepate dipotassium (Tranxene); diazepam (Valium); lorazepam (Ativan); meprobamate (Miltown); oxazepam (Serax)

Warning: If you are currently on a tranquilizer or antidepressant, you will need to work with a physician to get off the drug before taking any natural medicine for anxiety. Stopping the drug on your own can be dangerous—you absolutely must have proper medical supervision.

Natural Medicines

GABA
Effectiveness: C   Safety: C

***Kava* (Piper methysticum)**
Effectiveness: A   Safety: C

***St. John's wort* (Hypericum perforatum)**
Effectiveness: A   Safety: A

***Valerian* (Valeriana officinalis)**
Effectiveness: B   Safety: B

Commentary

Stress reduction and relaxation exercises are often recommended. Some of the most popular techniques are meditation, prayer, progressive relaxation, self-hypnosis, and biofeedback. The usual recommendation is to set aside at least five to ten minutes each day for the performance of a relaxation technique. St. John's wort is the best choice for mild anxiety associated with depression. Valerian is a good choice if the anxiety is also raising blood pressure or heart rate.

ARRHYTHMIA

Definition

Arrhythmia is a disturbance in the rhythm of the heartbeat. Some arrhythmias are very mild and nothing to worry about (such as atrial fibrillation and premature ventricular contractions); others are potentially life-threatening (such as ventricular tachycardia and severe ventricular arrhythmias). In atrial fibrillation, the atria (the upper chambers of the heart) beat irregularly and very rapidly (up to 300 to 500 beats a minute). This arrhythmia is minor because the atrium's job is simply to fill the ventricle—the lower chamber. In premature ventricular contractures, the heartbeat is irregular, as opposed to ventricular tachycardia, in which the beat is too fast (120 to 200 per minute). Other ventricular arrhythmias tend to be even more serious, such as ventricular fibrillation—rapid, uncontrolled, and ineffective contractions of the heart.

Signs and Symptoms

Many mild arrhythmias go unnoticed, or a person may feel the heart is beating out of pace or too rapidly (palpitations). In contrast, more serious arrhythmias can represent a medical emergency and can be associated with a heart attack.

Causes

Arrhythmias are primarily the result of a disturbance in the electrical system that stimulates the heart to beat. They can also occur when areas of heart muscle develop their own beat. Magnesium and potassium deficiencies are well-known nutritionally related causes of arrhythmia.

Dietary Factors

Usual recommendations are to eliminate salt (sodium chloride) intake; eat a high-potassium diet rich in fiber and complex carbohydrates; increase dietary consumption of celery, garlic, and onions; reduce or eliminate the intake of saturated fats; and increase the intake of magnesium-rich foods such as legumes, tofu, seeds, nuts, whole grains, and green leafy vegetables.

Caffeine may have the potential to cause cardiac arrhythmia. As a precaution, it is recommended that caffeine be avoided by individuals with a history of cardiac arrhythmia and/or palpitations and during the first month after suffering a heart attack.

Conventional Drugs

- *Antiarrhythmics:* amiodarone (Cordarone); disopyramide phosphate (Norpace); flecainide acetate (Tambocor); mexiletine (Mexitil); moricizine (Ethmozine); procainamide (Procanbid); propafenone (Rythmol); quinidine gluconate (Quinaglute); quinidine polygalacturonate (Cardioquin); quinidine sulfate (Quinidex); tocainide (Tonocard)

- *Beta-adrenergic blocking agents:* acebutolol (Sectral); propranolol (Inderal); sotalol (Betapace)
- *Calcium channel blocking agents:* verapamil (Calan)

Natural Medicines

Carnitine
Effectiveness: B+   Safety: B

Coenzyme Q_{10} (CoQ_{10})
Effectiveness: B+   Safety: A

Fish oils (eicosapentaenoic acid and docosahexaenoic acid)
Effectiveness: B+   Safety: A

Hawthorn (Crataegus *spp.*)
Effectiveness: A   Safety: A

Magnesium
Effectiveness: A   Safety: A

Commentary

Any person with an arrhythmia or any other heart disease should have an extensive cardiovascular evaluation, including a complete physical exam to look for signs of poor blood flow; an electrocardiogram, which assesses the electrical function of the heart; an echocardiogram, an ultrasound procedure to assess how the heart is functioning from a mechanical perspective as well as determine the heart's shape and size; and a complete laboratory assessment, including red or white blood cell magnesium level determination.

Natural medicines such as hawthorn and magnesium are often quite effective in minor arrhythmias but are not strong enough for moderate to severe cases. In these cases, the natural medicines can be used as supportive therapy.

ASTHMA

Definition

Asthma is an allergic disorder characterized by spasm of the bronchi (the airway tubes), swelling of the mucous lining of the lungs, and excessive production of a thick, viscous mucus. The major concern with asthma is that it can lead to respiratory failure—the inability to breathe.

Warning: An acute asthma attack can be a medical emergency. If you are suffering from an acute attack consult your physician or go to an emergency room immediately.

Signs and Symptoms

Chronic asthma is associated with recurrent attacks of shortness of breath, cough, wheezing, and excessive production of mucus. Typically the asthma patient will show laboratory signs of allergy (increased levels of eosinophils in blood, increased serum IgE levels, positive food and/or inhalant allergy tests).

Causes

Asthma has typically been divided into two major categories: extrinsic and intrinisic. Extrinsic, or atopic, asthma is generally considered an allergic condition, with a characteristic increase in levels of serum IgE, an antibody. Intrinsic asthma is associated with a bronchial reaction that is due not to allergy but rather to such factors as toxic chemicals, cold air, exercise, infection, and emotional upset. Both extrinsic and intrinsic factors trigger the release of chemicals such as histamine, which is involved in inflammation, from mast cells—specialized white blood cells that reside in various body tissues, including the lining of the respiratory passages.

The rate of asthma in the United States is rising rapidly, especially among children. Reasons often given to explain the rise in asthma include increased stress on the immune system due to greater chemical pollution in the air, water, and food; earlier weaning and earlier introduction of solid foods to infants; food additives; and genetic manipulation of plants, resulting in food components with greater allergenic tendencies.

Dietary Factors

The important dietary recommendations in asthma are the elimination of food allergies and food additives. Many studies have indicated that food allergies play an important role in asthma, particularly in children. It is also important to eliminate salt (sodium chloride), as there is strong evidence that increased salt intake increases the severity of and mortality from asthma.

Conventional Drugs

- *Beta-adrenergic agents:* albuterol (Airet, Albuterol, Proventil, Respirol, Ventolin, Volmax); metaproterenol sulfate (Alupent); terbutaline sulfate (Brethine)
- *Bronchodilators:* ipratropium bromide (Atrovent)
- *Corticosteroids:* beclomethasone dipropionate (Beclovent); flunisolide (Aerobid); fluticasone (Flonase, Flovent); triamcinolone acetonide (Azmacort); prednisone (Apo-Prednisone, Deltasone, Liquid Pred, Meticorten, Orasone, Prednicen, Sterapred, Winpred)
- *Leukotriene receptor antagonists:* zafirlukast (Accolate)
- *Theophylline* (Aerolate)

Natural Medicines

Adrenal cortex extracts
Effectiveness: C   Safety: C

***Alfalfa* (Medicago sativa)**
Effectiveness: D   Safety: A

Aloe vera *gel*
Effectiveness: B   Safety: C

Bee pollen
Effectiveness: C   Safety: F

***Boswellic acids* (Boswellia serrata)**
Effectiveness: B+   Safety: B

Caffeine
Effectiveness: B+   Safety: C

***Cat's claw* (Uncaria tomentosa)**
Effectiveness: B   Safety: C

Ephedra sinica *(ma huang)*
Effectiveness: B+ Safety: D

Fish oils (eicosapentaenoic acid and docosahexaenoic acid)
Effectiveness: B Safety: A

***Ivy* (Hedera helix)**
Effectiveness: B+ Safety: C

Magnesium
Effectiveness: B Safety: A

Procyanidolic oligomers
Effectiveness: C Safety: A

Vitamin B_6
Effectiveness: B Safety: A

Vitamin C
Effectiveness: B+ Safety: A

Commentary

Asthma can be a serious medical emergency. Proper medical care is essential. In severe cases the best treatment is a combined approach using natural measures to reduce the allergic threshold and prevent acute attacks along with proper drug treatment of acute attacks. Here is a suggested hierarchy of medical treatment for asthma.

1. Avoid airborne allergens and allergy-proof the house. Specifically, reduce exposure to airborne allergens, such as pollen, dander, and dust mites by removing dogs, cats, carpets, rugs, upholstered furniture, and other surfaces that can collect these allergens.
2. Eliminate food allergies and food additives from the diet.

3. Follow a vegetarian diet.
4. Support the body's antiallergy mechanisms with vitamin C, other antioxidants, quercetin, and vitamin B_6.
5. Cromolyn can be inhaled for preventing asthma attacks.
6. Take herbal products such as ephedra-based products or boswellic acids.
7. Bronchodilators can control acute attacks.
8. Use inhaled corticosteroids for acute asthma.
9. Try theophylline-containing products.
10. Oral corticosteroids are a last resort because of their serious side effects when used in the long term.

ATHEROSCLEROSIS

Definition

Atherosclerosis is the process of the hardening of an artery due to the buildup of cholesterol-containing plaque. Atherosclerosis is responsible for coronary artery disease—the leading cause of death in America—and many cases of stroke. All together, atherosclerosis is responsible for at least 43 percent of all deaths in the United States.

Signs and Symptoms

Atherosclerosis is sometimes referred to as the "silent killer" because often there are no symptoms or signs before what may be a fatal heart attack or stroke. Most people with significant atherosclerosis

have a history of elevated cholesterol levels and
may also experience angina.

Causes

The initial step in the development of atherosclerosis is damage to the lining of an artery. This damage
is usually the result of free radicals (highly reactive
toxic chemicals most often produced by body
processes). Once the artery lining has been damaged, the site of injury attracts monocytes (large
white blood cells) and platelets (small blood cells involved in the formation of blood clots), which adhere to the damaged area, where they release
growth factors that stimulate plaque formation and
the accumulation of fat and cholesterol deposits.

Reducing premature death from heart disease and
strokes involves reducing—and when possible eliminating—the following major risk factors:

- Smoking
- Elevated blood cholesterol levels
- High blood pressure
- Diabetes
- Physical inactivity
- Obesity

Dietary Factors

The key dietary recommendations to reduce the risk
for atherosclerosis are:

- Reduce the amount of saturated fat, cholesterol,
  and total fat in the diet by eating fewer animal
  products and more plant foods.
- Increase your intake of omega-3 oils by consum-

ing cold-water fish, walnuts, and flaxseed oil. There is considerable evidence that people who consume a diet rich in omega-3 oils from either fish or vegetable sources have a significantly reduced risk of developing atherosclerosis. Cold-water fish such as salmon, mackerel, herring, and halibut are good sources of the long-chain omega-3 fatty acids eicosapentaenoic acid (EPA) and docosahexaenoic acid (DHA). Walnuts and flaxseed oil are good sources of alpha-linolenic acid.

- Eat five or more servings daily of a combination of vegetables and fruits, especially green, orange, and yellow vegetables; berries; and citrus fruits. Antioxidant compounds in these plant foods such as carotenes, flavonoids, selenium, vitamin E, and vitamin C are important in protecting against the development of atherosclerosis.

- Increase your intake of fiber. A diet high in fiber, particularly the soluble fiber found in legumes, fruit, and vegetables, is effective in lowering cholesterol levels and thus preventing atherosclerosis.

- Limit the intake of sugar and other refined carbohydrates, which are a significant factor in the development of atherosclerosis. When consumed, these elevate levels of the hormone insulin. Elevated insulin levels, in turn, are associated with increased cholesterol, triglycerides, blood pressure, and risk of death from cardiovascular disease.

Conventional Drugs

See **cholesterol.**

Natural Medicines

Folic acid
Effectiveness: B   Safety: A

Lycopene
Effectiveness: B   Safety: A

Procyanidolic oligomers
Effectiveness: B   Safety: A

Selenium
Effectiveness: B+   Safety: D

Tocotrienols
Effectiveness: B   Safety: A

Vitamin B_6
Effectiveness: B   Safety: A

Vitamin C
Effectiveness: B   Safety: A

Vitamin E
Effectiveness: A   Safety: A

Commentary

Vitamin E appears to offer the greatest antioxidant protection against heart disease because of its ability to be easily incorporated into the LDL cholesterol molecule and prevent free-radical damage. Damaged LDL cholesterol is a major factor in the initial damage to arteries and progression of arterial plaque. Several large population studies have demonstrated that vitamin E levels may be more predictive of developing a heart attack or stroke than total cholesterol levels.

BOILS (FURUNCULES)

Definition

A boil (furuncle) is a deep-seated infection (abscess) involving the entire hair follicle and adjacent tissue. The most commonly involved sites are the hairy parts of the body that are exposed to friction, pressure, or moisture, such as the neck, armpits, and buttocks. Since the boil can spread, several boils are often found at one location. When several furuncles join together, they are called a carbuncle.

Signs and Symptoms

Boils are characterized by painful inflammatory swelling of a hair follicle that forms an abscess. They typically appear as a small rounded or conical nodule surrounded by redness, progressing to a localized pus pocket with a white center. There is tenderness and pain and, if severe, mild fever. Most lesions will resolve within one to two weeks.

Causes

There is no particular cause of boils, although occasionally they may indicate poor immune function. Recurrent boils may indicate a highly infective form of bacteria, poor hygiene, exposure to harmful chemicals, or chronic depression of the immune system.

Dietary Factors

Depressed immune system function may be caused by nutritional deficiencies, food allergies, and/or ex-

cessive consumption of sugar and other concentrated refined carbohydrates (see **low immunity and
immune support** for further discussion).

Conventional drugs

- *Topical antibiotics:* gentamicin sulfate (Gara-
  mycin)

Natural Medicines

See **low immunity and immune support**.

Tea tree oil
Effectiveness: B+   Safety: A

Commentary

If a boil is severe or does not appear to be getting
better after two or three days, consult a physician
immediately, since the infection can spread through
the subcutaneous (under the skin) tissues, causing
cellulitis (inflammation of the connective tissue), or
it may enter the bloodstream, causing bacteremia
(bacteria in the blood). Cleanliness should be rigorously maintained.

BRONCHITIS AND PNEUMONIA

Definition

Bronchitis is an infection or irritation of the bronchi, the passageways from the windpipe (trachea) to the lungs. Pneumonia, by contrast, is an infection or irritation of the lungs themselves. Both of these conditions are much more common in the winter, as they usually follow an upper respiratory infection (cold).

Warning: Symptoms of pneumonia, including a persistent cough, may indicate a serious condition. Consult your physician if you have symptoms suggestive of pneumonia or if a cough persists for more than one week, if it recurs, or if it is accompanied by high fever, rash, or persistent headache.

Signs and Symptoms

Bouts of coughing, shaking, chills, fever, and chest pain are usually preceded by an upper respiratory tract infection (cold). Pneumonia shows classic signs of lung involvement (shallow breathing, cough, and abnormal breath sounds), and a chest X ray shows infiltration of fluid and lymph into the lungs.

Causes

Bronchitis and pneumonia can be caused by a variety of viruses and bacteria. In healthy individuals, pneumonia and bronchitis most often follow an insult to the immune system. Viral infection (especially influenza or the common cold), cigarette smoke and other noxious fumes, loss of consciousness (which depresses the gag reflex, allowing the breathing in or aspiration of fluids), cancer, or hospitalization (which results in increased exposure to organisms that can cause pneumonia) are all risk factors for bronchitis and pneumonia.

Dietary Factors

Optimal immune function requires a healthy diet that (1) is rich in whole, natural foods, such as fruits, vegetables, grains, beans, seeds, and nuts, (2) is low in fats and refined sugars, and (3) contains adequate but not excessive amounts of protein.

Conventional drugs:

- *Antibiotics:* aztreonam (Azactam); cefixime (Suprax); ceftibuten (Cedax); cefuroxime (Axetil, Ceftin); cefprozil (Cefzil); cephalexin (Cephalexin); clarithromycin (Biaxin); dirithromycin (Dynabac); imipenem/cilastatin sodium (Primaxin); lomefloxacin (Maxaquin); loracarbef (Lorabid); bacampicillin (Spectrobid); ofloxacin (Floxin, Ocuflox); sulfamethoxazole/trimethoprim (Bactrim, Septra)
- *Beta-adrenergic agents:* terbutaline sulfate (Brethine)

Natural Medicines

See **low immunity and immune support.**

Bromelain
Effectiveness: A   Safety: A

Guaifenesin
Effectiveness: A   Safety: A

Commentary

One of the main treatment goals in cases of bronchitis and pneumonia is to help the lungs and air passages get rid of excessive mucus. Perform postural drainage by lying facedown with the top half of the body off the bed, using the forearms as support. The position should be maintained for five to fifteen minutes, while you try to cough and expectorate into a basin or newspaper on the floor.

CANDIDIASIS, CHRONIC

Definition

Chronic candidiasis, or yeast syndrome, is a complex medical syndrome attributed to an overgrowth in the gastrointestinal tract of the usually benign yeast *Candida albicans.*

Signs and Symptoms

Fatigue, allergies, immune system malfunction, depression, chemical sensitivities, and digestive disturbances are just some of the symptoms patients with yeast syndrome have been reported to experience. Laboratory tests, such as stool cultures for candida and measurement of antibody levels to candida or candida antigens in the blood, can help confirm the diagnosis.

Causes

Prolonged antibiotic use is believed to be the most important factor in the development of chronic candidiasis. Antibiotics suppress the immune system and the normal intestinal bacteria that prevent yeast overgrowth, strongly promoting the proliferation of candida. Other factors predisposing to candida overgrowth include decreased digestive secretions; immunosuppressive drugs such as corticosteroids; and impaired immunity.

Dietary Factors

A number of dietary factors may promote the overgrowth of candida. The most important of these factors are high intakes of sugar, milk and other dairy products, foods with a high content of yeast or mold (e.g., alcoholic beverages, cheeses, dried fruits, peanuts), and food allergies.

Conventional Drugs

- *Antifungal drugs:* fluconazole (Diflucan); flucytosine (Ancobon); ketoconazole (Nizoral); itraconazole (Sporanox); miconazole (Monistat); nystatin (Mycostatin, Nilstat, Nystex, Nystop)

Natural Medicines

Lactobacillus acidophilus
Effectiveness: C   Safety: C

Commentary

Since recurrent or chronic infections, including chronic candidiasis, are characterized by a depressed immune system, see **low immunity and immune support** for more recommendations.

CANKER SORES

Definition

Canker sores (aphthous stomatitis) are single or clustered shallow, painful ulcers found anywhere in the oral cavity. The sores usually resolve in seven to twenty-one days but are recurrent in many people.

Signs and Symptoms

Single or clustered shallow, painful ulcers found anywhere in the oral cavity.

Causes

Recurrent canker sores appear to be related to trauma, food sensitivities (especially milk and gluten sensitivity), stress, and/or nutrient deficiency. Stress is often a precipitating factor in recurrent canker sores.

Dietary Factors

There is considerable evidence that sensitivity to gluten (a protein found in grains) is the primary cause of recurrent canker sores in many cases. Withdrawing gluten from the diet results in complete remission of recurrent canker sores in many people.

Conventional Drugs

- Benzocaine (Anbesol, Num-Zit, Vicks Chloraseptic, Zilactin-B); chlorhexidine gluconate (Peridex, Periogard); amlexanox (Aphthasol)

Natural Medicines

Deglycyrrhizinated licorice (DGL)
Effectiveness: B   Safety: A

Commentary

The lining of the mouth and throat is often the first place where nutritional deficiency becomes visible because of the high turnover rate of the cells that line the surface. There are several studies that show nutrient deficiencies to be much more common among recurrent canker sore sufferers than in the general population, especially for thiamin, folic acid, B_{12}, B_6, and iron. When nutrient deficiencies were corrected, the majority of subjects with recurrent canker sores experienced complete remission. Taking a high-potency multiple vitamin and mineral formula will ensure adequate intake of all nutrients linked to recurrent canker sores.

CARPAL TUNNEL SYNDROME

Definition

Carpal tunnel syndrome (CTS) is a common, painful disorder caused by compression of the median nerve, which passes between the bones and ligaments of the wrist.

Signs and Symptoms

Compression of the median nerve causes weakness, pain when gripping, and burning, tingling, or aching that may radiate to the forearm and shoulder. Symptoms may be occasional or constant.

Causes

Carpal tunnel syndrome is caused most frequently by repetitive minor injury. This injury occurs most commonly in people who perform repetitive, strenuous work with their hands (e.g., carpenters) but may also occur in people who do light work (e.g., typists and keyboard operators). It may also follow more serious injuries of the wrist. Carpal tunnel syndrome can also be caused by anything that produces inflammation or swelling of the tissues of the wrist, such as rheumatoid arthritis, diabetes, and hypothyroidism.

Dietary Factors

The increased frequency of carpal tunnel syndrome since 1950 parallels the increased presence of compounds that interfere with vitamin B_6 in the body. Particularly incriminating is tartrazine (yellow dye #5). Tartrazine is added to almost every packaged food. In the United States, the average daily per capita consumption of certified dyes is 15 mg, of which 85 percent is tartrazine. Elimination of tartrazine from the diet may help alleviate carpal tunnel syndrome.

Conventional drugs

No prescription drugs are available with FDA-approved labeling for this indication.

Natural medicines

Vitamin B_6
Effectiveness: B   Safety: A

Bromelain
Effectiveness: C   Safety: A

Commentary

Studies have shown that simple stretching exercises for the wrist can be quite helpful in relieving carpal tunnel syndrome. Hold your arms out with your palms down, and then flex your wrists slowly so that your fingers point up toward the ceiling and then down toward the floor. Continue for up to five minutes. This sustained movement helps prepare the carpal tunnel nerve for repetitive actions. This exercise should be done before work starts and during every break.

CATARACTS

Definition

Cataracts are white, opaque blemishes on the normally transparent lens of the eye. They occur as a result of free-radical or oxidative damage to the protein structure of the lens, similar to the damage that occurs to the protein of egg whites when eggs are boiled or fried. Cataracts are the leading cause of impaired vision and blindness in the United States.

Signs and Symptoms

Clouding or opacity in the crystalline lens of the eye and gradual loss of vision.

Causes

Age-related cataracts form when the normal protective mechanisms of the eye are unable to prevent free-radical damage. The lens, like many other tissues of the body, is dependent on adequate levels and activities of the antioxidant nutrients and enzymes. When these normal protective mechanisms are overwhelmed or deficient, cataracts form. For example, exposure to cigarette smoke or sunlight increases the risk of cataracts.

Dietary Factors

Individuals with higher dietary intakes of antioxidant nutrients such as vitamins C and E, selenium, and carotenes have a much lower risk of developing cataracts. Increase consumption of high-antioxidant foods such as leafy greens, yams, carrots, broccoli, and other highly colored vegetables, and fresh fruits. Salt and saturated fat consumption have been linked to cataract formation. It is also important to avoid fried foods, rancid foods, and other sources of free radicals.

Conventional Drugs

No prescription drugs are available with FDA-approved labeling for this indication.

Natural Medicines

Bilberry (Vaccinium myrtillus)
Effectiveness: B+   Safety: A

Procyanidolic oligomers
Effectiveness: C   Safety: A

Riboflavin
Effectiveness: C   Safety: A

Selenium
Effectiveness: B+   Safety: D

Vitamin C
Effectiveness: B+   Safety: A

Commentary

While cataract formation can be stopped and even reversed in its early stages, significant reversal of well-developed cataracts does not appear possible at this time. In cases of marked vision impairment, surgical cataract removal and lens implant may be the only alternative. As with most diseases, prevention or treatment at an early stage is most effective.

CELLULITE

Definition

Cellulite is a cosmetic defect of the skin characterized by pitting and bulging. Women comprise 90 to
98 percent of the cases, reflecting differences between men and women in the supportive tissue
structures of the skin.

Signs and Symptoms

The basic appearance of cellulite is well described as
the "mattress phenomenon." Symptoms of cellulite
include feelings of tightness and heaviness in areas
affected, particularly the legs. Tenderness of the skin
is quite apparent when the skin is pinched, pressed,
or vigorously massaged. The areas of the body involved are typically the buttocks and thigh regions,
and, to a lesser extent, the lower abdomen, the nape
of the neck, and the upper arms. These are the areas
of the body usually affected in female obesity.

Causes

In cellulite, tissue just below the surface of the skin
that binds the skin loosely to underlying tissue or
bones (the subcutaneous tissue) is disturbed. The
subcutaneous tissue of the thighs is composed of
three layers of fat, with two planes of connective tissue (ground substance) between them. In women,
the uppermost subcutaneous layer consists of what
are termed large standing fat cell chambers, which
are separated by radial and arching dividing walls of
connective tissue anchored to the overlying connec-

tive tissue of the skin. In contrast, the corresponding tissue in men is thinner and has a network of criss-crossing connective tissue walls. In addition, the connective tissue (the corium) between the dermis and subcutaneous tissue is stronger in men than in women. These basic differences are the reason cellulite is seen almost exclusively in women. Increased size of the fat cells or weakened connective tissue can lead to cellulite.

Dietary Factors

Reducing the size of the fat cells through diet and exercise is a primary goal. Weight reduction should be gradual, especially in women over the age of forty. Rapid weight loss in individuals whose skin and connective tissues are already undergoing changes from aging will often make cellulite more apparent.

Conventional Drugs

No prescription drugs are available with FDA-approved labeling for this indication.

Natural Medicines

Gotu kola (Centella asiatica)
Effectiveness: B+   Safety: A

Cellasene
Effectiveness: C   Safety: C

Commentary

Some of the physical treatments for cellulite such as endodermologie (a mechanical method of deep massage) seem to be effective. See **varicose veins** for some other possible measures to help cellulite, as the two conditions are often found together and have much in common.

CEREBRAL VASCULAR INSUFFICIENCY

Definition

Cerebral vascular insufficiency refers to decreased blood supply to the brain. It is extremely common among the elderly in developed countries due to the high prevalence of atherosclerosis (hardening of the arteries). The arteries affected in most cases are the carotid arteries—one on each side of the neck, running parallel to the jugular vein—which are the main arteries that supply blood to the brain.

Typically, the problem develops at the carotid bifurcation—the splitting of the carotid artery into the internal (supplying the brain) and external (supplying the face and scalp) branches. This bifurcation is similar to a stream splitting into two branches, and just as in a stream, debris and sediment can accumulate at the split. Significant symptoms begin to appear in most cases only when the blockage of the artery has reached 90 percent.

Signs and Symptoms

Symptoms of cerebral vascular insufficiency are caused by reduced blood flow and oxygen supply to the brain. Severe disruption of blood and oxygen supply results in a stroke. The official definition of a stroke is loss of nerve function for at least twenty-four hours due to lack of oxygen. Some strokes are quite mild; others can leave a person paralyzed, in a coma, or unable to talk, depending on which part of the brain is affected. Smaller ministrokes, or transient ischemic attacks (TIAs), may result in loss of nerve function for an hour or more, but less than twenty-four hours. TIAs may produce transient symptoms of cerebral vascular insufficiency: dizziness, ringing in the ears, blurred vision, and confusion.

Causes

In most cases, cerebral vascular insufficiency is a consequence of atherosclerosis.

Dietary Factors

The dietary factors given in the section on **atherosclerosis** are recommended. It may also be appropriate to consult the sections on **cholesterol** and **high blood pressure**.

Conventional Drugs

- Isoxsuprine (Vasodilan)

Natural Medicines

Aortic glycosaminoglycans
Effectiveness: A   Safety: A

Ginkgo biloba extract
Effectiveness: A   Safety: A

Commentary

Anyone who experiences signs and symptoms of cerebral vascular insufficiency should consult a physician immediately for proper evaluation. The modern evaluation of blood flow to the brain involves the use of ultrasound techniques. These techniques determine the rate of blood flow and the degree of blockage by using sound waves.

CERVICAL DYSPLASIA

Definition

Cervical dysplasia indicates the appearance of abnormal cells on the surface of the cervix. These abnormal cells are detected by a Pap smear—a sampling of cells collected from the surface of the cervix. Cervical dysplasia is generally regarded as a precancerous lesion; in other words, it is not a cancerous state, but if untreated, it could lead to cancer of the cervix.

Signs and Symptoms

Cervical dysplasia does not have any symptoms. It is discovered in a Pap smear. It is the presence of cells that are abnormal but not yet cancerous.

Causes

Recent attention has focused on the role of the human papillomavirus (HPV) as the major cause. The risk factors for becoming infected with HPV and developing cervical dysplasia include early age at first intercourse, multiple sexual partners, herpes simplex type 2, smoking, oral contraceptive use, and many nutritional factors.

Dietary factors

A high fat intake has been associated with increased risk for cervical cancer, while a diet rich in fruits and vegetables offers significant protection against carcinogenesis, probably due to the higher intake of fiber, beta-carotene, and vitamin C. Eat five or more servings daily of a combination of vegetables and fruits, especially green, orange, and yellow vegetables; berries; and citrus fruits. Folic acid deficiency is also a risk factor for cervical dysplasia.

Conventional Drugs

No prescription drugs are available with FDA-approved labeling for this indication.

Natural Medicines

Folic acid
Effectiveness: B+   Safety: A

Commentary

Cigarette smoking is a major risk factor for cervical cancer and/or cervical dysplasia. The incidence of cervical dysplasia in smokers is two to three times greater than that in nonsmokers. Smoking depresses immune functions, allowing HPV to promote abnormal cellular development; it depletes body stores of vitamin C; and cervical cells may concentrate carcinogenic compounds from inhaled smoke.

CHOLESTEROL, ELEVATED

Definition

Cholesterol is a fatty substance in the body that serves several vital roles. It is a building block for various hormones and bile acids; and it plays a major role in stabilizing cell membranes. While proper cholesterol levels are important to good health, the evidence overwhelmingly demonstrates that elevated blood cholesterol levels greatly increase the risk of death due to heart disease. See also **atherosclerosis**.

Cholesterol is transported in the blood by lipoproteins. The major categories of lipoproteins are very-low-density lipoprotein (VLDL), low-density lipoprotein (LDL), and high-density lipoprotein (HDL). VLDL and LDL are responsible for transporting fats (primarily triglycerides and cholesterol) from the liver to body cells, and elevations of either VLDL or LDL are associated with an increased risk of developing atherosclerosis, the primary cause of a heart attack or stroke. In contrast, HDL is responsible for returning fats to the liver, and a high HDL is associated with a low risk of heart attack.

Signs and Symptoms

Elevated blood cholesterol is usually without symptoms but may be associated with conditions such as high blood pressure, angina, and heart disease. It is currently recommended that total blood cholesterol level be less than 200 mg/dl. In addition, it is recommended that LDL cholesterol be less than 130 mg/dl, HDL cholesterol be greater than 35 mg/dl, and triglyceride levels be less than 150 mg/dl.

Causes

Elevated cholesterol levels are usually reflective of dietary and lifestyle factors, such as high saturated fat intake and lack of physical exercise, although it can also be due to genetic factors.

Dietary Factors

See **atherosclerosis**.

Conventional Drugs

- Niacin
- Probucol
- *Bile salt sequestrants:* cholestyramine (Questran); colestipol (Colestid)
- *Statins (HMG-CoA reductase inhibitors):* atorvastatin (Lipitor); cerivastatin (Baycol); fluvastatin (Lescol); lovastatin (Mevacor); pravastatin (Pravachol); simvastatin (Zocor)

Natural Medicines

Alfalfa (Medicago sativa)
Effectiveness: C   Safety: A

Artichoke (Cynara scolymus)
Effectiveness: B   Safety: C

Beta-sitosterol
Effectiveness: B–   Safety: A

Carnitine
Effectiveness: B+   Safety: B

Chitosan
Effectiveness: B   Safety: B

Chromium
Effectiveness: B–   Safety: B

Fenugreek seed powder (Trigonella fornum-graecum)
Effectiveness: B+   Safety: C

Fiber
Effectiveness: A   Safety: A

Fructooligosaccharides
Effectiveness: B   Safety: A

Gamma-oryzanol
Effectiveness: B   Safety: B

Garlic
Effectiveness: A   Safety: A

Ginseng (Panax ginseng and Panax quinquefolius)
Effectiveness: B   Safety: C

Guggul (Commiphora mukul)
Effectiveness: A   Safety: B

Niacin
Effectiveness: A   Safety: D

Pantethine
Effectiveness: A   Safety: A

Phosphatidylcholine
Effectiveness: B   Safety: A

Policosanol
Effectiveness: A   Safety: A

Red yeast rice extract
Effectiveness: A   Safety: D

Royal jelly
Effectiveness: A   Safety: D

Soy isoflavones
Effectiveness: B   Safety: B

Tocotrienols
Effectiveness: B+   Safety: A

Commentary

Neither niacin nor red yeast rice extract should be used by patients with preexisting liver disease or elevated levels of liver enzymes. For these patient groups, guggul preparations, garlic, or pantethine is recommended.

For most people, niacin is the most cost-effective way to lower blood cholesterol levels. Typically, niacin will produce reductions in total cholesterol of 50 to 75 mg/dl in patients with initial total cholesterol levels above 250 mg/dl within the first two months. In cases where the initial cholesterol level is above 300 mg/dl it may take four to six months before cholesterol levels begin to reach recommended levels. Once the cholesterol level is reduced below 200 mg/dl, reduce the dosage of niacin to 500 mg three times daily for two months. If the cholesterol levels creep up above 200 mg/dl, then raise the dosage of niacin back to 1,000 mg three times daily. If the cholesterol level remains below 200 mg/dl, then withdraw the niacin completely and check the cholesterol levels in two months. Reinstitute niacin therapy if levels have crept up over 200 mg/dl.

CHRONIC FATIGUE SYNDROME

Definition

Chronic fatigue syndrome (CFS) is a defined syndrome that describes a varying combinations of symptoms, one of which is recurrent fatigue.

Signs and Symptoms

Chronic fatigue syndrome was formally defined in 1988 by a consensus panel convened by the Centers for Disease Control (CDC). The major criterion is the presence of new onset of fatigue causing 50 percent reduction in activity for at least six months, and exclusion of other illnesses that can cause fatigue. The minor criteria required are eight of the eleven symptoms listed below, or six of the eleven symptoms plus two of the three signs listed.

Symptoms: mild fever, recurrent sore throat, painful lymph nodes, muscle weakness, muscle pain, prolonged fatigue after exercise, recurrent headache, migratory joint pain, neurological or psychological complaints, sensitivity to bright light, forgetfulness, confusion, inability to concentrate, excessive irritability, depression, sleep disturbance (hypersomnia or insomnia), sudden onset of symptom complex
Signs: low-grade fever, sore throat, palpable or tender lymph nodes

Causes

Many research studies have focused on identifying an infectious agent as the cause of CFS. The Epstein-Barr virus (EBV), a member of the herpes group of viruses and the virus that causes infectious mononucleosis, emerged as the leading yet controversial candidate. In addition to EBV, a number of other viruses have been investigated as possible causes of CFS. But rather than being the result of an infectious organism per se, CFS is more likely due to a disturbed immune system. While no specific immunological dysfunction has been recognized, the most consistent abnormality is a decreased number or activity of natural killer (NK) cells. NK cells received their name because of their ability to destroy cells that have become cancerous or infected with viruses.

Dietary Factors

Eliminate or restrict intake of refined sugar and caffeine. Sugar is a major contributor to hypoglycemia, and caffeine stresses the adrenal glands. Although caffeine consumption provides temporary stimulation, regular caffeine intake may actually lead to chronic fatigue.

Eliminate food allergies. As far back as 1930, chronic fatigue was recognized as a key feature of food allergies. Between 55 and 85 percent of individuals with CFS have food allergies. For more information, see **food allergy.**

Conventional Drugs

Most often used are antidepressants in low dosages. See **depression** for list.

Natural Medicines

Magnesium
Effectiveness: B   Safety: A

NADH (Niacinamide adenine dinucleotide)
Effectiveness: B   Safety: A

Siberian ginseng (Eleutherococcus senticosus)
Effectiveness: B   Safety: C

Commentary

Depression is often an underlying factor in individuals with CFS.

COMMON COLD

Definition

The common cold is an upper respiratory tract infection that is caused by a virus.

Signs and Symptoms

Typically, the individual with a cold will experience general malaise, fever, headache, and upper respiratory tract congestion. Initially, there is usually a watery nasal discharge and sneezing, followed by thicker secretions containing mucus, white blood cells, and dead organisms. The throat may be red, sore, and quite dry. The common cold typically lasts anywhere from four to ten days.

Causes

We are all constantly exposed to many of these viruses, yet the majority of us experience the discomfort of a cold once or twice a year at the most. This scenario suggests that a decrease in resistance or immune function is the major factor in catching a cold.

Dietary Factors

Increasing fluid consumption maintains a moist respiratory tract that repels viral infection. Drinking plenty of liquids will also improve the function of white blood cells by decreasing the concentration of compounds that are in solution in the blood. The type of liquids you consume is very important. Studies have shown that consuming concentrated sources of sugars, such as glucose, fructose, sucrose, honey, or orange juice, greatly reduces the ability of the white blood cells to kill bacteria. Before being consumed, fruit juices should be greatly diluted. Keep daily intake to four to eight ounces of undiluted fruit juices.

Conventional Drugs

- *Antihistamines:* fexofenadine (Allegra); pseudoephedrine/triprolidine (Actifed)
- *Nasal vasoconstrictors:* oxymetazoline (Afrin)

Natural Medicines

Andrographis paniculata
Effectiveness: B+   Safety: C

Cat's claw **(Uncaria tomentosa)**
Effectiveness: B   Safety: A

Echinacea
Effectiveness: B+   Safety: A

Elderberry **(Sambucus nigra)**
Effectiveness: B+   Safety: A

Esberitox
Effectiveness: A   Safety: A

Licorice **(Glycyrrhiza glabra)**
Effectiveness: C   Safety: C

Olive leaf **(Olea europa)**
Effectiveness: C   Safety: C

Peppermint **(Mentha piperita)**
Effectiveness: C   Safety: A

Sinupret
Effectiveness: A   Safety: A

Vitamin C
Effectiveness: A   Safety: A

Zinc
Effectiveness: A   Safety: A

Commentary

Once a cold develops, there are several things that
can speed up recovery. If you start soon enough,
you may be able to quickly shed the cold. However,
if the virus has already established a firm foothold,
it may take a couple of days to completely throw it
off. Do not expect immediate relief in most instances when using natural substances. In fact,
since most natural therapies for colds involve as-
sisting the body rather than the familiar drug action

of suppressing the symptoms, the symptoms of the cold may temporarily worsen when using natural remedies. How can this be? Many cold symptoms are a result of our body's defense mechanisms. For example, the potent immune-stimulating compound interferon, released by our blood cells and other tissues during infections, is responsible for many flu-like symptoms. Another example is the beneficial effect of fever on the course of infection. While an elevated body temperature can be uncomfortable, suppression of fever is thought to counteract a major defense mechanism and prolong the infection. In general, fever should not be suppressed during an infection unless it is dangerously high (>104°F). For these and other reasons it is not uncommon for individuals treating themselves for the common cold with natural medicines to experience a greater degree of discomfort due to the immune-enhancing effects of these compounds. Of course, the illness is generally much shorter-lived.

CONGESTIVE HEART FAILURE

Definition

Congestive heart failure (CHF) refers to an inability of the heart to effectively pump enough blood.

Signs and Symptoms

Weakness, fatigue, and shortness of breath are the most common symptoms of CHF.

Causes

Chronic CHF is most often due to the long-term effects of high blood pressure, previous myocardial infarction, disorder of a heart valve or the heart muscle, or chronic lung disease such as asthma or emphysema.

Dietary Factors

Since CHF is most often due to chronic high blood pressure, the same dietary factors that alleviate that condition apply in CHF. Most notably, eliminate salt (sodium chloride) intake; follow a high-potassium diet rich in fiber and complex carbohydrates; increase dietary consumption of celery, garlic, and onions; and reduce or eliminate the intake of saturated fats.

Conventional Drugs

See also **high blood pressure.**

- *Digitalis glycosides:* digitoxin (Crystodigin); digoxin (Lanoxin)
- *Inotropic drugs:* amrinone lactate (Inocor); milrinone lactate (Primacor)
- *Alpha-adrenergic blocking agents:* phentolamine mesylate (Regitine)
- *Alpha/beta-adrenergic blocking agents:* carvedilol (Coreg)
- *Hypotensives, ACE blocking type:* benazepril (Lotensin); captopril (Capoten); captopril/hydrochlorothizaide (Capozide); enalapril maleate (Vasotec); fosinopril sodium (Monopril); lisinopril (Prinivil, Zestril); quinapril/magnesium carbonate (Accupril); ramipril (Altace); trandolapril (Mavik)

- *Hypotensives, miscellaneous:* nitroprusside sodium (Nipride, Nitropress)
- *Hypotensives, vasodilators:* hydralazine (Apresoline); prazosin (Minipress)
- *Loop diuretics:* bumetanide (Bumex); ethacrynic acid (Edecrin); furosemide (Furoside, Lasix, Uritol)
- *Potassium-sparing diuretics:* amiloride (Midamor); spironolactone (Aldactone); triamterene (Dyrenium)
- *Thiazide diuretics:* bendroflumethiazide (Naturetin); benzothiazide (Exna, Hydrex); chlorothiazide (Diuril); chlorthalidone (Hydone, Hygroton, Novo-Thalidone, Thalitone, Uridon); cyclothiazide (Anhydron); hydrochlorothiazide (Apo-Hydro, Diuchlor H, Esidrix, Hydro-chlor, HydroDIURIL, Neo-Codema, Novo-Hydrazide, Oretic, Urozide); hydroflumethiazide (Diucardin, Saluron); methyclothiazide (Aquatensen, Duretic, Enduron); metolazone (Diulo, Mykrox, Zaroxolyn); polythiazide (Renese); quinethazone (Hydromox); trichlormethiazide (Aquazide, Diurese, Metahydrin, Naqua, Trichlorex)

Natural Medicines

Carnitine
Effectiveness: B+   Safety: B

Coenzyme Q₁₀ (CoQ₁₀)
Effectiveness: A   Safety: A

Hawthorn (Crataegus spp.)
Effectiveness: A   Safety: A

Magnesium
Effectiveness: A   Safety: A

Thiamin
Effectiveness: B+　　　Safety: A

Commentary

Moderate to severe cases of CHF usually require conventional medical approaches. However, the natural medicines listed have been shown to assist conventional drugs used in CHF.

CONSTIPATION

Definition

Constipation refers to the inability to defecate. The frequency of defecation and the consistency and volume of stools vary so greatly from individual to individual that it is difficult to determine normal function. In general, most nutritionally oriented physicians recommend at least one bowel movement a day.

Signs and Symptoms

Hard, small, and difficult-to-pass stools are the most frequent complaint.

Causes

There are a number of possible causes of constipation, but the most common is a low-fiber diet. Other common causes include inadequate fluid intake, lack of physical activity, various medications (e.g., anesthetics, antacids, diuretics), low thyroid function, and irritable bowel syndrome.

Dietary Factors

A high-fiber diet, plentiful fluid consumption, and exercise are an effective prescription in most cases of constipation. High levels of dietary fiber increase both the frequency and quantity of bowel movements, decrease the transit time of stools (the amount of time between consumption of a food and its elimination in the feces) and the absorption of toxins from the stool, and appear to be a preventive factor in several diseases. Particularly effective in relieving constipation are bran and prunes. The typical recommendation for bran is ½ cup of bran cereal per day, increasing to 1½ cups over several weeks. When using bran, make sure to consume enough liquids. Drink at least six to eight glasses of water per day. Whole prunes as well as prune juice also possess good laxative effects; 8 ounces is usually an effective dose.

Conventional Drugs

- *Bulk-forming laxatives:* calcium polycarbophil (FiberCon, Konsyl); biscadoyl (Correctol Laxative, Dulcolax); lactulose (Duphalac); methylcellulose (Citrucel, Fiberease); psyllium (Metamucil, Perdiem)
- *Stimulant laxatives:* castor oil (Purge Concentrate); magnesium sulfate (Epsom salts); mineral oil (Kondremul); phenolphthalein (Ex-Lax, Fletcher's); polyethylene glycol 3350 (Miralax); senna (Correctol Herbal Tea, Fletcher's Castoria, Senokot)

- *Stool softeners:* docusate calcium (Surfak); docusate calcium/phenolphthalein (Doxidan); docusate sodium (Colace, Correctol Extra Gentle, Dialose, Fleet Sof-Lax); docusate sodium/phenolphthalein (Dialose Plus, Extra Gentle Ex-Lax)

Natural Medicines

Aloin
Effectiveness: A   Safety: D

Artichoke (Cynara scolymus)
Effectiveness: B   Safety: C

Cascara sagrada
Effectiveness: A   Safety: C

Fiber
Effectiveness: A   Safety: A

Maltsupex
Effectiveness: A   Safety: A

Senna (Cassia senna)
Effectiveness: A   Safety: C

Commentary

If you have been using stimulant laxatives, even natural ones such as senna or *Cascara sagrada,* you will need to retrain your bowels to get them to function normally without the stimulant laxative. Here is the program that I recommend for reestablishing bowel regularity. It usually takes four to six weeks.

- Find and eliminate known causes of constipation.
- Never repress an urge to defecate.
- Add bran cereal to the diet and eat more high-fiber foods such as whole grains, fruits, and vegetables.

- Drink six to eight glasses of fluid per day.
- Sit on the toilet at the same time every day (even when the urge to defecate is not present), preferably immediately after breakfast or exercise.
- Exercise for at least twenty minutes three times per week.
- Week one: Every night before bed, take a stimulant laxative containing either cascara or senna. Take the lowest amount necessary to reliably ensure a bowel movement every morning.
- Weekly: Each subsequent week, decrease the laxative dosage by half. If constipation recurs, go back to the previous week's dosage. Decrease the dosage if diarrhea occurs.

DEPRESSION

Definition

Depression is characterized by feelings of low self-esteem, pessimism, and despair. It can range from a transient low mood to a potentially life-threatening severe clinical depression.

Signs and Symptoms

Clinical depression is more than feeling depressed. The official definition of clinical depression is based on the following eight primary criteria:

1. Poor appetite accompanied by weight loss, or increased appetite accompanied by weight gain
2. Insomnia or excessive sleep habits (hypersomnia)
3. Physical hyperactivity or inactivity

4. Loss of interest or pleasure in usual activities, or decrease in sexual drive
5. Loss of energy, feelings of fatigue
6. Feelings of worthlessness, self-reproach, or inappropriate guilt
7. Diminished ability to think or concentrate
8. Recurrent thoughts of death or suicide

The presence of five of these eight symptoms definitely indicates clinical depression; an individual with four is probably depressed. The symptoms must be present for at least one month to be called clinical depression.

Causes

Depression can be the result of psychological as well as physiological factors. The most significant psychological theory is the learned-helplessness model, which theorizes that depression is the result of habitual feelings of pessimism and hopelessness. The chief physiological theory is the monoamine hypothesis, which stresses imbalances of monoamine neurotransmitters such as serotonin, epinephrine, and norepinephrine. Serotonin deficiency is the most common biochemical cause.

It is important to rule out the simple organic factors that are known to contribute to depression, such as nutrient deficiency, drugs (including many prescription and illicit drugs, alcohol, caffeine, and nicotine), hypoglycemia, and hypothyroidism.

Dietary Factors

A deficiency of any single nutrient can alter brain function and lead to depression, anxiety, and other mental disorders. Since the brain requires a constant

supply of blood sugar to function properly, hypoglycemia must be avoided. Symptoms of hypoglycemia can range from mild to severe and include
depression, anxiety, irritability, and other psychological disturbances; fatigue; headache; blurred vision;
excessive sweating; mental confusion; incoherent
speech; bizarre behavior; and convulsions. Several
studies have shown hypoglycemia to be very common in depressed individuals. Simply eliminating refined carbohydrates from the diet is sometimes all
that is needed for effective therapy in patients whose
depression results from reactive hypoglycemia.

Conventional Drugs

- *Selective serotonin reuptake inhibitors (SSRIs):*
  paroxetine (Paxil); fluoxetine (Prozac); sertraline
  (Zoloft)
- *Tricyclic antidepressants:* amitriptyline (Elavil,
  Endep, Vanatrip); amitriptyline/chlordiazepoxide
  (Limbitrol); Amitriptyline/perphenazine (Etrafon,
  Triavil); amoxapine (Asendin); Clomipramine
  (Anafranil); desipramine (Norpramin); doxepin
  (Adapin, Sinequan, Zonalon); imipramine
  (Tofranil, Tofranil-PM); maprotiline (Ludiomil);
  nortriptyline (Pamelor); protriptyline (Vivactil);
  trimipramine maleate (Surmontil)
- *Miscellaneous antidepressants:* bupropion
  (Wellbutrin, Zyban); mirtazapine (Remeron); ne-
  fazodone (Serzone); selegiline (Atapryl, Carbex,
  Eldepryl); trazodone (Desyrel, Trazodone); ven-
  lafaxine (Effexor)
- *Monoamine oxidase inhibitors:* furazolidone
  (Furoxone); isocarboxazid (Marplan); pargyline
  HCL (Eutonyl); phenelzine sulfate (Nardil); pro-
  carbazine (Matulane); tranylcypromine sulfate
  (Parnate)

Natural Medicines

DHEA
Effectiveness: A   Safety: C

D,L-phenylalanine
Effectiveness: B+   Safety: C

Fish oils (eicosapentaenoic acid and docosahexanoic acid)
Effectiveness: B   Safety: A

Folic acid
Effectiveness: B   Safety: A

Ginkgo biloba
Effectiveness: B+   Safety: A

Hydroxytryptophan (5-HTP)
Effectiveness: A   Safety: D

Inositol
Effectiveness: A   Safety: A

Phosphatidylserine
Effectiveness: B+   Safety: A

S-adenosylmethionine (SAMe)
Effectiveness: A   Safety: A

St. John's wort (Hypericum perforatum)
Effectiveness: A   Safety: A

Tyrosine
Effectiveness: B   Safety: C

Vitamin B_6
Effectiveness: B   Safety: A

Vitamin B_{12}
Effectiveness: B+   Safety: A

Commentary

If you are currently on a prescription antidepressant drug, you will need to work with a physician to get off the drug. Stopping the drug on your own can be dangerous to your health. Although St. John's wort, 5-HTP, and other natural approaches to depression have been shown to be comparable in efficacy to standard drugs in mild to moderate depression, in severe cases the value of supervised medical care and the appropriate use of conventional antidepressants cannot be overstated.

DIABETES MELLITUS

Definition

Diabetes mellitus is a chronic disorder of carbohydrate, fat, and protein metabolism characterized by fasting elevations of blood sugar (glucose) levels and a greatly increased risk of heart disease, stroke, kidney disease, retinopathy, and loss of nerve function. Diabetes can occur when the pancreas does not secrete enough insulin or when the cells of the body become resistant to insulin. In either case, the blood sugar cannot get into the cells for storage, which then leads to serious complications.

Diabetes is divided into two major categories: type 1 and type 2. Type 1, or insulin-dependent diabetes mellitus (IDDM), occurs most often in children and adolescents and is associated with complete destruction of the beta cells of the pancreas, which manufacture the hormone insulin. Type 1 diabetics require lifelong insulin for the control of blood sugar levels. Type 2, or non-insulin-dependent diabetes mellitus (NIDDM), usually has an onset after forty years of age. About 90 percent of all diabetics are type 2. Initially, their insulin levels are typically elevated, indicating a loss of sensitivity to insulin by the cells of the body, otherwise known as insulin resistance.

Other types of diabetes include:

- *Secondary diabetes:* a form of diabetes that is secondary to conditions such as pancreatic disease, hormone disturbances, drugs, and malnutrition).
- *Gestational diabetes:* glucose intolerance that occurs during pregnancy.
- *Impaired glucose tolerance:* a condition that includes prediabetic or borderline diabetes. Individuals with impaired glucose tolerance have blood glucose levels and glucose tolerance test results that are intermediate between normal and clearly abnormal.

Signs and Symptoms

The classic symptoms of type 1 diabetes are frequent urination, excessive thirst, and excessive appetite. In type 2 diabetes, these symptoms may also be present but are usually much milder than in type 1. When symptoms are mild, many people do not seek medical care. In fact, of the more than ten million Americans with diabetes, fewer than half know they have it. The following criteria are used for diagnosing diabetes:

- *Fasting (overnight):* serum glucose (blood sugar) concentration greater than or equal to 140 mg/dl on at least two separate occasions

- *Following ingestion of 75 g of glucose:* serum glucose concentration greater than or equal to 200 mg/dl at two hours postingestion and at least one other sample during the two-hour test

Causes

Although the exact cause of type 1 diabetes is unknown, current theory suggests an autoimmune process leads to destruction of the insulin-producing beta cells in the pancreas. Antibodies for beta cells are present in 75 percent of all cases of type 1 diabetes, compared to 0.5 to 2 percent of nondiabetics. The antibodies to the beta cells appear to develop in response to cell destruction due to other mechanisms (chemicals, free radicals, viruses, food allergies, etc.).

On the other hand, obesity is a major contributing factor to the development of insulin resistance; approximately 90 percent of individuals with type 2 diabetes are obese. In most cases, achieving ideal body weight is associated with restoration of normal blood sugar levels in these patients.

Dietary Factors

Weight loss, in particular a significant decrease in body fat percentage, is a prime objective in treating the majority of type 2 diabetics. It improves all aspects of diabetes and may result in cure.

All simple, processed, and concentrated carbohydrates must be avoided. Foods high in complex carbohydrates and fiber should be stressed, and saturated fats should be kept to a minimum. Legumes, onions, and garlic are particularly useful. Since diabetics have a higher incidence of death from cardiovascular disease (60 to 70 percent, versus 20 to 25 percent in people without diabetes), the dietary recommendations given in the section on **atherosclerosis** are equally appropriate here.

Conventional Drugs

- Insulin (Humulin, Novolin)
- *Oral hypoglycemics:*
  - *Alpha-glucosidase inhibitors:* acarbose (Precose); miglitol (Glyset)
  - *Biguanide type (non-sulfonylureas):* metformin (Glucophage)
  - *Sulfonylureas:* acetohexamide (Dymelor); chlorpropamide (Diabinese, Insulase); glimepiride (Amaryl); glipizide (Glipizide, Glucotrol); glyburide (Diabeta, Micronase); repaglinide (Prandin); tolazamide (Tolinase); tolbutamide (Orinase)
  - *Insulin-response enhancers:* pioglitazone (actos); rosiglitazone maleate (Avandia); troglitazone (Rezulin)

Natural Medicines

Aloe vera
Effectiveness: B   Safety: C

Bilberry* (Vaccinium myrtillus) *(for retinopathy)
Effectiveness: B   Safety: A

Biotin
Effectiveness: C   Safety: A

***Bitter melon* (Momardica charantia)**
Effectiveness: B+   Safety: B

Capsaicin (topical use for neuropathy)
Effectiveness: A   Safety: A

Chromium
Effectiveness: B   Safety: B

Coenzyme Q₁₀ (CoQ₁₀)
Effectiveness: B   Safety: A

Fenugreek seed powder (Trigonella foenum-graecum)
Effectiveness: B+   Safety: C

Fiber
Effectiveness: A   Safety: A

Fructooligosaccharides
Effectiveness: B–   Safety: A

Gamma-linolenic acid (for neuropathy)
Effectiveness: B+   Safety: A

Garlic (Allium sativum)
Effectiveness: B+   Safety: A

Ginseng (Panax ginseng *and* P. quinquefolius)
Effectiveness: B   Safety: C

Gymnema sylvestre
Effectiveness: B+   Safety: B

Lipoic acid
Effectiveness: A   Safety: A

Magnesium
Effectiveness: B   Safety: A

Manganese
Effectiveness: C   Safety: C

Niacinamide (a form of vitamin B₃)
Effectiveness: B+   Safety: B

Olive leaf (Olea europa)
Effectiveness: C   Safety: C

Procyanidolic oligomers
Effectiveness: B   Safety: A

Vanadium
Effectiveness: B   Safety: C

Vitamin B₆ (prevention of complications)
Effectiveness: B+   Safety: A

Vitamin B₁₂ (neuropathy)
Effectiveness: B+   Safety: A

Vitamin C
Effectiveness: B+   Safety: A

Vitamin E
Effectiveness: B+   Safety: A

Zinc
Effectiveness: C   Safety: A

Commentary

If you have diabetes and utilize nutritional and herbal products, you must monitor blood sugar levels using a home glucose monitoring kit, especially if you are on insulin or have relatively uncontrolled diabetes. Typically, insulin and drug dosages will have to be adjusted after employing natural medicines. Under no circumstances should you suddenly stop taking insulin or oral diabetic drugs without consulting your physician.

Poor blood sugar control dramatically raises the risk of developing the complications of diabetes. The availability of easy-to-use home glucose monitoring kits has resulted in a major improvement in the care of diabetes. Another major improvement is the measurement of the level of glycosylated hemoglobin (Hgb A1c), which can tell you how your blood

sugar levels have been maintained over a long period of time (three months). Hgb A1c should be
measured every three months in poorly controlled
diabetes, and every year in well-controlled cases. If
a diabetic can keep the Hgb A1c between 6 and 7
percent, the risk for developing complications is dramatically reduced.

DIARRHEA

Definition

Diarrhea refers to an increase in frequency, fluidity,
and volume of bowel movements.

Definition

Diarrhea is usually a mild, temporary event.
However, it may also be the first suggestion of a serious underlying disease or infection.

Causes

Diarrhea is divided into four major types: osmotic,
secretory, exudative, and inadequate contact.

Osmotic diarrhea can be the result of carbohydrate malabsorption (e.g., lactose intolerance), magnesium salts, and excess vitamin C intake.

Secretory diarrhea can be the result of toxin-
producing bacteria, hormone-producing tumors, fat
malabsorption (e.g., lack of bile output), laxative
abuse, and surgical resection of the small intestine.

Exudative diarrhea can be caused by inflamma-

tory bowel disease (Crohn's disease or ulcerative colitis), pseudomembranous colitis (a postantibiotic
diarrhea caused by an overgrowth of the bacteria
Clostridium difficile), and bacterial infection.

Inadequate contact diarrhea is the result of surgical removal of sections of the small intestine.

Dietary Factors

Here are the key dietary recommendations for people with diarrhea:

- Don't eat solid foods. During the acute phase of
  diarrhea, no solid foods should be consumed.
  Instead the focus should be on liquids.
- Replace water and electrolytes by consuming herbal
  teas, vegetable broths, fruit juices, and electrolyte
  replacement drinks. An old naturopathic remedy is
  to sip a drink made of equal parts of sauerkraut juice
  and tomato juice.
- Avoid dairy products. Acute intestinal illnesses,
  whether viral or bacterial, frequently injure the
  cells that line the small intestine. This results in a
  temporary deficiency of lactase, the enzyme responsible for digesting milk sugar (lactose) from
  dairy products. Avoid dairy products (with the
  possible exception of yogurt containing live cultures) while experiencing diarrhea.
- Avoid food allergens. Food allergy is one of the
  most common causes of chronic diarrhea. The ingestion of an allergenic food can result in the release of histamine and other allergic compounds
  from most cells, specialized white blood cells that
  reside in the lining of the intestines. These allergic
  compounds can produce a powerful laxative effect.

Conventional Drugs

- *Antidiarrheal agents:* bismuth subsalicylate (Pepto-Bismol); difenoxin/atropine sulfate (Motofen); diphenoxylate/atropine sulfate (Lomotil, Lonox); loperamide (Imodium A-D, Maalox Anti-Diarrheal, Pepto Diarrhea Control)
- *Intestinal adsorbents and protectives:* attapulgite (Donnagel, Kaopectate, Rheaban)

Natural Medicines

Berberine-containing plants
Effectiveness: B+   Safety: B

Bismuth subcitrate
Effectiveness: B+   Safety: D

Bovine colostrum
Effectiveness: B   Safety: C

Carob
Effectiveness: B+   Safety: A

Lactobacillus acidophilus
Effectiveness: A   Safety: A

Commentary

A high-potency multiple vitamin and mineral formula is required due to the decreased absorption of micronutrients that results from the diarrhea.

Although most acute cases of diarrhea are self-limiting, a physician should be consulted immediately if any of the following apply: diarrhea in a child under six years of age, severe or bloody diarrhea, diarrhea that lasts more than three days, and significant signs of dehydration (sunken eyes, severe dry mouth, strong body odor, etc.).

EAR INFECTIONS
(OTITIS MEDIA)

Definition

In acute otitis media, the middle ear, including the eardrum, becomes inflamed and infected. Otitis media is usually preceded by an upper respiratory infection or allergy. Chronic otitis media (also known as serous otitis media) refers to a constant swelling of the middle ear that can serve as a fertile breeding ground for an acute ear infection. Recurrent bouts of acute otitis media are responsible for more office visits by children to pediatricians than any other reason.

Signs and Symptoms

An acute ear infection is characterized by earache or irritability; history of recent upper respiratory tract infection or allergy; red, opaque, bulging eardrum; and fever and chills. Since an ear infection can be quite serious, it is necessary that any individual with symptoms of an acute ear infection be seen by a physician. Chronic inflammation of the middle ear (serous otitis media) is characterized by painless hearing loss and a dull, immobile eardrum.

Causes

The primary risk factors for an ear infection in children are day care attendance, wood-burning stoves, parental smoking (or exposure to other secondhand smoke), and not being breast-fed. Aside from day care, all of the other factors have something in common: they lead to abnormal eustachian tube function, the underlying cause in virtually all cases of otitis media. The eustachian tube regulates gas pressure in the middle ear, protects the middle ear from nose and throat secretions and bacteria, and clears fluids from the middle ear. Swallowing causes active opening of the eustachian tube due to the action of the surrounding muscles. Infants and small children are particularly susceptible to eustachian tube problems since theirs are smaller in diameter and more horizontal.

Obstruction of the eustachian tube leads first to fluid buildup and then, if bacteria start to grow, bacterial infection. Obstruction results from collapse of the tube (due to weak tissues holding the tube in place and/or an abnormal opening mechanism), blockage with mucus in response to allergy or irritation, or infection.

Dietary Factors

The role of allergy as the major cause of chronic otitis media has been firmly established in the medical literature. Elimination of food allergens has been shown to produce a dramatic effect in the treatment of chronic otitis media in over 90 percent of children in some studies. Since it is usually not possible to determine the exact allergen during an acute attack, the most common allergenic foods should be eliminated from the diet: milk and dairy products, eggs, wheat, corn, oranges, and peanut butter. The diet should also eliminate concentrated simple carbohydrates (sugar, honey, dried fruit, concentrated fruit juice, etc.) since they inhibit the immune system.

Conventional Drugs

- *Antibiotics*
  - *Cephalosporins:* cefaclor (Ceclor); cefazolin; cefdinir (Omnicef); cefixime (Suprax); cefpodoxime (Proxetil, Vantin); cefprozil (Cefzil); ceftibuten dihydrate (Cedax); ceftriaxone sodium (Rocephin); cefuroxime axetil (Ceftin); cephalexin hydrochloride (Keftab); cephalexin (Biocef, Keflex, Zartan); cephradine (Velosef)
  - *Macrolides:* azithromycin (Zithromax); clarithromycin (Biaxin); erythromycin base (EryTab); erythromycin ethylsuccinate (E.E.S., EryPed); erythromycin ethylsuccinate/sulfisoxazole acetyl (Eryzole, Pediazole, Sulfimycin); erythromycin stearate (Erythrocin Stearate)
  - *Miscellaneous:* ofloxacin (Floxin); clindamycin (Cleocin); loracarbef (Lorabid)
  - *Penicillins:* amoxicillin trihydrate (Amoxicillin, Amoxil, Trimox); amoxicillin trihydrate/clavulanic potassium (Augmentin); ampicillin trihydrate (Omnipen, Principen, Totacillin); bacampocillin (Spectrobid)
  - *Sulfonamides:* sulfamethoxazole (Apo-Sulfamethoxazole, Gantanol, Urobak); sulfamethoxazole/trimethoprim (Bactrim, Bethaprim, Cotrim, Septra, Sulfaprim, Sulfatrim, Sultrex); sulfisoxazole (Apo-Sulfisoxizole, Gantrisin, Novo-Soxazole, Sulfizole)

- *Local anesthetics:* benzocaine (Americaine); antipyrine/benzocaine/glycerin (Auralgan, Aurodex, Benzopirin, Rx-Otic); benzocaine/antipyrine/phenylephrine (Tympagesic)

Natural Medicines

See **low immunity and immune support**.

Commentary

Low humidity often contributes to ear infections by causing nasal swelling and reduced ventilation of the eustachian tube, or it may dry the eustachian tube lining, which could lead to increased secretions and an inability to clear fluid. Increasing the humidity level with the help of a humidifier is an important goal in the treatment of ear infections.

ECZEMA (ATOPIC DERMATITIS)

Definition

Eczema is an allergic disorder of the skin.

Signs and Symptoms

Eczema is characterized by chronic itchy, inflamed skin. The skin tends to be very red and scaly. Scratching and rubbing lead to darkened and hardened areas of thickened skin with accentuated furrows, most commonly seen on the inside of the wrist and elbows, face, and the back of the knees.

Causes

Food allergy is the most frequent cause of chronic eczema.

Dietary Factors

Elimination of food allergy is the primary goal in dealing with eczema. Although any food can trigger eczema, milk, eggs, and peanuts appear to be the most common food allergens. In one study, these three foods accounted for roughly 81 percent of all cases of childhood eczema. For more information on dealing with food allergies, see **food allergy**.

Conventional Drugs

- *Antihistamines:* astemizole (Hismanal); azatadine maleate/pseudoephedrine sulfate (Trinalin Repetabs); azelastine (Astelin); diphenhydramine (Benadryl); hydroxyzine (Atarax, Vistaril); fexofenadine (Allegra); loratadine (Claritin); terfenadine (Seldane)
- *Corticosteroids for oral or topical use:* betamethasone (Alphatrex, Beben, Betaderm, Betatrex, Beta-Val, Betnovate, Celestoderm, Celestone, Dermabet, Diprolene, Ectosone, Maxivate, Metaderm, Prevex B, Teladar, Topilene, Topisone, Uticort, Valisone, Valnac); clobetasol (Dermovate, Temovate); desonide (DesOwen, Tridesilon); dexamethasone (Aeroseb-Dex, Decaderm, Decadron); diflorasone (Florone, Maxiflor); fluocinolone (Bio-Syn, Fluocet, Fluoderm, Fluolar, Fluonid, Fluonide, Flurosyn, Synalar, Synamol, Synemol); fluocinonide (Fluocin, Licon, Lidemol, Lidex, Lyderm, Topsyn); flurandrenolide (Cordran,

Drenison); halcinonide (Halog); hydrocortisone
(Acticort, Aeroseb-HC, Ala-Cort, Allercort, Alpha-
derm, Bactine, Cetacort, Cortacet, Cortaid,
Cortate, Cortef, Corticaine, Cortiment, Cortoderm,
Cortril, Delacort, Dermacort, DermiCort, Emo-
Cort, Hi-Cor, Hyderm, Hydro-Tex, Hytone, Lana-
cort, Locoid, MyCort, Nutracort, Penecort,
Pentacort, Prevex HC, Sential, Synacort, Texa-
cort, Unicort, Westcort); mometasone (Elocom,
Elocon); prednisone (Apo-Prednisone, Deltasone,
Liquid Pred, Meticorten, Orasone, Prednicen,
Sterapred, Winpred); triamcinolone (Aristocort,
Flutex, Kenac, Kenalog, Kenonel, Oracort,
Oralone, Triacet, Trianide, Triderm)

Natural Medicines

**Fish oils (eicosapentaenoic acid and
docosahexaenoic acid)**
Effectiveness: B   Safety: A

Gamma-linolenic acid
Effectiveness: B–   Safety: A

Glycyrrhetinic acid (topical use)
Effectiveness: B   Safety: A

Quercetin
Effectiveness: C   Safety: B

Witch hazel (Hamamelis virginiana) (topical use)
Effectiveness: B+   Safety: A

Zinc
Effectiveness: C   Safety: B

Commentary

It is also important to avoid rough-textured clothing
wash clothing with mild soaps only and rinse thor
oughly; and avoid exposure to chemical irritants and
any other agents that might cause skin irritation.

FIBROCYSTIC BREAST DISEASE

Definition

Fibrocystic breast disease (FBD), also known as cys
tic mastitis, is a benign breast condition associated
with the presence of multiple cysts in the breast tis
sue. FBD is usually a component of premenstrual
syndrome (PMS) and is considered a risk factor for
breast cancer. It is not, however, as significant a fac
tor as the classic breast cancer risk factors: family
history, early onset of menstruation (menarche), and
late or no first pregnancy.

Signs and Symptoms

FBD is characterized by the presence of multiple cyst
of varying sizes, giving the breast a nodular consis
tency. FBD tends to worsen premenstrually and may
be associated with breast pain and tenderness.

Causes

FBD is apparently the result of an increased estrogen
to-progesterone ratio. However, other hormones are

also important. For example, the changes within the breast in FBD may be due to the hormone prolactin. Typically, significantly elevated levels of prolactin are found in women with FBD—the levels are higher than normal, but not so high as to cause loss of menstruation (amenorrhea). The increase in prolactin is thought to be the result of higher estrogen levels.

Dietary Factors

The diet should emphasize whole, unprocessed foods: whole grains, legumes, vegetables, fruits, nuts, and seeds. Drink at least 48 fluid ounces of water daily. These recommendations can help promote regular bowel movements. Women who have fewer than three bowel movements per week have a 4.5 times greater rate of FBD than women who have at least one bowel movement a day. This association is probably due to the bacterial flora in the large intestine transforming excreted steroids into toxic derivatives or allowing these excreted steroids to be reabsorbed (see **calcium D-glucarate** for more information).

Eliminate caffeine. Population studies, experimental evidence, and clinical evaluations indicate a strong association between caffeine consumption and FBD. In one study, limiting sources of coffee, tea, cola, chocolate, and caffeinated medications resulted in improvement in 97.5 percent of the 45 women who completely abstained and in 75 percent of the 28 who limited their consumption.

Conventional Drugs

- Danazol (Danocrine)

Natural Medicines

Vitamin E
Effectiveness: B   Safety: A

Commentary

It is important to consult a physician immediately if you notice a lump of any kind. Although pain, cyclic variations in size, high mobility, and multiplicity of nodules are indicative of FBD, further steps are usually necessary to rule out breast cancer. Noninvasive procedures, such as ultrasound, can help to aid differentiation further, but at this time definitive diagnosis depends upon biopsy. It is better to be safe than sorry, as the effective treatment for most types of breast cancer is dependent upon early diagnosis.

FIBROMYALGIA

Definition

Fibromyalgia is a recently recognized disorder that is regarded as a common cause of chronic musculoskeletal pain and fatigue.

Signs and Symptoms

Fibromyalgia is characterized by generalized aches or stiffness of at least three anatomical sites for at least three months and six or more typical, reproducible tender points. It is also associated with fatigue; chronic headache; sleep disturbance; depression; numbing or tingling sensations in the extremities; irritable bowel syndrome; and variation of symptoms in relation to activity, stress, and weather changes (i.e., symptoms tend to get worse with increased activity, stress, and cold weather).

Causes

The cause of fibromyalgia is unknown. The primary treatment goals in fibromyalgia are to raise serotonin levels, improve sleep quality, and ensure adequate magnesium levels.

Dietary Factors

Eliminate or restrict intake of refined sugar (see **hypoglycemia**) and food allergies (see **food allergy**). Increase the dietary intake of magnesium. The best food sources of magnesium are legumes, tofu, seeds, nuts, whole grains, and green leafy vegetables. Fish, meat, milk, and most commonly eaten fruits are low in magnesium. Most Americans consume a low-magnesium diet because their diet is high in refined foods, meat, and dairy products.

Conventional Drugs

Most often used are antidepressants in low dosages. See **depression** for list.

Natural Medicines

Capsaicin (topical use)
Effectiveness: B+   Safety: C

Guaifenesin
Effectiveness: D   Safety: C

Hydroxytryptophan (5-HTP)
Effectiveness: A   Safety: D

Magnesium
Effectiveness: B+   Safety: A

S-adenosylmethionine (SAMe)
Effectiveness: A   Safety: A

Commentary

One of the key findings in patients with fibromyalgia is an altered sleep pattern—presumably as a result of the low serotonin levels. The main problem is that the deeper levels of sleep (stages 3 and 4) are not achieved for long enough periods. As a result, people with fibromyalgia wake up feeling tired, worn out, and in pain. The severity of the pain of fibromyalgia correlates with the rating of sleep quality; when patients with fibromyalgia get a good night's sleep, they have less pain.

FOOD ALLERGY

Definition

A food allergy or sensitivity occurs when there is an adverse reaction to the ingestion of a food. The allergic reaction may or may not involve the immune system. The allergic reaction may be caused by a protein, starch, or other food component, or by food additives (e.g., colorings, flavoring agents, or preservatives).

Signs and Symptoms

Food allergies are associated with a multitude of symptoms and health conditions.

* *Gastrointestinal:* canker sores, celiac disease, chronic diarrhea, duodenal ulcer, gastritis, irritable bowel syndrome, malabsorption, ulcerative colitis
* *Genitourinary:* bed-wetting, chronic bladder infections, nephrosis
* *Immune:* chronic infections, frequent ear infections
* *Mental/emotional:* anxiety, depression, hyperactivity, inability to concentrate, insomnia, irritability, mental confusion, personality change, seizures
* *Musculoskeletal:* bursitis, joint pain, low back pain
* *Respiratory:* asthma, chronic bronchitis, wheezing
* *Skin:* acne, eczema, hives, itching, skin rash
* *Miscellaneous:* arrhythmia, edema, fainting, fatigue, headache, hypoglycemia, itchy nose or throat, migraines, sinusitis

Causes

Food allergy is often inherited. When both parents have allergies, there is a 67 percent chance that the children will also have allergies. Where only one parent is allergic, the chance of a child being prone to allergies drops to 33 percent.

Repetitious exposure to a food, improper digestion, and poor integrity of the intestinal barrier are additional factors that can lead to the development and maintenance of food allergy.

A classic food allergy occurs when an ingested food molecule acts as an antigen—a foreign substance that triggers the release of an antibody (immunoglobulin E), by white blood cells. When the IgE and food antigen bind to specialized cells known as mast cells, it causes the release of histamine and other allergic compounds, leading to swelling and inflammation.

Dietary Factors

An allergy elimination diet is valuable in identifying food allergies. In an allergy elimination diet, many commonly eaten foods are eliminated and replaced with either hypoallergenic foods or special hypoallergenic formulas. The fewer the allergenic foods eaten, the greater the ease of establishing a diagnosis. The standard elimination diet consists of lamb, chicken, potatoes, rice, bananas, apples, and a cabbage-family vegetable (cabbage, Brussels sprouts, broccoli, etc.). Variations of this diet may be suitable; the key point is that no allergenic foods are consumed.

The individual stays on the elimination diet for at least one week and up to one month. If the symptoms are related to food sensitivity, they will typically disappear by the fifth or sixth day of the diet. If the symptoms do not disappear, it is possible that a reaction to a food in the elimination diet is responsible. In that case, an even more restricted diet must be utilized.

After the elimination-diet period, individual foods are reintroduced every two days. Methods range from reintroducing only a single food every two days to reintroducing a food every one or two meals. Usually after the one-week cleansing period the patient will develop an increased sensitivity to offending foods.

Reintroduction of allergenic foods will typically

produce a more severe or recognizable symptom
than before. A careful, detailed record must be kept
describing when foods were reintroduced and what
symptoms appeared upon reintroduction. It can be
very useful to track the pulse during reintroduction,
as pulse changes may occur when an allergenic
food is consumed.

Conventional Drugs

- Promethazine (Anergan, Histantil, Pentazine,
  Phenazine, Phencen, Phenergan, Phenerzine,
  Phenoject, Promacot, Promet, Prorex, Shogan,
  V-Gan); cromolyn sodium (Gastrocrom)

Natural Medicines

Pancreatin
Effectiveness: B   Safety: A

Quercetin
Effectiveness: C   Safety: B

Commentary

Do not rely on the skin-prick test or skin-scratch test
commonly employed by many allergists to determine food allergies. Skin-prick tests test solely for
IgE-mediated allergies. Since only about 10 to 15
percent of all food allergies are mediated by IgE,
skin-prick tests are of little value in diagnosing most
food allergies. If you don't want to do an elimination
diet, most nutritionally oriented physicians now employ blood tests to diagnose food allergies. The best
laboratory test appears to be the ELISA (enzyme-
linked immunosorbent assay).

GALLSTONES

Definition

Gallstones are round or oval, smooth or faceted lumps of solid matter found in the gallbladder, the sac under the liver where bile is stored and concentrated.

Signs and Symptoms

Gallstones may be without symptoms or may be associated with periods of intense pain in the abdomen that radiates to the upper back. Symptoms begin only when a gallstone gets stuck in the duct leading from the gallbladder to the intestine. An ultrasound exam provides definitive diagnosis of gallstones.

Causes

Gallstones arise when there is an imbalance among the bile components. Bile is composed of bile salts, bilirubin, cholesterol, phospholipids, fatty acids, water, electrolytes, and other substances. The most common stones are mixed, containing cholesterol and inorganic salts of calcium.

A low-fiber diet is one of the main causes of gallstones. Such a diet, which is typically high in refined carbohydrates and fat and low in fiber, leads to a reduction in the synthesis of bile acids by the liver, which in turn significantly reduces the solubility of the bile. A high intake of refined sugar is also a risk factor for gallstones.

The frequency of gallstones is two to four times greater in women than in men. Women are predisposed to gallstones because of either increased cholesterol synthesis or suppression of bile acids by estrogens. Pregnancy, use of oral contraceptives, or other causes of elevated estrogen levels greatly increase the incidence of gallstones. Obesity is also associated with a significant increase in risk.

Dietary Factors

For prevention and treatment of gallstones, increase intake of vegetables, fruits, and dietary fiber, especially the gel-forming or mucilaginous fibers (oat bran, guar gum, pectin, etc.); reduce consumption of saturated fats, cholesterol, sugar, and animal proteins; avoid all fried foods; and drink at least six 8-fluid-ounce glasses of water each day to maintain the proper water content of the bile.

Food allergies have long been known to trigger gallbladder attacks. A 1968 study revealed that 100 percent of a group of patients with gallstones were free from symptoms while they were on a basic elimination diet (consisting of beef, rye, soybeans, rice, cherries, peaches, apricots, beets, and spinach). Foods that induced symptoms of gallstones, in decreasing order of their occurrence, were eggs, pork, onions, poultry, milk, coffee, citrus, corn, beans, and nuts. Adding eggs to the diet caused gallbladder attacks in 93 percent of the patients.

A vegetarian diet has been shown to be protective against gallstone formation. While this may simply be a result of the increased fiber content of the vegetarian diet, other factors may be equally important. Animal proteins, such as casein from dairy products, have been shown to increase the formation of gallstones in animals, while vegetable proteins, such as soy, were shown to be preventive against gallstone formation.

Coffee (both regular and decaffeinated) induces gallbladder contractions, so if you have gallstones, avoid coffee until the stones are resolved.

Conventional Drugs

• Ursodiol (Actigall, Urso)

Natural Medicines

Milk thistle (Silybum marianum)
Effectiveness: B   Safety: A

Commentary

A commercial product, Rowachol, that contains a natural terpene combination (menthol, menthone, pinene, borneol, cineole, and camphene) has demonstrated an ability to dissolve gallstones in several studies. Rowachol is not available in the United States at this time. However, as menthol is the major component of this formula, enteric-coated peppermint oil may offer similar benefits. The dosage is 1 to 2 capsules (0.2 ml/capsule) three times per day between meals. Although terpenes are effective alone, the best results appear to be achieved when used in combination with usodiol (available only by prescription).

GLAUCOMA

Definition

Glaucoma is increased pressure within the eye (intraocular pressure), which results from greater production than outflow of the fluid of the eye (the aqueous humor). The normal intraocular pressure (IOP) is about 10 to 21 mm Hg. In chronic glaucoma, the IOP is usually mildly to moderately elevated (22 to 40 mm Hg). In acute glaucoma, the IOP is greater than 40 mm Hg.

Signs and Symptoms

Since patients in the early stages of chronic glaucoma rarely have symptoms, it is important that regular eye exams be included in their annual checkup after the age of sixty. Chronic glaucoma can mean the gradual loss of peripheral vision, eventually resulting in tunnel vision.

Signs and symptoms of acute glaucoma include extreme pain, blurring of vision, reddened eyes, and a fixed and dilated pupil. Acute glaucoma is a medical emergency. If you are showing any signs of glaucoma, consult an ophthalmologist immediately. Unless acute glaucoma is adequately treated within twelve to forty-eight hours, it results in permanent blindness within two to five days.

Causes

The cause of glaucoma appears to be an abnormality in the composition of the supportive structures of the eye. Specifically, structural changes reflecting poor collagen integrity and function are the hallmarks of glaucoma. These changes lead to blockage in the flow of the aqueous humor and result in elevated IOP readings.

Dietary Factors

For chronic glaucoma, a generally healthful diet is recommended, with a focus on foods high in vitamin C and flavonoids, such as fresh fruits and vegetables. In addition, regular consumption of cold-water fish (e.g., salmon, mackerel, herring, and halibut) is also encouraged due to their high content of omega-3 fatty acids. Animal studies have shown that an increased consumption of omega-3 fatty acids can lower IOP.

Chronic glaucoma has been successfully treated by eliminating allergies. In one study, an immediate rise in IOP of up to 20 mm Hg was noted in some people when exposed to a food or airborne allergen. To treat glaucoma by eliminating food allergens, follow the guidelines given in **food allergies**.

Conventional Drugs

- *Beta-adrenergic blocking agents:* timolol maleate (Blocadren, Timoptic)
- *Carbonic anhydrase inhibitors:* acetazolamide (Diamox); dichlorphenamide (Daranide); methazolamide (GlaucTabs, Mzm, Neptazane)
- *Miotics:* apraclonidine (Lopidine); betaxolol (Betoptic, Kerlone); brimonidine tartrate (Alphagan); brinzolamide (Azopt); carbachol (Isopto Carbachol, Miostat); dorzolamide (Trusopt); ephinephryl borate (Epinal); metipranolol (Op-

tipranolol); latanoprost (Xalatan); physostigmine salicylate (Antilirium)
- *Mydriatics:* dipivefrin (Akpro, Propine)

Natural Medicines

Bilberry **(Vaccinium myrtillus)**
Effectiveness: B   Safety: A

Ginkgo biloba
Effectiveness: B   Safety: A

Magnesium
Effectiveness: B   Safety: A

Vitamin C
Effectiveness: B   Safety: A

Commentary

Corticosteroid drugs such as prednisone, used in severe allergic and inflammatory conditions, weaken
collagen structures throughout the body, including
the eye. Use of corticosteroid drugs is a major risk
for glaucoma. The individual with glaucoma should
do everything possible to avoid corticosteroid
drugs. If you must take corticosteroids, it is advis-
able to supplement with vitamin C and flavonoids to
support collagen integrity.

GOUT

Definition

Gout is a common type of arthritis caused by an increased concentration of uric acid (the final breakdown product of purine, one of the units of DNA and RNA) in biological fluids. In gout, uric acid crystals are deposited in joints, tendons, kidneys, and other tissues, where they cause considerable inflammation and damage. Gout may lead to debilitation from the uric acid deposits around the joints and tendons, and kidney involvement may result in kidney failure.

Signs and Symptoms

The first attack of gout is characterized by intense pain, usually involving only one joint. The first joint of the big toe is affected in nearly half of first attacks, and is at some time involved in over 90 percent of individuals with gout. If the attack progresses, fever and chills will appear. First attacks usually occur at night and are usually triggered by a specific event, such as dietary excess, alcohol ingestion, trauma, certain drugs (mainly chemotherapy drugs, certain diuretics, and high dosages of niacin), or surgery.

Causes

Gout is the result of either increased synthesis of uric acid, reduced ability to excrete uric acid, or both. Several dietary factors are known to trigger gout, including consumption of alcohol, high-purine-content foods (such as organ meats, meat, yeast, and poultry), fats, refined carbohydrates, and excessive calories.

Dietary Factors

Alcohol increases uric acid production by accelerating purine breakdown. It also reduces uric acid excretion by increasing lactate production, which impairs kidney function. Elimination of alcohol is all that is needed to reduce uric acid levels and prevent gouty arthritis in many individuals.

A low-purine diet has long been the mainstay of dietary therapy for gout. Foods with high purine levels should be entirely omitted. These include organ meats, meats, shellfish, yeast (brewer's and baker's), herring, sardines, mackerel, and anchovies. Intake of foods with moderate levels of purine should be reduced as well. These include legumes, spinach, asparagus, fish, poultry, and mushrooms.

Obesity is associated with an increased rate of gout. Weight reduction in obese individuals significantly reduces serum uric acid levels. Weight reduction should involve the use of a high-fiber, low-fat diet, as this type of diet will help manage the elevated cholesterol and triglyceride levels that are also common with obesity.

Refined carbohydrates, fructose, and saturated fat intake should be kept to a minimum. Simple sugars (refined sugar, honey, maple syrup, corn syrup, fructose, etc.) increase uric acid production, while saturated fats decrease uric acid excretion. The diet should focus on complex carbohydrates such as legumes, whole grains, and vegetables rather than on simple sugars.

Liberal fluid intake keeps the urine diluted and promotes the excretion of uric acid. Furthermore, dilution of the urine reduces the risk of kidney stones. Drink at least 48 fluid ounces of water each day.

Conventional Drugs

- Colchicine
- *Nonsteroidal anti-inflammatory drugs:* indomethacin (Indocin); naproxen sodium (Aleve, Anaprox, Naprelan)
- *Purine inhibitors:* allopurinol (Zyloprim)
- *Uricosuric agents:* probenecid (Benemid); probenecid/colchicine (ColBenemid)

Natural Medicines

Devil's claw (Harpagophytum procumbens)
Effectiveness: B   Safety: C

Folic acid
Effectiveness: B   Safety: A

Quercetin
Effectiveness: C   Safety: C

Procyanidolic oligomers
Effectiveness: C   Safety: C

Commentary

The pain of an acute attack of gout is absolutely excruciating. In this situation heroic measures are clearly appropriate. The standard medical treatment for acute gout is administration of colchicine, an anti-inflammatory drug. Colchicine has no effect on uric acid levels, but it does stop the inflammatory process. Studies indicate that over 75 percent of patients with gout show major improvement in symptoms within the first twelve hours after receiving colchicine. Long-term treatment of gout with colchicine, however, is not appropriate, as colchicine can cause serious side effects such as bone marrow depression, hair loss, liver damage, depression, seizures, respiratory depression, and even death. Fortunately, most cases of gout can be adequately controlled with diet alone.

HAY FEVER

Definition

Hay fever is characterized by a watery nasal discharge, sneezing, and itchy eyes and nose. It is usually associated with a particular season because of pollen or another allergen. As hay fever and asthma share similar causes and mechanisms as well as natural medicine treatments, see **asthma** for more information.

Conventional Drugs

- *Antihistamines:* acrivastine/pseudoephedrine (Semprex-D); astemizole (Hismanal); azatadine maleate/pseudoephedrine sulfate (Trinalin Repetabs); azelastine (Astelin); brompheniramine maleate/phenylpropanolamine (Dimetapp); brompheniramine maleate/pseudoephedrine (Bromfed); cetirizine (Zyrtec); chlorpheniramine maleate/phenylephrine (Novahistine Elixir, Ryna Liquid); chlorpheniramine maleate/phenylpropanolamine (Ornade Spansule); chlorpheniramine maleate/methscopalomine nitrate/ phenylephrine (Extendryl); cyproheptadine (Periactin); diphenhydramine

(Benadryl); hydroxyzine (Atarax); hydroxyzine
pamoate (Vistaril); fexofenadine (Allegra);
loratadine (Claritin); phenindamine tartrate
(Nolahist); pseudoephedrine/chlorpheniramine
(Codimal, Chlor-Trimeton); pseudoephedrine/
triprolidine (Actifed); terfenadine (Seldane)

- *Antihistamines for intranasal application:* azelastine (Astelin); pseudoephedrine sulfate (Afrin)
- *Nasal allergy preparations:* beclomethasone
dipropionate (Beconase, Vancenase); budes-
onide (Rhinocort); cromolyn sodium (Crolom,
Gastrocrom, Intal, Nasalcrom, Opticrom); flunisolide (Aerobid, Nasarel); fluticasone pro-
pionate (Flonase, Flovent); triamcinolone
acetonide (Nasacort)

HEADACHE (TENSION TYPE)

Definition

The two most common types of headache are tension headaches and migraine headaches. Tension
headaches usually have a steady, constant, dull
pain, while migraine headaches are characterized by
a throbbing or pounding sharp pain (see **migraine**).

Signs and Symptoms

Tension headaches are characterized by a steady,
constant, dull pain that starts at the back of the head
or in the forehead and spreads over the entire head,

giving the sensation of pressure or a feeling that a
vise grip has been applied to the skull.

Cause

A tension headache is usually caused by tightening
in the muscles of the face, neck, or scalp as a result
of stress or poor posture. These tight muscles pinch
the nerve or its blood supply, creating the sensation
of pain and pressure. Relaxation of the muscle usually brings about immediate relief. Often a tension
headache can be worsened (or improved) by applying hand pressure to trigger points on the neck muscles. A trigger point is the central area of tension in
the muscle.

Conventional Drugs

- Aspirin (Ascriptin Enteric, Bayer, Bufferin,
  Ecotrin); aspirin/caffeine/acetaminophen (Ex-
  cedrin); acetaminophen (Panadol, Tylenol);
  ibuprofen (Advil, Motrin, Nuprin); ketoprofen
  (Actron, Orudis)

Natural Medicines

Please see **migraine**, as the recommendations
there are also appropriate for tension headache.

Menthol (topical use)
Effectiveness: B+   Safety: A

Commentary

Since tension headaches are primarily a mechanical
event, it is important to address any structural problem. They often respond to physical treatments,

such as massage, chiropractic, and other forms of bodywork. Learning how to relax the muscles with progressive relaxation exercises or other techniques has been shown in clinical studies to provide exceptional benefits without side effects.

HEART DISEASE

Definition

The general term "heart disease" is most often used to describe atherosclerosis (hardening of the artery walls due to a buildup of plaque, which contains cholesterol, fatty material, and cellular debris) of the blood vessels that supply the heart—the coronary arteries. For other specific diseases, see **angina, arrhytmia, congestive heart failure,** and **mitral valve prolapse.**

HEMORRHOIDS

Definition

Hemorrhoids are enlarged or painful varicose veins in the anal/rectal area.

Signs and Symptoms

The symptoms most often associated with hemorrhoids include itching, burning, pain, inflammation, irritation, swelling, bleeding, and seepage. Pain is usually worse with defecation. A person with hemorrhoids may also notice bright red bleeding on the surface of the stool, on the toilet tissue, and/or in the toilet bowl.

Causes

The causes of hemorrhoids are similar to the causes of varicose veins (see **varicose veins**). Because the venous system that supplies the rectal area contains no valves, factors that increase venous congestion in the region can lead to hemorrhoid formation. These factors include increased intra-abdominal pressure (caused by defecation, pregnancy, coughing, sneezing, vomiting, physical exertion, or cirrhosis of the liver), an increase in straining during defecation due to a low-fiber diet, diarrhea, and standing or sitting for prolonged periods of time.

Dietary Factors

A low-fiber diet, high in refined foods, contributes greatly to the development of hemorrhoids. Individuals who consume a low-fiber diet tend to strain more during bowel movements since their smaller, harder stools are more difficult to pass. This straining raises the pressure in the abdomen, which obstructs venous blood flow, increases pelvic congestion, and may significantly weaken the veins, causing hemorrhoids to form.

A high-fiber diet is perhaps the most important component in the prevention of hemorrhoids. A diet rich in vegetables, fruits, legumes, and grains promotes peristalsis, the normal rhythmic contractions of the intestines. Furthermore, many fiber components attract water and form a gelatinous mass that keeps the feces soft, bulky, and easy to pass. The net

effect of a high-fiber diet is significantly less straining during defecation.

The diet should also contain liberal amounts of
flavonoid-rich foods, such as blackberries, citrus
fruits, cherries, and blueberries, to strengthen vein
structures.

Conventional Drugs

- *Corticosteroids:* hydrocortisone acetate (Anu-
  cort-HC, Anumed-HC, Anusol-HC, Hemril-HC,
  Proctocort, Proctosol-HC, Rectosol-HC)
- *Hemorrhoidal preparations:* phenylephrine/
  shark liver oil/glycerin (Preparation H); phenyle-
  phrine/pramoxine (Hemorid); pramoxine/zinc
  oxide (Anusol)
- *Local anesthetics:* benzocaine (Americaine);
  dibucaine (Nupercainal); pramoxine (Pramagel,
  Prax, Tronolane, Tronothane); tetracaine (Ponto-
  caine)

Natural Medicines

Aortic glycosaminoglycans
Effectiveness: A   Safety: A

Bilberry (Vaccinium myrtillus)
Effectiveness: B+   Safety: A

Butcher's broom (Ruscus aculeatus)
Effectiveness: A   Safety: B

Citrus bioflavonoids
Effectiveness: A   Safety: A

Fiber
Effectiveness: A   Safety: A

Gotu kola **(Centella asiatica)**
Effectiveness: B+   Safety: B+

Horse chestnut **(Aesculus hippocastanum)**
Effectiveness: A   Safety: C

Procyanidolic oligomers
Effectiveness: A   Safety: A

Commentary

Another useful treatment for temporary relief of hemorrhoids is the warm sitz bath—a partial-immersion bath of the pelvic region. The temperature of the water should be between 100 and 105° F.

HEPATITIS

Definition

Hepatitis is an inflammation of the liver. Hepatitis can be caused by many drugs and toxic chemicals, but in most instances it is caused by a virus.

Signs and Symptoms

A loss of appetite, nausea, vomiting, fatigue, and flulike symptoms can occur two weeks to one month before liver involvement, depending on the incubation period of the virus. Once the liver is involved, a person with hepatitis shows a tender and enlarged liver, fever, jaundice (yellow appearance of the skin), and markedly elevated liver enzymes (aminotransaminases) and bilirubin levels in the blood.

Acute viral hepatitis can be an extremely debilitating disease requiring bed rest. It can take anywhere from two to sixteen weeks to recover. Most patients recover completely (usually by nine weeks for type A and sixteen weeks for types B, C, D, and G). However, about one out of one hundred will die, and 10 percent of hepatitis B and 10 to 40 percent of hepatitis C cases develop into chronic viral hepatitis (hepatitis C contracted from a transfusion is associated with a 70 to 80 percent chance of developing chronic hepatitis). The symptoms of chronic hepatitis vary. The symptoms may be virtually nonexistent or they may include chronic fatigue, serious liver damage, and even death due to cirrhosis of the liver or liver cancer.

Causes

Hepatitis can be caused by many drugs and toxic chemicals, but in most instances it is caused by a virus. Viral types A, B, and C are the most common. Hepatitis A occurs sporadically or in epidemics and is transmitted primarily through fecal contamination. Hepatitis B is transmitted through infected blood or blood products as well as through sexual contact (the virus is shed in saliva, semen, and vaginal secretions). Hepatitis C (formerly known as hepatitis non-A, non-B) historically has a primary route of transmission through blood transfusion (blood supplies are now screened for the presence of hepatitis C virus) but is now transmitted via the same factors as hepatitis B. Other viral causes of hepatitis include hepatitis viruses D, E, and G, as well as herpes simplex, cytomegalovirus, and Epstein-Barr virus.

Dietary Factors

During the acute phase, the focus should be on replacing fluids through consumption of vegetable broths, diluted vegetable juices (diluted by half with water), and herbal teas. Solid foods should be restricted to brown rice, steamed vegetables, and moderate intake of lean protein sources.

In chronic cases, a general healthful diet should be followed. The diet should be low in saturated fats, simple carbohydrates (sugar, white flour, fruit juice, honey, etc.), oxidized fatty acids (fried foods), and animal products to help aid the liver's detoxification mechanisms. A diet that focuses on plant foods has been shown to increase the elimination of bile acids, drugs, and toxic bile substances from the system.

Conventional Drugs

- *Bile salts:* ursodiol (Actigall, Urso)
- *Immune-modifying drugs:* interferon-beta-1a (Avonex); interferon-beta-1b (Betaseron); interferon-alpha-2a (Roferon); interferon-alpha-2b (Intron).
- Prednisone (Apo-Prednisone, Deltasone, Liquid Pred, Meticorten, Orasone, Prednicen, Sterapred, Winpred)

Natural Medicines

Lemon balm (Melissa officinalis) *(topical use)*
Effectiveness: B+   Safety: A

Licorice (Glycyrrhiza glabra)
Effectiveness: B+   Safety: C

Liver extracts
Effectiveness: B   Safety: C

Milk thistle (Silybum marianum)
Effectiveness: B+   Safety: A

Reishi (Ganoderma lucidum)
Effectiveness: B   Safety: C

Thymus extracts
Effectiveness: B+   Safety: B

Vitamin C
Effectiveness: B   Safety: A

Commentary

In chronic hepatitis, effective treatment is essential due to the increased risk of liver cancer and cirrhosis. Talk to your doctor about using the drug alpha-interferon. It has side effects and is not perfect, but it has been shown to be helpful in improving chronic hepatitis. It can be used in conjunction with the natural products listed above.

HERPES

Definition

Herpes simplex is a virus that is responsible for cold sores and genital herpes. There are two types of herpes simplex viruses: type 1 (HSV-1) is most often responsible for cold sores (also referred to as fever blisters), while type 2 (HSV-2) is responsible for nearly 90 percent of cases of genital herpes (the remaining 10 percent are caused by HSV-1).

Signs and Symptoms

In some people (mostly children) an initial HSV-1 infection may cause fever, painful swelling and open sores on the gums and inside the cheeks, or a painful, sore throat. When these herpes symptoms do develop, they usually begin two to twelve days after exposure to someone with HSV-1.

Symptoms of a first episode of HSV-2 usually appear within two to ten days of exposure to the virus and last an average of two to three weeks. Early symptoms can include an itching or burning sensation; pain in the legs, buttocks, or genital area; vaginal discharge; or a feeling of pressure in the abdominal region. Within a few days, sores (lesions) appear at the site of infection. Lesions also can occur on the cervix in women or in the urinary passage in men. These small red bumps may develop into blisters or painful open sores. Over a period of days, the sores become crusted and then heal without scarring. Other symptoms that may accompany a primary episode of genital herpes can include fever, headache, muscle aches, painful or difficult urination, vaginal discharge, and swollen glands in the groin area.

After the initial infection in the skin or mucous membranes, the virus travels to the sensory nerves at the end of the spinal cord and makes a home. In most people, the virus becomes dormant (inactive). In others, however, it can be reactivated by trauma or stress, and whenever the immune system fails to keep it in check. When the virus becomes reactivated, it travels along the nerves to the skin, where it multiplies on the surface at or near the site of the original herpes sores, causing new sores to erupt. It also can reactivate without causing any visible sores.

Causes

Herpes is caused by an infection with the herpes simplex virus and is spread via direct contact with infected lesions.

Dietary Factors

A diet high in the amino acid lysine and low in arginine can be an effective measure in preventing HSV infections, especially if used in conjunction with lysine supplementation. This dietary approach arose from research showing that lysine exerts antiviral activity in vitro by blocking arginine. HSV replication requires the manufacture of proteins rich in arginine, and arginine itself has been suggested as a stimulator of HSV replication. From a theoretical perspective, this approach should be effective, since studies have shown that HSV replication is dependent on adequate levels of arginine and low levels of lysine. Foods high in arginine are chocolate, peanuts, seeds, and almonds and other nuts. Foods high in lysine include most vegetables, legumes, fish, turkey, and chicken.

Conventional Drugs

- *Oral antiviral agents:* acyclovir (Zovirax); famciclovir (Famvir); foscarnet sodium (Foscavir); valacyclovir (Valtrex)
- *Topical antiviral agents:* acyclovir (Zovirax); penciclovir (Denavir)

Natural Medicines

Glycyrrhetinic acid (topical use)
Effectiveness: B   Safety: A

Lemon balm (topical use)
Effectiveness: B+   Safety: A

Lysine
Effectiveness: B+   Safety: B

Vitamin C
Effectiveness: B   Safety: A

Commentary

Enhancement of the immune status is key to the prevention and control of herpes infection, and recurrent herpes attacks are a clear sign that the immune system needs support. See **low immunity and immune support**.

HIGH BLOOD PRESSURE

Definition

High blood pressure is a major risk factor for a heart attack or stroke. The blood pressure reading measures the resistance produced each time the heart beats and sends blood coursing through the arteries. The peak reading of the pressure exerted by this contraction is the systolic pressure. Between beats the heart relaxes and blood pressure drops. The lowest reading is referred to as the diastolic pressure. A normal blood pressure reading for an adult is 130 (systolic)/85 (diastolic) mm Hg. High blood pressure is divided into different levels:

Borderline (130–139/85–89)
Stage I (140–159/90–99)

Stage II (160–179/100–109)
Stage III (180+/110+)

Signs and Symptoms

Borderline to moderate high blood pressure is generally without symptoms. Severe hypertension may be associated with increased sleepiness, confusion, headache, nausea, and vomiting.

Causes

Although medical textbooks state that the cause is unknown in 95 percent of cases, genetics definitely play a role, and high blood pressure is closely related to lifestyle and dietary factors. Important lifestyle factors include coffee consumption, alcohol intake, lack of exercise, stress, and smoking. Dietary factors include obesity; high sodium-to-potassium ratio; low-fiber, high-sugar diet; high intake of saturated fat and low intake of essential fatty acids; and a diet low in calcium, magnesium, and vitamin C.

Dietary Factors

Achieving ideal body weight is the most important recommendation for those with high blood pressure. However, overweight people who lose even modest amounts of weight experience a reduction in blood pressure.

Vegetarians generally have a lower incidence of high blood pressure and other cardiovascular diseases than nonvegetarians. While dietary levels of sodium do not differ significantly between these two groups, a vegetarian's diet typically contains more potassium, complex carbohydrates, essential fatty acids, fiber, calcium, magnesium, and vitamin C, and less saturated fat and refined carbohydrates, all of which have a favorable influence on blood pressure.

A diet high in sodium and low in potassium is associated with high blood pressure. Conversely, a diet high in potassium and low in sodium can lower blood pressure. Numerous studies have shown that sodium restriction alone does not improve blood pressure control in most people; it must be accompanied by a high potassium intake. Most Americans have a potassium-to-sodium ratio of less than 1:2, meaning they ingest more than twice as much sodium as potassium. By contrast, researchers recommend a dietary potassium-to-sodium ratio of greater than 5:1 to maintain health. The easiest way to lower sodium intake is to avoid prepared foods and table salt—use potassium chloride salt substitutes, such as the popular brands NoSalt and Nu-Salt, instead. The best way to boost potassium levels is to increase the intake of fruits, vegetables, whole grains, and legumes.

Conventional Drugs

- *ACE inhibitors:* benazepril (Lotensin); captopril (Capoten); captopril/hydrochlorothizaide (Capozide); enalapril maleate (Vasotec); fosinopril sodium (Monopril); lisinopril (Prinivil, Zestril); quinapril/magnesium carbonate (Accupril); ramipril (Altace); trandolapril (Mavik)
- *Alpha/beta-adrenergic blocking agents:* labetalol (Labetalol, Normodyne, Trandate)
- *Angiotensin receptor antagonists:* candesartan cilexetil (Atacand); eprosartan mesylate (Teveten); irbesartan (Avapro); losartan potassium (Cozaar); telmisartan (Micardis); valsartan (Diovan)

- *Beta-adrenergic blocking agents:* acebutolol (Acebutolol, Sectral); atenolol (Senormin, Tenormin); bisoprolol fumarate (Zebeta); carteolol (Cartrol, Ocupress); metoprolol succinate (Toprol-XL); metoprolol tartrate (Lopressor); nadolol (Corgard); penbutolol sulfate (Levatol); pindolol (Visken); propranolol (Betachron, Inderal, Pronol); timolol maleate (Blocadren, Timoptic)
- *Calcium channel blocking agents:* diltiazem (Cardizem CD, Cartia, Dilacor XR, Diltia XT, Tiazac); nifedipine (Adalat CC, Procardia XL); verapamil (Calan, Covera-HS, Isoptin, Verelan)
- *Hypotensives, miscellaneous:* nitroprusside sodium (Nipride, Nitropress)
- *Hypotensives, vasodilators:* hydralazine (Apresoline); prazosin (Minipress)
- *Loop diuretics:* bumetanide (Bumex); ethacrynic acid (Edecrin); furosemide (Furoside, Lasix, Uritol)
- *Potassium-sparing diuretics:* amiloride (Midamor); spironolactone (Aldactone); triamterene (Dyrenium)
- *Thiazide diuretics:* bendroflumethiazide (Naturetin); benzothiazide (Exna, Hydrex); chlorothiazide (Diuril); chlorthalidone (Hydone, Hygroton, Novo-Thalidone, Thalitone, Uridon); cyclothiazide (Anhydron); hydrochlorothiazide (Apo-Hydro, Diuchlor H, Esidrix, Hydro-chlor, HydroDIURIL, Neo-Codema, Novo-Hydrazide, Oretic, Urozide); hydroflumethiazide (Diucardin, Saluron); methyclothiazide (Aquatensen, Duretic, Enduron); metolazone (Diulo, Mykrox, Zaroxolyn); polythiazide (Renese); quinethazone (Hydromox); trichlormethiazide (Aquazide, Diurese, Metahydrin, Naqua, Trichlorex)

Natural Medicines

Calcium
Effectiveness: B+ Safety: A

Coenzyme Q$_{10}$ (CoQ$_{10}$)
Effectiveness: A Safety: A

Fish oils (eicosapentaenoic acid and docosahexaenoic acid)
Effectiveness: B+ Safety: A

Flaxseed oil
Effectiveness: B Safety: A

***Garlic* (Allium sativum)**
Effectiveness: A Safety: A

Hawthorn (*Crataegus *spp.)
Effectiveness: B+ Safety: A

Magnesium
Effectiveness: B Safety: A

***Olive leaf* (Olea europa)**
Effectiveness: B Safety: C

Potassium
Effectiveness: A Safety: A

Taurine
Effectiveness: B Safety: C

Vitamin C
Effectiveness: B+ Safety: A

Commentary

High blood pressure should not be taken lightly. By keeping your blood pressure in the normal range, you will not only lengthen your life but improve its quality as well. A healthy lifestyle goes a long way in lowering blood pressure. Be sure to get enough exercise. Also, relaxation techniques, such as deep breathing exercises, biofeedback, meditation, yoga, progressive muscle relaxation, and hypnosis, have all been shown to have some value in lowering blood pressure.

HIVES (URTICARIA)

Definition

Hives (urticaria) are an allergic reaction in the skin.

Signs and Symptoms

Hives are characterized by white or pink welts or large bumps surrounded with redness. These lesions are known as wheal and flare lesions and are caused primarily by the release of histamine in the skin. Hives tend to be quite itchy. About 50 percent of patients with chronic hives develop angioedema, a deeper, more serious form involving the tissue below the surface of the skin.

Causes

While the basic cause of hives involves the release of histamine from mast cells or basophils—white blood cells that play a key role in allergies—what actually triggers this release can be a variety of factors, such as physical contact or pressure (dermographism), heat (cholinergic urticaria or prickly heat rash), cold (cold urticaria), water (aquagenic urticaria), autoimmune reactions, allergies or sensitivities to drugs (especially antibiotics and aspirin), allergies or sensitivities to foods and food additives, and infectious organisms (e.g., hepatitis B, *Candida albicans,* and streptococcal bacteria).

Dietary Factors

Food allergy is a common cause of hives, especially in chronic cases. The foods that most commonly trigger hives are milk, eggs, chicken, cured meat, alcoholic beverages, cheese, chocolate, citrus fruits, shellfish, and nuts. Food additives that trigger hives include colorants (azo dyes), flavorings (salicylates), artificial sweeteners (aspartame), preservatives (benzoates, nitrites, sorbic acid), antioxidants (BHT, hydroxytoluene, sulfite, gallate), and emulsifiers/stabilizers (polysorbates, vegetable gums). Numerous clinical studies demonstrate that diets that are free of food allergies and/or food additives typically produce significant reductions in roughly 50 to 75 percent of people with chronic hives.

The best dietary recommendation appears to be an allergy elimination diet, or at the very least a diet that excludes all common food allergies and all food additives. The strictest allergy elimination diet allows only water, lamb, rice, pears, and vegetables. The individual stays on this limited diet for at least one week. If the hives are related to food allergy or food additives, they will typically disappear by the fifth or sixth day of the diet. After one week, individual foods are reintroduced at a rate of one new food every two days. Reintroduction of sensitive foods will typically produce a more severe or recognizable symptom than before.

Conventional Drugs

* *Antihistamines:* acrivastine/pseudoephedrine
  (Semprex-D); astemizole (Hismanal); azatadine
  maleate/pseudoephedrine sulfate (Trinalin
  Repetabs); azelastine (Astelin); brompheniramine maleate (Dimetapp); brompheniramine
  maleate/pseudoephedrine (Bromfed); cetirizine
  (Zyrtec); chlorpheniramine maleate/phenyle-
  phrine (Novahistine Elixir, Ryna Liquid); chlorpheniramine maleate/methscopalomine nitrate/
  phenylephrine (Extendryl); cyproheptadine
  (Periactin); diphenhydramine (Benadryl); hydroxyzine (Atarax); hydroxyzine pamoate
  (Vistaril); fexofenadine (Allegra); loratadine
  (Claritin); phenindamine tartrate (Nolahist);
  pseudoephedrine/chlorpheniramine (Codimal,
  Chlor-Trimeton); pseudoephedrine/triprolidine
  (Actifed); terfenadine (Seldane)

Natural Medicines

Quercetin
Effectiveness: C   Safety: B

Vitamin C
Effectiveness: B   Safety: A

Commentary

Psychological stress is often reported as a triggering
factor in patients with chronic hives. Stress may
play an important role by decreasing the effectiveness of immune system mechanisms that block allergies. In a small study of fifteen patients with
chronic hives, relaxation therapy and hypnosis were
shown to provide significant benefit. Patients were

given an audiotape and asked to use the relaxation techniques described on the tape at home. At a follow-up examination five to fourteen months after the initial session, six patients were free of hives and an additional seven reported improvement.

HYPOGLYCEMIA

Definition

Hypoglycemia is low blood sugar. Normally, the body maintains blood sugar levels within a narrow range through the coordinated effort of several glands and their hormones. If these control mechanisms are disrupted, hypoglycemia (low blood sugar) or diabetes (high blood sugar) may result.

Signs and Symptoms

Symptoms of hypoglycemia can range from mild to severe, including headache; depression, anxiety, irritability, and other psychological disturbances; blurred vision; excessive sweating; mental confusion; incoherent speech; bizarre behavior; and convulsions.

The standard methods of diagnosing hypoglycemia, as well as diabetes, involve the measurement of blood glucose levels. The normal fasting blood glucose level is between 70 and 105 mg/dl. A fasting blood glucose measurement greater than 140 mg/dl on two separate occasions is diagnostic of diabetes. At levels below 50 mg/dl, the diagnosis is fasting hypoglycemia.

Causes

Dietary carbohydrates play a central role in the cause, prevention, and treatment of hypoglycemia. Simple carbohydrates, or sugars, are quickly absorbed by the body, resulting in a rapid elevation in blood sugar level; this stimulates a corresponding excessive elevation in serum insulin levels, which can then lead to hypoglycemia.

Dietary Factors

All simple, processed, and concentrated carbohydrates must be avoided. Virtually all of the fiber, vitamin and trace mineral content has been removed from white sugar, white breads and pastries, and many breakfast cereals. When these refined carbohydrates are eaten, blood sugar levels rise quickly, producing a strain on blood sugar control. Eating foods high in simple sugars in any form—sucrose, honey, or maple syrup—can lead to hypoglycemia.

Conventional Drugs

No prescription drugs are available with FDA-approved labeling for this indication.

Natural Medicines

Chromium
Effectiveness: B   Safety: B

Commentary

Alcohol consumption severely stresses blood sugar control and is often a contributing factor to hypoglycemia. Alcohol induces reactive hypoglycemia by interfering with normal glucose utilization and increasing the secretion of insulin. The resultant drop in blood sugar produces a craving for food, particularly foods that quickly elevate blood sugar levels, as well as a craving for more alcohol. The increased sugar consumption aggravates the reactive hypoglycemia, particularly in the presence of more alcohol.

INSOMNIA

Definition

Insomnia is difficulty in achieving or maintaining normal sleep.

Signs and Symptoms

There are two basic forms of insomnia. In sleep-onset insomnia a person has a difficult time falling asleep. In sleep-maintenance insomnia a person suffers from frequent or early awakening.

Causes

The most common causes of insomnia are psychological: depression, anxiety, and tension. If psychological factors do not seem to be the cause, various foods, drinks, and medications may be responsible. There are numerous compounds in food and drink (most notably caffeine) that can interfere with normal sleep. There are also over three hundred drugs that interfere with normal sleep.

Dietary Factors

In dealing with insomnia, it is essential that the diet be free of stimulants such as caffeine and related compounds. Coffee, as well as less obvious caffeine sources such as soft drinks, chocolate, coffee-flavored ice cream, hot cocoa, and tea, must all be eliminated. Even small amounts of caffeine such as those found in decaffeinated coffee or chocolate may be enough to cause insomnia in some people.

Conventional Drugs

- *Antihistamines:* diphenhydramine (Sleepinal, Sominex)
- *Benzodiazepine drugs:* alprazolam (Xanax); buspirone (BuSpar); chlordiazepoxide (Librium); chlormezanone (Trancopal); chlorazepate dipotassium (Tranxene); diazepam (Valium); flurazepam (Dalmane); lorazepam (Ativan); meprobamate (Miltown); oxazepam (Serax); quazepam (Doral); temazepam (Restoril); triazolam (Halcion)
- *Barbiturates:* butabarbitol (Butisol); pentobarbital (Nembutal); phenobarbital; secobarbital (Seconal)
- *Sedative-hypnotics, nonbarbiturate:* doxylamine succinate (Nytol, Unisom); estazolam (Prosom); ethchloryvnol (Placidyl); zolpidem tartrate (Ambien)

Warning: If you have taken a prescription sleeping pill regularly for more than four weeks, do not stop taking the drug suddenly. It is important to work with your physician to taper off the drug gradually to avoid potentially dangerous withdrawal symptoms. Symptoms of withdrawal can include anxiety, irritability, panic, insomnia, nausea, headache, impaired concentration, memory loss, depression, extreme sensitivity to the environment, seizures, hallucinations, and paranoia.

Natural Medicines

Chamomile (Matricaria chamomilla)
Effectiveness: C   Safety: C

GABA (gamma-aminobutyric acid)
Effectiveness: C   Safety: C

Hydroxytryptophan (5-HTP)
Effectiveness: B+   Safety: D

Kava (Piper methysticum)
Effectiveness: B   Safety: C

Melatonin
Effectiveness: B+   Safety: A

Passionflower (Passiflora incarnata)
Effectiveness: C   Safety: C

Valerian (Valeriana officinalis)
Effectiveness: A   Safety: B

Commentary

Avoid over-the-counter and prescription pills. While effective in the short term, they can cause significant problems in the long term. Benzodiazepines and barbiturates are not designed to be used for the long term, as they are addictive, have numerous side effects, and cause abnormal sleep patterns. Antihistamines also interfere with normal sleep patterns. As a result, people who take sleeping pills enter a vicious cycle. They take the drug to induce sleep, but the drug causes further disruption of normal sleep. In the morning, in an attempt to get going, they will typically drink large quantities of coffee, which further worsens insomnia.

IRRITABLE BOWEL SYNDROME

Definition

Irritable bowel syndrome (IBS) is a functional disorder of the large intestine with no evidence of accompanying structural defect.

Signs and Symptoms

IBS is characterized by some combination of the following symptoms: abdominal pain or distension; altered bowel function, constipation, or diarrhea; hypersecretion of colonic mucus; dyspeptic symptoms (flatulence, nausea, anorexia); and varying degrees of anxiety or depression. If you have symptoms suggestive of IBS, please consult a physician for an accurate diagnosis.

Causes

There appear to be four main causes of IBS: stress, insufficient intake of dietary fiber, food allergies, and meals too high in sugar. Stress increases intestinal motility (the rhythmic contractions of the intestine that propel food through the digestive tract) and leads to abdominal pain and irregular bowel function.

Dietary Factors

Dietary fiber promotes proper colon function. Patients with constipation are much more likely to respond to dietary fiber than are those with diarrhea. Increasing intake of dietary fiber from fruit and vegetable sources rather than cereal sources may offer more benefit to some individuals.

Food allergy as a cause of IBS has been recognized since the early 1900s. More recent studies have shown the majority of patients with IBS (approximately two-thirds) have at least one food allergy, and some have multiple allergies. The most common allergens are dairy products (40 to 44 percent) and grains (40 to 60 percent). Many patients have noted marked clinical improvement when using elimination diets (see **food allergy** for further discussion).

Meals high in refined sugar can contribute to IBS by decreasing intestinal motility. When blood sugar levels rise too rapidly, the normal rhythmic contractions of the gastrointestinal tract slow down and in some portions stop altogether. A diet high in refined sugar may be the key factor that makes IBS far more common in the United States compared to other countries.

Conventional Drugs

- *Anticholinergics/antispasmodics:* dicyclomine (Antispas, Bentyl, Pasmin)
- *Belladonna alkaloids:* hyoscyamine (Cytospaz, Hyospaz); hyoscyamine sulfate (Anaspaz, Levbid, Levsin, Spacol, Spasdel)
- *Laxatives:* calcium polycarbophil (Equalactin, Fibercon, Konsyl Fiber, Mitrolan); psyllium (Metamucil)

Natural Medicines

Artichoke (Cynara scolymus)
Effectiveness: B   Safety: C

Chamomile (Matricaria chamomilla)
Effectiveness: C   Safety: C

Fiber
Effectiveness: A   Safety: A

Fructooligosaccharides
Effectiveness: F   Safety: A

Grapefruit seed extract
Effectiveness: B   Safety: C

Iberogast
Effectiveness: B+   Safety: C

Peppermint (Mentha piperita)
Effectiveness: A   Safety: B

Commentary

Clinical studies have documented that psychological approaches such as relaxation therapy, biofeedback, hypnosis, counseling, or stress management training significantly improve the symptoms of IBS. Many people with IBS find that daily leisurely walks markedly reduce symptoms, probably due to the well-known stress-reduction effects of exercise.

KIDNEY STONES

Definition

Kidney stones are lumps of solid matter usually composed of calcium oxalate, uric acid, or other crystals.

Signs and Symptoms

Kidney stones usually do not produce symptoms until a stone becomes dislodged. A dislodged stone can produce excruciating intermittent radiating pain originating in the flank or kidney; nausea, vomiting, and abdominal distension; and chills, fever, and urinary frequency.

Causes

Components in human urine normally remain in solution due to pH control and the secretion of inhibitors of crystal growth. However, when there is an increase in stone components or a decrease in protective factors, kidney stones can develop. The high frequency of calcium-containing stones in affluent societies is directly associated with the following dietary patterns: low intake of fiber, high intake of refined carbohydrates, high alcohol consumption, large amounts of animal protein, and high fat intake.

Dietary Factors

Increase intake of fiber, complex carbohydrates, and green leafy vegetables, and decrease intake of simple carbohydrates. Increase intake of high-magnesium-

to-calcium-ratio foods (barley, bran, corn, buck-
wheat, rye, soy, oats, brown rice, avocado, banana,
cashew, coconut, peanuts, sesame seeds, lima
beans, potato). If there are oxalate stones, reduce
oxalate-containing foods (e.g., black tea, cocoa,
spinach, rhubarb).

Vegetarians have a decreased risk of developing
stones. Studies have shown that, even among meat
eaters, those who ate higher amounts of fresh fruits
and vegetables had a lower incidence of stones. The
simple change from white to whole wheat bread can
result in a lowering of urinary calcium levels.

Sugar consumption contributes to kidney stones.
The ingestion of sucrose and other simple sugars
causes an exaggerated increase in the urinary calcium oxalate content in approximately 70 percent of
people with recurrent kidney stones.

Salt (sodium chloride) consumption contributes to
kidney stones by increasing calcium excretion.
People who tend to form kidney stones have an
even greater increase in urinary calcium with an increase in salt intake.

It is not necessary to restrict calcium intake, as calcium actually inhibits oxalate absorption, according
to recent studies. Calcium supplementation has also
been shown to significantly reduce oxalate absorption.

Conventional Drugs

- *Ammonia inhibitors:* acetohydroxamic acid (Litho-
  stat)
- *Antiurolithics:* cellulose sodium phosphate (Cal-
  cibind); tiopronin (Thiola)
- *Carbonic anhydrase inhibitors:* acetazolamide
  (Diamox)

- *Purine inhibitors:* allopurinol (Zyloprim)
- *Urinary pH alkalizers:* citric acid/sodium citrate (Bicitra, Oracit); potassium citrate (Urocit-K); potassium citrate/sodium citrate (Citrolith); tricitrates (Polycitra)

Natural Medicines

Cranberry (Vaccinium macrocarpon)
Effectiveness: B   Safety: A

Magnesium
Effectiveness: A   Safety: A

Vitamin B$_6$
Effectiveness: B+   Safety: A

Commentary

For prevention of kidney stones, increasing urine flow to dilute the urine is essential. A person with a history of kidney stones should consume enough fluid to produce a daily urinary volume of at least 2,000 ml (roughly 2 quarts).

LOW IMMUNITY AND IMMUNE SUPPORT

Definition

Immune support is often used to correct an underactive and/or poorly performing immune system. The immune system's prime function is to protect the body against infection and the development of cancer. Support and enhancement of the immune system is perhaps the most important step in achieving resistance to disease and reducing susceptibility to colds, the flu, and cancer. Supporting the immune system involves a health-promoting lifestyle, stress management, exercise, diet, and the appropriate use of nutritional supplements and herbal medicines.

Signs and Symptoms

If you answer yes to any of the following questions, it is a sign that your immune system may need support:

- Do you catch colds easily?
- Do you get more than two colds a year?
- Are you suffering from any chronic infection?
- Do you get frequent cold sores or have recurrent genital herpes?
- Are your lymph glands sore and swollen at times?
- Do you now have or have you ever had cancer?

Recurrent or chronic infections—even very mild colds—occur only when the immune system is weakened. Under such circumstances, there is a repetitive cycle that makes it difficult to overcome the tendency toward infection: A weakened immune system leads to infection, and infection causes damage to the immune system, which further weakens resistance. Enhancing the immune system can help to break the cycle.

Causes

The health of the immune system is greatly impacted by your emotional state, level of stress,

lifestyle, dietary habits, and nutritional status.
Nutrient deficiency is the most frequent cause of a
depressed immune system. An overwhelming number of clinical and experimental studies indicate that
deficiency in any single nutrient can profoundly impair the immune system.

Dietary Factors

Optimal immune function requires a healthy diet
that (1) is rich in whole, natural foods, such as fruits,
vegetables, grains, beans, seeds, and nuts, (2) is low
in fats and refined sugars, and (3) contains adequate
but not excessive amounts of protein.

   Dietary factors that depress immune function include nutrient deficiency, excessive consumption of
sugar, and consumption of allergenic foods.

Conventional Drugs

No prescription drugs are available with FDA-
approved labeling for this indication.

Natural Medicines

Aloe vera
Effectiveness: B   Safety: C

Astragalus membranaceus
Effectiveness: B   Safety: C

Beta-carotene
Effectiveness: B+   Safety: A

Cat's claw **(Uncaria tomentosa)**
Effectiveness: B   Safety: C

Cordyceps sinensis
Effectiveness: C   Safety: B

Echinacea
Effectiveness: B+   Safety: A

Garlic **(Allium sativum)**
Effectiveness: B   Safety: C

Ginseng **(Panax ginseng** *or* **P. quinquefolium)**
Effectiveness: B   Safety: C

Kombucha
Effectiveness: C   Safety: C

Kyolic
Effectiveness: B   Safety: C

Noni fruit **(Morinda citrifolia)**
Effectiveness: C   Safety: C

Propolis
Effectiveness: C   Safety: D

Selenium
Effectiveness: A   Safety: D

Shiitake **(Lentinus edodes)**
Effectiveness: B   Safety: C

Siberian ginseng **(Eleutherococcus senticosus)**
Effectiveness: B   Safety: C

Thymus extracts
Effectiveness: B+   Safety: A

Vitamin A
Effectiveness: B+   Safety: A

Vitamin C
Effectiveness: A   Safety: A

Vitamin E
Effectiveness: A   Safety: A

Zinc
Effectiveness: A   Safety: A

Commentary

A high-potency multiple vitamin and mineral formula is an important step in supporting the immune system, as it will address any underlying nutritional deficiencies.

MACULAR DEGENERATION

Definition

The macula is the area of the retina where images are focused. It is the portion of the eye responsible for fine vision. Age-related degeneration of the macula is the leading cause of severe visual loss in the United States in persons fifty-five years and older.

Signs and Symptoms

Individuals with macular degeneration may experience blurred vision. Also, straight objects may appear distorted or bent; there may be a dark spot near or around the center of the visual field; and while reading, parts of words may be missing. People with macular degeneration generally have good peripheral vision; they just can't see directly in front of them.

Causes

The major risk factors for macular degeneration are smoking, aging, atherosclerosis (hardening of the arteries), and high blood pressure. Apparently the degeneration is a result of free-radical damage, similar to the type of damage that induces cataracts. However, decreased blood and oxygen supply to the retina is the key factor leading to macular degeneration.

The two most common types of age-related macular degeneration (ARMD) are the atrophic (dry) form, by far the more frequent, and the neovascular (wet) form. Between 80 and 95 percent of people with ARMD have the dry form of the disease. The primary cause of dry ARMD is related to oxidative (free-radical) damage to the innermost layer of the retina. Wet ARMD is characterized by the growth of abnormal blood vessels.

Dietary Factors

A diet rich in fruits and vegetables is associated with a lowered risk for ARMD. Presumably, this protection is the result of increased intake of antioxidant vitamins and minerals. However, various nonessential food components, such as carotenes (lutein, zeaxanthin, and lycopene) and flavonoids, are proving to be even more significant in protecting against ARMD than traditional nutritional antioxidants such as vitamin C, vitamin E, and selenium. The macula, especially the central portion (the fovea), owes its yellow color to its high concentration of lutein and zeaxanthin. These yellow carotenes function in preventing oxidative damage to the area of the retina responsible for fine vision and obviously play a central role in protecting against the development of macular degeneration. Focusing on dietary sources of these carotenes appears to be more practical than looking to supplements.

Conventional Drugs

No prescription drugs are available with FDA-approved labeling for this indication.

Natural Medicines

Bilberry (Vaccinium myrtillus)
Effectiveness: B+   Safety: A

Ginkgo biloba
Effectiveness: B   Safety: A

Lutein
Effectiveness: B   Safety: B

Procyanidolic oligomers
Effectiveness: B   Safety: A

Zinc
Effectiveness: B   Safety: A

Commentary

Wet ARMD can be treated quite effectively with laser photocoagulation therapy; dry ARMD cannot. Because wet ARMD can rapidly progress to a point where surgery cannot be utilized, the surgery should be performed as soon as possible. Anyone with any vision loss should see a physician for complete evaluation, especially if the loss is progressing rapidly.

MENOPAUSE

Definition

Menopause denotes the cessation of menstruation in women, which usually occurs when a woman reaches the age of fifty, but may occur as early as forty and as late as fifty-five years of age. Six to twelve months without a menstrual period is the commonly accepted rule for diagnosing menopause. The time period prior to menopause is referred to as perimenopause, while the time period after menopause is referred to as postmenopause. During the perimenopausal period, many women have irregular periods.

Signs and Symptoms

The most common complaints of menopause are hot flashes, headaches, atrophic vaginitis (vaginal dryness and irritation due to lack of estrogen), frequent urinary tract infections, cold hands and feet, forgetfulness, and an inability to concentrate. In the United States, 65 to 80 percent of menopausal women experience hot flashes to some degree.

Causes

Menopause occurs when there are no longer any active eggs left in the ovaries due to normal aging or as a result of chemotherapy or surgery. At birth, there are about one million eggs (ova). This number drops to around three hundred thousand to four hundred thousand at puberty, but only about four hundred of these ova will actually mature during reproductive years. By the time a woman reaches the age of fifty, few eggs remain. With menopause, the absence of active follicles (the cellular housing of the egg) results in reduced production of estrogen and progesterone. In response to this drop in estrogen, the pituitary gland increases secretion of follicle-stimulating hormone (FSH) and luteinizing hormone (LH).

Dietary Factors

The key dietary recommendation is to increase the amount of plant foods, especially those high in phytoestrogens, while reducing the amount of animal foods in the diet. Phytoestrogens are plant compounds that are capable of binding to estrogen receptors. Foods high in phytoestrogens include soy, flaxseed and flaxseed oil (highest sources of lignans), nuts, whole grains, apples, fennel, celery, parsley, and alfalfa. A high intake of phytoestrogens is thought to explain why hot flashes and other menopausal symptoms rarely occur in cultures in which people consume a predominantly plant-based diet. Increasing the intake of dietary phytoestrogens helps decrease hot flashes, increase maturation of vaginal cells, and inhibit osteoporosis. In addition, a diet rich in phytoestrogens results in a decreased frequency of breast, colon, and prostate cancer. An especially important dietary recommendation is to increase the consumption of soy foods. Clinical studies have shown eating soy foods (the equivalent of ⅔ cup of soybeans daily) to be effective in relieving hot flashes and vaginal atrophy.

Conventional Drugs

- *Estrogen/androgen combinations:* methyltestosterone/esterified estrogens (Estratest, Menogen)

- *Estrogens:* estradiol (Alora, Climara, Esclim, Estrace, Estraderm, Fempatch, Gynodiol, Vivelle); estradiol valerate (Delestrogen, Dioval, EstroSpan, Valergen); conjugated estrogens, equine (Premarin); conjugated estrogens, synthetic (Cenestin); esterified estrogens (Estratab, Menest); estropipate (Ogen, Ortho-Est); ethinyl estradiol (Estinyl)
- *Estrogen/progesterone combinations:* conjugated estrogens/medroxyprogesterone acetate (Premphase, Prempro)
- *Progestins:* medroxyprogesterone acetate (Amen, Curretab, Cycrin, Depo-Provera, Prodoxy-10, Provera)
- Progesterone (Crinone, Progestasert, Prometrium)

Natural Medicines

Alfalfa (Medicago sativa)
Effectiveness: C   Safety: A

Black cohosh (Cimicifuga racemosa)
Effectiveness: A   Safety: A

Citrus bioflavonoids
Effectiveness: B   Safety: A

Dong quai (Angelica sinensis)
Effectiveness: C   Safety: C

Gamma-oryzanol
Effectiveness: B+   Safety: B

Ginseng (Panax ginseng *or* P. quinquefolium)
Effectiveness: C   Safety: C

Mexican wild yam (Dioscorea villosa)
Effectiveness: C   Safety: C

Red clover **(Trifolium pratense)**
Effectiveness: B   Safety: C

Soy isoflavones
Effectiveness: B+   Safety: B

Vitamin C
Effectiveness: B   Safety: A

Vitamin E
Effectiveness: B   Safety: A

Commentary

Women with atrophic vaginitis (vaginal drying and irritation) should also avoid substances that tend to dry the mucous membranes, including antihistamines, alcohol, caffeine, and diuretics.

MIGRAINE HEADACHE

Definition

A migraine is a vascular-type headache characterized by a sharp, pounding pain located within one side of the head.

Signs and Symptoms

The pain of a migraine is characterized as a throbbing or pounding sharp pain. It is typically noticed on just one side of the head. Although some migraines come on without warning, many migraine sufferers have warning symptoms (auras) before the onset of pain. Typical auras last a few minutes and include blurring or bright spots in the vision, anxiety, fatigue, disturbed thinking, and numbness or tingling on one side of the body.

Causes

Considerable evidence supports an association between migraine headache and instability of blood vessels. The mechanism of migraine can be described as a three-stage process: initiation, prodrome (time between initiation and appearance of headache), and headache. Although a particular stressor may be associated with the onset of a specific attack, it appears that initiation is dependent on the accumulation of several stressors over time. These stressors ultimately affect serotonin metabolism. Once a critical point of susceptibility (or threshold) is reached, a cascade event is initiated—a dominolike effect that ultimately produces a headache. Food allergies, histamine-releasing foods, alcohol (especially red wine), stress, hormonal changes (e.g., menstruation, ovulation, birth control pills) and weather changes—especially barometric pressure changes—are examples of some common triggers of migraines.

Dietary Factors

Food allergy or sensitivity plays a role in many cases of migraine headache. Many double-blind, placebo-controlled studies have demonstrated that the detection and removal of allergenic or untolerated foods will eliminate or greatly reduce migraine symptoms in the majority of patients. Food allergy/intolerance induces a migraine attack largely as a result of platelets releasing serotonin and histamines. In addition, foods such as chocolate, cheese, beer, and wine contain histamines and/or other compounds that can trigger migraines in sensitive individuals by causing blood vessels to expand. Red wine is much more likely than white wine to cause a headache because it contains twenty to two hundred times as much histamine.

Conventional Drugs

- *Antimigraine preparations:* dihydroergotamine mesylate (D.H.E. 45, Migranal); ergotamine tartrate (Ergomar, Ergomax); ergotamine tartrate/caffeine (Cafergot, Ercaf, Wigraine); isometheptene mucate/acetaminophen/dichloralphenazone (Amidrine, Duradrin, Isocom, Midrin, Migquin, Migratine, Migrazone, Mitride, Va-Zone); methysergide maleate (Sansert); sumatriptan succinate (Imitrex), zolmitriptan (Zomig)
- *Beta-adrenergic blocking agents:* propanolol (Betachron, Inderal, Pronol); timolol maleate (Blocadren)
- Dovalproex sodium (Depakote)

Natural Medicines

Feverfew (Tanacetum parthenium)
Effectiveness: B–   Safety: B

Ginger (Zingiber officinalis)
Effectiveness: B   Safety: A

Hydroxytryptophan (5-HTP)
Effectiveness: A   Safety: D

Magnesium
Effectiveness: B   Safety: A

Riboflavin
Effectiveness: B+　　　Safety: A

S-adenosylmethionine (SAMe)
Effectiveness: B　　　Safety: A

Commentary

In addition to the dietary and supplement strategies, biofeedback and relaxation training can also be helpful. The effectiveness of biofeedback and relaxation training in reducing the frequency and severity of recurrent migraine headaches has been the subject of over thirty-five clinical studies. When the results from these studies were compared with those of studies using prescription drug therapy, it was apparent that the nondrug approach was as effective as the drug approach but was without side effects. Ask your doctor about these therapies.

MITRAL VALVE PROLAPSE

Definition

Mitral valve prolapse refers to a loss of tone or a slight deformity of the mitral valve of the heart—the valve that blocks off the left upper chamber (the left atrium) from the left ventricle. This deformity causes leakage of the valve and produces a heart murmur that can be heard by a stethoscope.

Signs and Symptoms

Most cases of mitral valve prolapse go unnoticed until a heart murmur is discovered during a physical exam. In more severe cases of mitral valve prolapse, an individual may experience shortness of breath (especially with exertion), palpitations, fatigue, and a chronic unproductive cough. It can also lead to arrhythmia (a disturbance in heartbeat).

Causes

Mitral valve prolapse is associated with a magnesium deficiency. It can also simply be the result of a mechanical abnormality in the shape of the heart or valve due to trauma, rheumatic heart disease, infection in the heart, or other factor that can damage the heart.

Dietary Factors

A diet designed to support healthy heart function is indicated. Reduce salt (sodium chloride) intake; eat a high-potassium diet rich in fiber and complex carbohydrates; increase dietary consumption of celery, garlic, and onions; and reduce or eliminate the intake of saturated fats.

Conventional Drugs

- *Beta-adrenergic blocking agents:* acebutolol (Acebutolol, Sectral); atenolol (Atenolol, Senormin, Tenormin); bisoprolol fumarate (Zebeta); carteolol (Cartrol); metoprolol succinate (Toprol-XL); metoprolol tartrate (Lopressor); nadolol (Corgard); penbutolol sulfate (Levatol); pindolol (Visken); propranolol (Betachron, Inderal, Pronol); timolol maleate (Blocadren)

Natural Medicines

Coenzyme Q₁₀ (CoQ₁₀)
Effectiveness: B+   Safety: A

*Hawthorn (*Crataegus *spp.)*
Effectiveness: B   Safety: A

Magnesium
Effectiveness: B+   Safety: A

Commentary

Anyone with mitral valve prolapse or any other heart disease should have an extensive cardiovascular evaluation, including a complete physical exam to look for signs of poor blood flow; an electrocardiogram, which assesses the electrical function of the heart; an echocardiogram, an ultrasound procedure to assess how the heart is functioning from a mechanical perspective as well as determine the heart's shape and size; and a complete laboratory assessment.

MULTIPLE SCLEROSIS

Definition

Multiple sclerosis (MS) is a syndrome of progressive nerve disturbances that usually occurs early in adult life. It is caused by gradual loss of the myelin sheath that surrounds the nerve cell. This process is called demyelination. One of the key functions of this myelin sheath is to facilitate the transmission of the erve impulse. Without the myelin sheath, nerve unction is lost. Symptoms correspond to the nerves hat have lost their myelin sheath.

Signs and Symptoms

Sudden transient motor and sensory disturbances, including blurred vision, dizziness, muscle weakness, and tingling sensations, suggest MS. The diagnosis is confirmed by the detection of evidence of demyelination on magnetic resonance imaging (MRI).

Causes

The cause of MS remains to be identified conclusively. It is thought that MS is an autoimmune disease, where the immune system attacks body tissues as foreign proteins. What triggers this process in MS is unknown.

Dietary Factors

Dr. Roy Swank, professor of neurology at the University of Oregon Medical School, has provided convincing evidence that a diet low in saturated fats, maintained over a long period of time, tends to retard the disease process of MS and reduce the number of attacks. Swank began successfully treating patients with his low-fat diet in 1948. Dr. Swank recommends:

A saturated fat intake of no more than 10 g per day
A daily intake of 40 to 50 g of polyunsaturated oils per day (margarine, shortening, and hydrogenated oils are not allowed)
At least 1 tsp of cod liver oil per day

- A normal allowance of protein
- Consumption of fish three or more times per week

The Swank diet was originally thought to help patients with MS by overcoming an essential fatty acid deficiency. Currently it is thought that the beneficial effects are probably a result of (1) decreasing platelet aggregation, (2) decreasing an autoimmune response, and (3) normalizing the decreased essential fatty acid levels found in patients with MS.

A high intake of saturated fatty acids and animal fat are linked to MS. Consumption of saturated fat increases the requirements for the essential fatty acids, creating a relative deficiency state. Making matters worse is that individuals with MS are also thought to have a defect in essential fatty acid absorption and/or transport, which results in a functional deficiency state. Without the essential fatty acids the myelin sheath does not form or function properly.

Food allergy has been implicated in the progression of MS, in particular the consumption of two common allergens—gluten and milk. While there is no convincing clinical evidence that gluten-free or allergy-elimination diets are universally beneficial in the management of MS, it certainly is generally healthful to eliminate food allergens (as long as other dietary measures are also included, such as in the Swank diet); there is anecdotal evidence that specific individuals have been helped.

Conventional Drugs

- *Immune-modulating drugs:* glatiramer acetate (Copaxone); interferon beta-1b (Avonex); interferon beta-1a (Betaseron)
- *Corticosteroids:* betamethasone sodium phos

phate (Adbeon, Celestone); cortisone acetate (Cortisone, Cortone); dexamethasone (Decadron); dexamethasone acetate (Dalalone DP); hydrocortisone (Hydrocortone); methylprednisolone; prednisolone (Prelone); prednisolone tebutate (Hydeltra-TBA); prednisone (Apo-Prednisone, Deltasone, Liquid Pred, Meticorten, Orasone, Prednicen, Sterapred, Winpred)

Natural Medicines

Fish oils (eicosapentaenoic acid and docosahexaenoic acid)
Effectiveness: C   Safety: C

Pancreatin
Effectiveness: B   Safety: A

Vitamin B$_{12}$ (prevention of deficiency)
Effectiveness: B   Safety: A

Commentary

Synthetically produced beta-interferon (Avonex, Betaseron) is emerging as the most popular medical treatment for multiple sclerosis. However, alpha-interferon (Roferon, Intron) may prove to be a better choice. In preliminary studies of patients receiving 5 million to 30 million IU of alpha-interferon per week, 83 percent improved or stabilized in the first year, and in year two 76 percent remained improved or stabilized. This remission rate for alpha-interferon is better than the 30 percent rate reported for beta-interferon. Further studies are needed to confirm these comparative remission rates.

NONULCER DYSPEPSIA

Definition

Nonulcer dyspepsia (NUD) is a medical term often used to label indigestion and/or heartburn that is not related to an ulcer. Another common term for similar symptoms is gastroesophageal reflux disease (GERD). The main symptoms of GERD are heartburn and/or upper abdominal pain.

Signs and Symptoms

Symptoms of NUD include symptoms of GERD (heartburn and/or upper abdominal pain) as well as difficulty swallowing, feelings of pressure or heaviness after eating, sensations of bloating after eating, and stomach or abdominal pains and cramps, as well as all of the symptoms of irritable bowel syndrome (IBS). About three out of ten patients with NUD also meet the criteria for IBS.

Causes

NUD and GERD are most often caused by the flow of gastric juices up the esophagus, leading to a burning discomfort that radiates upward and is made worse by lying down. This reflux of gastric juice can be the result of factors that increase intraabdominal pressure (e.g., overeating, obesity) or factors that decrease the tone of the esophageal sphincter (e.g., hiatal hernias, coffee).

Dietary Factors

Common dietary causes of NUD and GERD include overeating, obesity, coffee, chocolate, fried foods, carbonated beverages (soft drinks), and alcohol.

Conventional Drugs

- *Antacids:* aluminum carbonate (Basaljel); aluminum hydroxide (ALternaGEL, Amphojel, Nephrox); aluminum hydroxide/magnesium hydroxide (Maalox, Mylanta); calcium carbonate (Alka-Mint, Titralac, Tums); calcium carbonate/magnesium hydroxide (Rolaids); magaldrate (Losopan, Ri Mag, Riopan); magnesium carbonate/calcium carbonate (Marblen); magnesium hydroxide (Phillips' Milk of Magnesia); magnesium oxide (Mag-Ox, Uro-Mag); magnesium trisilicate/aluminum hydroxide (Gaviscon Antacid); sodium bicarbonate (Alka-Seltzer, Arm & Hammer)
- *Histamine-2 receptor antagonists:* cimetidine (Tagamet); famotidine (Mylanta Ar, Pepcid); nizatidine (Axid); ranitidine (Zantac)
- *Proton pump inhibitors:* lansoprazole (Prevacid); omeprazole (Prilosec)

Natural Medicines

***Artichoke* (Cynara scolymus)**
Effectiveness: B   Safety: C

Betaine hydrochloride
Effectiveness: C   Safety: C

Calcium (for antacid effects)
Effectiveness: A   Safety: A

Iberogast
Effectiveness: A   Safety: A

Commentary

In the person with chronic heartburn or indigestion, rather than focus on blocking the digestive process with antacids, many alternative medicine practitioners utilize betaine hydrochloride to aid digestion.

OBESITY

Definition

Obesity is defined as a state of being more than 20 percent above normal weight, or having a body fat percentage greater than 30 percent for women and 25 percent for men.

Signs and Symptoms

Obesity is divided into several categories based on how the fat is distributed in the body. Fat primarily distributed around the waist is referred to as male-pattern or android obesity, since it is typically seen in obese males. In android obesity, the waist is bigger around than the hips (apple-shaped). In gynecoid obesity, the hips are larger (pear-shaped). Android obesity carries with it a greater risk for cardiovascular disease and diabetes, while gynecoid obesity increases the risk of hormone-sensitive cancers such as breast cancer.

Causes

Theories of the underlying causes of obesity are tied to brain serotonin levels (see discussion of **hydroxytryptophan (5-HTP)**, diet-induced thermogenesis, and the inner workings of fat cells. All of these models support the notion that obesity is not just a matter of overeating. They explain why some people can eat large quantities of food and not increase their weight substantially, while for others just the reverse is true. For example, a certain amount of the food we consume is converted immediately to heat. This is known as diet-induced thermogenesis (heat production). There is evidence that the level of diet-induced thermogenesis is what determines whether an individual is likely to be overweight. In lean individuals, a meal may stimulate up to a 40 percent increase in heat production. In contrast, overweight individuals often display only a 10 percent or less increase in heat production. The food energy is stored as fat instead of being converted to heat.

Dietary Factors

There are literally hundreds of diets and diet programs that claim to be the answer to obesity. However, the basic equation for losing weight never changes. In order for an individual to lose weight, energy intake must be less than energy expenditure. This goal can be achieved by decreasing caloric intake (dieting) or by increasing the rate at which calories are burned (exercising). Most individuals will begin to lose weight if they decrease their caloric intake below 1,500 calories per day and do aerobic exercise for fifteen to twenty minutes three to four times per week. Starvation and crash diets usually result in

rapid weight loss (largely muscle and water) but
cause rebound weight gain. The most successful approach to weight loss is gradual weight reduction
(½ to 1 pound per week) through adopting long-term
dietary and lifestyle modifications.

Conventional Drugs

- *Appetite suppressants:* benzophetamine (Didrex);
  dexfenfluramine (Redux); diethylproprion (Ten-
  uate); fenfluramine (Pondimin); mazindo
  (Sanorex); phendimetrazine tartrate (Adipost,
  Appecon, Bontril, Obezine, Phendiet, Plegin,
  Prelu-2); phentermine (Adipex-P, Fastin, Oby-Cap,
  Zantryl); phentermine resin (Ionamin)
- *Fat absorption blocking agents:* orlistat
  (Xenical)
- *Stimulants:* dextroamphetamine sulfate (Dexe-
  drine); methamphetamine (Desoxyn)

Natural Medicines

Bitter orange (Citrus aurantium)
Effectiveness: C   Safety: C

Cayenne pepper (Capsicum frutescens)
Effectiveness: B+   Safety: A

Chitosan
Effectiveness: B–   Safety: B

Chromium
Effectiveness: B–   Safety: B

Coenzyme Q$_{10}$
Effectiveness: B   Safety: A

Conjugated linoleic acid
Effectiveness: C   Safety: C

Ephedrine-caffeine combinations (thermogenic formulas)
Effectiveness: A   Safety: D

Fiber
Effectiveness: A   Safety: A

Garcinia (Garcinia cambogia)
Effectiveness: D   Safety: B

Hydroxytryptophan (5-HTP)
Effectiveness: A   Safety: D

7-keto DHEA
Effectiveness: B   Safety: B

Medium-chain triglycerides
Effectiveness: B+   Safety: A

Pyruvate
Effectiveness: B   Safety: B

Spirulina
Effectiveness: B   Safety: C

Commentary

A successful program to treat obesity is consistent with the basic tenets of good health: a positive mental attitude, a healthy lifestyle (especially important is regular exercise), a health-promoting diet, and supplementary measures. All of these components are interrelated, and no single component is more important than another. Improvement in one aspect may be enough to result in some weight loss, but the best approach is one that is comprehensive.

OSTEOARTHRITIS

Definition

Osteoarthritis (also known as degenerative joint disease) is a form of arthritis (inflammation of a joint) caused by degeneration of cartilage. Cartilage serves an important role in joint function. Its gel-like nature provides protection to the ends of bones by acting as a shock absorber. Without the cartilage in the joint, bone rubs against bone, leading to pain, deformity, inflammation, and limitation of motion in the joint.

Signs and Symptoms

The onset of osteoarthritis can be subtle. Morning joint stiffness is often the first symptom. As the disease progresses, there is pain on motion of the involved joint that is made worse by prolonged activity and relieved by rest. There is usually local tenderness, soft tissue swelling, joint crepitus (cracking sounds), bony swelling, restricted mobility, and bony nodules. X-ray findings show narrowing of the joint space (the area between the bones taken up by cartilage). The weight-bearing joints of the knees, hips, and spine as well as those in the hands are most often affected. These joints are under greater stress because of weight and use.

Causes

Osteoarthritis is divided into two categories, primary and secondary. In primary osteoarthritis, the degenerative "wear-and-tear" process occurs after a person turns forty years of age. The cumulative effects of decades of use leads to the degenerative changes by stressing the collagen matrix of the cartilage. Damage to the cartilage results in the release of enzymes that further destroy cartilage components. With aging, the ability to restore and manufacture normal cartilage structures decreases.

Secondary osteoarthritis is associated with some predisposing factor that is responsible for the degenerative changes. Predisposing factors in secondary osteoarthritis include inherited abnormalities in joint structure or function, trauma (fractures along joint surfaces, surgery, etc.), presence of abnormal cartilage, and previous inflammatory disease of joint (rheumatoid arthritis, gout, etc.).

Dietary Factors

It is critical that the diet be rich in fruits and vegetables. Their natural plant compounds can protect against cellular damage including damage to joints. Foods especially beneficial in osteoarthritis are flavonoid-rich fruits such as cherries, blueberries, and blackberries. Also important are sulfur-containing foods such as garlic, onions, Brussels sprouts, and cabbage; studies have shown that the sulfur content in fingernails of arthritis sufferers is lower than that of healthy subjects without arthritis, suggesting a link between low levels of sulfur and arthritis.

Conventional Drugs

- Acetaminophen (Panadol, Tylenol)
- *Aspirin and other nonsteroidal anti-inflammatory drugs:* aspirin (Ascriptin Enteric, Bayer,

Bufferin, Ecotrin); diclofenac sodium (Voltaren) diclofenac potassium (Cataflam); etodolac (Lodine); fenoprofen calcium (Nalfon); ibuprofen (Advil, IBU, Motrin, Nuprin); indomethacin (Indocin); ketoprofen (Actron, Orudis); nabumetone (Relafen); naproxen sodium (Aleve, Anaprox, Naprelan); oxaprozin (Daypro); piroxicam (Feldene); sulindac (Clinoril); tolmetin sodium (Tolectin)

- *Cox-2 inhibitors:* celecoxib (Celebrex), rofecoxib (Vioxx)

Natural Medicines

Boswellic acids (Boswellia serrata)
Effectiveness: B+   Safety: B

Capsaicin (topical use)
Effectiveness: A   Safety: D

Cetylmyristoleate (CMO)
Effectiveness: B   Safety: B

Chondroitin sulfate
Effectiveness: A   Safety: A

Glucosamine
Effectiveness: A   Safety: A

MSM (methylsulfonylmethane)
Effectiveness: C   Safety: C

Menthol (topical use)
Effectiveness: A   Safety: A

Niacinamide
Effectiveness: B+   Safety: B

Phytodolor
Effectiveness: B+   Safety: A

S-adenosylmethionine (SAMe)
Effectiveness: A   Safety: A

Shark cartilage
Effectiveness: C   Safety: C

***Stinging nettle* (Urtica dioica)**
Effectiveness: B   Safety: C

Vitamin E
Effectiveness: B   Safety: A

***White willow* (Salix alba)**
Effectiveness: B   Safety: C

Commentary

Nonsteroidal anti-inflammatory drugs (aspirin, ibuprofen, piroxicam, etc.) may produce short-term benefit, but as several clinical studies have shown, they actually accelerate the progression of the joint destruction. The way in which these drugs work is to inhibit enzymes involved in the production of inflammatory compounds. However, they also inhibit enzymes that manufacture cartilage components. A person may feel free from pain while on the NSAID, but their arthritis is silently getting worse.

OSTEOPOROSIS

Definition

The word *osteoporosis* literally means "porous bone." While many erroneously consider osteoporosis to be the result of the loss of calcium and other minerals of bone, it actually involves a loss of both the mineral (inorganic) and nonmineral (organic matrix, composed primarily of protein) components of bone. Bone is dynamic living tissue that is constantly being broken down and rebuilt, even in adults. Osteoporosis occurs when there is more bone breaking down than being formed.

Signs and Symptoms

Osteoporosis is usually without symptoms until severe backache (due to compression of the vertebrae) or fracture occurs. Osteoporosis may result in considerable loss of height. Osteoporosis is best diagnosed by dual-energy X-ray absorptiometry (DEXA), a technique that measures bone density.

Causes

Normal bone metabolism is dependent on an intricate interplay of many nutritional, lifestyle, and hormonal factors. Many dietary factors have been suggested as a cause of osteoporosis, including a low calcium intake combined with a high phosphorus intake, a high-protein diet, high salt intake, and trace-mineral deficiencies, to name a few. Osteoporosis is most common in postmenopausal Asian and white women. Other risk factors for osteoporosis include a family history of osteoporosis; alcoholism; smoking; physical inactivity; short stature, low body mass, and/or small bones; and never having been pregnant.

Dietary Factors

A vegetarian diet is associated with a lower risk of osteoporosis. Although bone mass in vegetarians does not differ significantly from that of omnivores in the third, fourth, and fifth decades of life, there are significant differences in the later decades. These findings indicate that the decreased incidence of osteoporosis among vegetarians is due not to increased initial bone mass but rather to decreased bone loss.

A high-protein diet is associated with increased excretion of calcium in the urine and increased risk for osteoporosis. Raising daily protein intake from 47 to 142 grams doubles the excretion of calcium in the urine. Refined sugar intake also increases the loss of calcium from the body.

Soft drinks containing phosphates (phosphoric acid) are linked to osteoporosis because they lead to lower calcium levels and higher phosphate levels in the blood. When phosphate levels are high and calcium levels are low, calcium is pulled out of the bones. The phosphate content of soft drinks like Coca-Cola and Pepsi is very high, and they contain virtually no calcium.

Green leafy vegetables (kale, collard greens, parsley, lettuce, etc.) as well as green tea offer significant protection against osteoporosis. These foods are a rich source of a broad range of vitamins and minerals that are important to maintaining healthy bones, including calcium, vitamin K_1, and boron. Vitamin K_1 is the form of vitamin K that is found in plants. A function of vitamin K_1 is to convert inactive osteocalcin to its active form. Osteocalcin is an important protein in bone. Its role is to anchor calcium molecules and hold them in place within the bone.

Soy foods such as tofu, soy milk, roasted soybeans, and soy extract powders may be beneficial in preventing osteoporosis. In several double-blind studies, taking 40 g of soy protein powder containing

80 to 90 mg isoflavones increased bone mineral density of the spine and hips in postmenopausal women.

Conventional Drugs

- *Bone resorption suppression agents:* alendronate sodium (Fosamax); calcitonin (Calcimir, Miacalcin); raloxifene (Evista)
- *Estrogens:* estradiol (Estrace, Estraderm, Estradiol, Fempatch), conjugated estrogens (Premarin); conjugated estrogens/medroxyprogesterone acetate (Premphase, Prempro); estropipate (Ogen, Ortho-Est)

Natural Medicines

Boron
Effectiveness: B+   Safety: B

Calcium
Effectiveness: A   Safety: A

Ipriflavone
Effectiveness: A   Safety: A

Silicon
Effectiveness: C   Safety: C

Soy isoflavones
Effectiveness: B+   Safety: B

Vitamin D
Effectiveness: B   Safety: A

Vitamin K
Effectiveness: B   Safety: A

Commentary

Although nutritional factors are important, the best way to strengthen the bones is to get physical activity. One hour of moderate activity (walking, weight lifting, dancing, etc.) three times a week has been shown to prevent bone loss and actually increase bone mass in postmenopausal women. In contrast, lack of physical activity doubles the rate of calcium lost from the system.

PARKINSON'S DISEASE

Definition

Parkinson's disease is a neurological disease resulting from damage to the nerves in the basal ganglia, the area of the brain that is responsible for controlling muscle tension and movement. The damaged cells are the ones needed to produce the neurotransmitter called dopamine. There is no cure for Parkinson's, but symptoms are often improved by drug therapy.

Signs and Symptoms

The disease usually begins as a slight tremor of one hand, arm, or leg. In the early stages the tremors are more apparent while the person is at rest, such as while sitting or standing, and are less noticeable when the hand or limb is being used. A typical early symptom of Parkinson's disease is "pill-rolling," in which the person appears to be rolling a pill back and forth between the fingers. As the disease progresses, symptoms often worsen. The tremors and weakness affect the limbs on both sides of the body. The hands and the head may shake continuously. The person may walk with stiff, shuffling steps. In many cases, the disease causes a permanent rigid, stooped posture and an unblinking, fixed expression.

Causes

The cause of Parkinson's disease is unknown, but it is thought that a neurotoxin causes oxidative damage to the basal ganglia in the brain. In the oxidative damage model, oxidation reactions lead to the generation of free radicals that are capable of destroying the cell membranes and nerve cells.

Dietary Factors

The value of a low-protein diet in enhancing the action of L-dopa therapy has been demonstrated in several clinical studies and is now a well-accepted supportive therapy. The usual recommendation is to eliminate good sources of dietary protein from breakfast and lunch, keeping daytime protein intake below 7 g, with no restriction at dinner. This simple recommendation can offer an effective method for the reduction of tremors and other symptoms of Parkinson's disease during working hours.

Conventional Drugs

- *Anticholinergic drugs:* benzotropine mesylate (Cogentin); biperiden (Akineton); trihexyphenidyl (Artane, Trihexane); procyclidine (Kemadrin)
- *Antiparkinson drugs:* amantadine (Symmetrel); carbidopa/levodopa (Atamet, Sinemet); enta-

capone (Comtan); levodopa (Dopar, L-Dopa, Larodopa); pergolide mesylate (Permax); pramipexole (Mirapex); ropinirole (Requip); selegiline (Atapryl, Deprenyl, Carbex); tolcapone (Tasmar)

- *Pituitary suppressive agents:* bromocriptine mesylate (Parlodel); cabergoline (Dostinex)

Natural Medicines

NADH (Niacinamide adenine dinucleotide)
Effectiveness: B   Safety: A

Phosphatidylserine
Effectiveness: B   Safety: A

Vitamin C (prevention)
Effectiveness: B   Safety: A

Vitamin E (prevention)
Effectiveness: B   Safety: A

Commentary

At this time, Parkinson's disease is best treated with prescription drug therapy. The dietary, nutritional, and herbal recommendations can be used to enhance the effectiveness of drug therapy. The most popular drug used is Sinemet, which contains two key ingredients, levodopa and carbidopa. Levodopa, or L-dopa, is the middle step in the conversion of the amino acid tyrosine into dopamine. L-dopa, but not dopamine, crosses the blood-brain barrier. Carbidopa is a drug that works by ensuring that more L-dopa is converted to dopamine within the brain, where it is needed, and not within the other tissues of the body.

PERIODONTAL DISEASE

Definition

Periodontal disease is an inclusive term used to describe an inflammatory condition of the gums (gingivitis) and/or support structures (periodontitis). The periodontal disease process typically progresses from gingivitis to periodontitis.

Signs and Symptoms

Gingivitis is characterized by redness, contour changes, and bleeding. Periodontitis is characterized by localized pain, loose teeth, dental pockets, redness, swelling, and/or signs of infection. X rays may reveal destruction of bone.

Causes

Periodontal disease can be caused by poor dental hygiene or may be a manifestation of a more systemic condition, such as diabetes mellitus, collagen diseases, anemia, vitamin deficiency states or leukemia, or other disorders of leukocyte function. An association with hardening of the arteries (atherosclerosis) has also been reported.

Dietary Factors

The key dietary recommendation is to avoid sugar. Sugar is known to significantly increase plaque accumulation while decreasing white blood cell function.

Conventional Drugs

- *Tetracycline antibiotics:* doxycycline hyclate (Bio-Tab, Doryx, Doxy Caps, Periostat, Vibra-Tabs, Vibramycin); tetracycline periodontal fibers (Actisite)

Natural Medicines

Coenzyme Q₁₀ (CoQ₁₀)
Effectiveness: A   Safety: A

Procyanidolic oligomers
Effectiveness: C   Safety: C

Vitamin C
Effectiveness: A   Safety: A

Zinc
Effectiveness: C   Safety: A

Commentary

Although oral hygiene is of great importance in treating and preventing periodontal disease, it is not sufficient in many cases. In addition to proper dental care (brushing after meals, daily flossing, and regular dental cleanings), nutritional status and immune system function must be normalized if development and progression of the disease are to be controlled. Bacterial plaque has long been considered the causative agent in most forms of periodontal disease. However, it is now widely accepted that people with poor nutritional status or immune function are likely to develop periodontal disease even with the best possible oral hygiene.

PREMENSTRUAL SYNDROME

Definition

Premenstrual syndrome (PMS) is a recurrent condition of women of childbearing age, characterized by troublesome symptoms seven to fourteen days before menstruation.

Signs and Symptoms

Typical symptoms include decreased energy level, tension, irritability, depression, headache, altered sex drive, breast pain, backache, abdominal bloating, and edema of the fingers and ankles. Severe PMS, with depression, irritability, and extreme mood swings, is referred to as premenstrual dysphoric disorder.

Causes

Although there is a wide spectrum of symptoms, there are common hormonal patterns among PMS patients compared to women who have no symptoms of PMS. The primary finding is that estrogen levels are elevated and plasma progesterone levels are reduced five to ten days before the menses, or the ratio of estrogen to progesterone is increased. In addition to this hormonal abnormality, hypothyroidism and/or elevated prolactin levels are common.

Dietary Factors

Reduce or eliminate the amount of animal products in the diet, and increase consumption of fiber-rich foods (fruits, vegetables, grains, and legumes). Vegetarian women have been shown to excrete two to three times more estrogen in their feces and have 50 percent lower levels of free estrogen in their blood than women who eat meat. These differences are thought to be a result of the lower fat intake and higher fiber intake of vegetarians.

Caffeine intake must be avoided by women with PMS. This recommendation is particularly important if anxiety, depression, or breast tenderness and fibrocystic breast disease are the major symptoms. There is considerable evidence that caffeine consumption is strongly related to the presence and severity of PMS. The effect of caffeine is particularly significant in the psychological symptoms associated with PMS, such as anxiety, irritability, insomnia, and depression.

Excessive salt (sodium chloride) consumption, coupled with diminished dietary potassium, greatly stresses the kidneys' ability to maintain proper fluid volume. As a result, some people are salt sensitive, in that high salt intake causes high blood pressure or water retention. In general, it is a good idea to avoid salt if you have PMS. If you tend to notice more water retention during the latter part of your menstrual cycle, reducing your salt intake is an absolute must.

Conventional Drugs

- *Analgesic preparations:* acetaminophen/pamabrom/pyrilamine maleate (Midol PMS); acetaminophen/pamabrom/vitamin B_6 (Lurline PMS)
- *Antianxiety drugs:* buspirone (BuSpar)
- *Antidepressant drugs:* fluoxetine (Prozac)

Natural Medicines

Calcium
Effectiveness: B+   Safety: A

Chaste berry (Vitex agnus-castus)
Effectiveness: A   Safety: C

Gamma-linolenic acid
Effectiveness: D   Safety: A

Ginkgo biloba
Effectiveness: B   Safety: A

Licorice (Glycyrrhiza glabra)
Effectiveness: C   Safety: C

Magnesium
Effectiveness: B+   Safety: A

Vitamin B$_6$
Effectiveness: B+   Safety: A

Vitamin E
Effectiveness: B   Safety: A

Commentary

Although supplementary progesterone is recommended by many physicians, controlled clinical trials have failed to consistently demonstrate the superiority of progesterone therapy over a placebo. The studies that demonstrate a beneficial effect of progesterone therapy have used dosages (200 to 400 mg twice daily as a vaginal or rectal suppository, from fourteen days before the expected onset of menstruation until the onset of vaginal bleeding) that far exceed the normal levels for progesterone and for the estrogen-to-progesterone ratio. Side effects, although generally mild, are common. Irregular menstruation, vaginal itching, and headache were reported more frequently by women who took the progesterone.

PROSTATE ENLARGEMENT (BENIGN PROSTATIC HYPERPLASIA)

Definition

The prostate is a doughnut-shaped gland about the size of a walnut that lies below the bladder and surrounds the urethra. The prostate secretes a thin, milky, alkaline fluid that increases sperm motility and lubricates the urethra to prevent infection. Prostate secretions are extremely important to successful fertilization of the egg. Benign (nonmalignant) enlargement of the prostate gland is known medically as benign prostatic hyperplasia, or BPH for short. Because an enlarged prostate can pinch off the flow of urine, BPH is characterized by symptoms of bladder obstruction, such as increased urinary frequency, nighttime awakening to empty the bladder, and reduced urinary force and speed of flow.

BPH is an extremely common condition. Current estimates are that it affects over 50 percent of men during their lifetime. The actual frequency increases with advancing age, from approximately 5 to 10 percent at age thirty to over 90 percent in men older than eighty-five.

Signs and Symptoms

The key symptoms relate to blockage of the bladder
outlet, such as progressive urinary frequency, urgency and increased nighttime urination, hesitancy
and intermittency, with reduced urinary force and
speed of flow.

Warning: Prostate disorders can only be diagnosed by a physician. Do not self-diagnose. If you
are experiencing any symptoms associated with
BPH, see your physician immediately for proper diagnosis.

Causes

BPH is largely the result of hormonal changes associated with aging. It is clearly dependent on the actions of male hormones (androgens) within the
prostate gland. These changes within the prostate
reflect the many significant changes in both male
(androgen), female (estrogen), and pituitary hormone levels in aging men. The ultimate effect of
these changes is that there is an increased concentration of testosterone within the prostate gland and
an increased conversion of this testosterone to an
even more potent form known as dihydrotestos-
terone (DHT).

Dietary Factors

Diet appears to play a critical role in the health of the
prostate. Focus on whole, unprocessed foods
(whole grains, legumes, vegetables, fruits, nuts, and
seeds). Eat ¼ cup of raw sunflower seeds or pumpkin seeds each day along with regular consumption
of soy foods and lycopene-rich vegetables and fruits
such as tomatoes, spinach, kale, mangoes, broccoli,

and berries. Reduce the intake of alcohol (especially beer), caffeine, and sugar.

Conventional Drugs

- *Antiandrogenic agents:* finasteride (Propecia, Proscar)
- *Bladder outlet relaxants:* doxazosin mesylate (Cardura); phenoxybenzamine (Dibenzyline); prazosin (Minipress); tamsulosin (Flomax); terazosin (Hytrin)

Natural Medicines

Beta-sitosterol
Effectiveness: B+   Safety: A

Cernilton
Effectiveness: A   Safety: A

Saw palmetto (Serenoa repens)
Effectiveness: A   Safety: A

Prostex
Effectiveness: B+   Safety: A

Pumpkin seed oil or extract (Cucurbita pepo)
Effectiveness: B   Safety: A

Pygeum africanum
Effectiveness: A   Safety: A

Stinging nettle (Urtica dioca)
Effectiveness: B+   Safety: C

Commentary

Even if symptoms of BPH are quite mild, it is important to treat it early. If left untreated, BPH can eventually obstruct the bladder outlet, resulting in the retention of urine and eventually kidney damage. As this situation is potentially life-threatening, proper treatment is crucial.

PSORIASIS

Definition

Psoriasis is a common skin disorder characterized by the appearance of silvery plaque-like, scaly lesions caused by a pileup of skin cells that have replicated too rapidly. In addition to affecting the skin, psoriasis can cause an inflammatory form of arthritis and affect the nails.

Signs and Symptoms

The lesions of psoriasis are usually sharply bordered reddened rash or plaques covered with overlapping silvery scales. Psoriasis usually affects the wrists, elbows, knees, buttocks, and ankles, as well as sites of repeated trauma. Nail involvement results in characteristic "oil drop" stippling (thimble-like appearance). Psoriasis can also affect the joints, producing psoriatic arthritis.

Causes

Psoriasis is caused by a pileup of skin cells that have replicated too rapidly. The rate at which skin cells divide in psoriasis is roughly one thousand times greater than in normal skin. This high rate of replication is simply too fast for the cells to be shed, so they accumulate, resulting in the characteristic silvery scale. Although psoriasis has a significant genetic component, a number of factors appear to cause or contribute to psoriasis, including incomplete protein digestion, bowel toxemia, impaired liver function, alcohol consumption, excessive consumption of animal fats, and stress.

Dietary Factors

Limit the consumption of sugar and increase the intake of high-fiber foods like vegetables, legumes, fruit, and whole grains. Dietary fiber helps bind gut-derived toxins that otherwise can be absorbed and trigger psoriasis.

Limit the consumption of meat and animal fats while increasing the intake of cold-water fish (salmon, mackerel, herring, halibut, etc.). In the skin of individuals who have psoriasis, the production of inflammatory compounds known as leukotrienes is many times greater than normal. These toxic compounds are produced from arachidonic acid. Since arachidonic acid is found only in animal tissues, it is necessary to limit intake of animal products, particularly meat, animal fats, and dairy products.

Eliminate alcohol. Alcohol is known to significantly worsen psoriasis because it increases the absorption of toxins from the gut that can stimulate psoriasis.

An allergy elimination diet can help psoriasis. Follow the recommendations given in the section on **food allergy.**

Conventional Drugs

- *Antimetabolites:* methotrexate sodium (Rheumatrex)

- *Antipsoriatic agents, vitamin A derivatives for oral use:* acitretin (Soriatane); etretinate (Tegison)
- *Antipsoriatic agents, topical:* calcipotriene (Dovonex); coal tar (DHS, Fotota, MG 217, Pentrax, Tegrin); tazarotene (Tazorac)
- *Corticosteroids for oral or topical use:* betamethasone (Alphatrex, Beben, Betaderm, Betatrex, Beta-Val, Betnovate, Celestoderm, Celestone, Dermabet, Diprolene, Ectosone, Maxivate, Metaderm, Prevex B, Teladar, Topilene, Topisone, Uticort, Valisone, Valnac) clobetasol (Dermovate, Temovate); desonide (DesOwen, Tridesilon) dexamethasone (Aeroseb-Dex, Decaderm, Decadron); diflorasone (Florone, Maxiflor); fluocinolone (Bio-Syn, Fluocet, Fluoderm, Fluolar, Fluonid, Fluonide, Flurosyn, Synalar, Synamol, Synemol); fluocinonide (Fluocin, Licon, Lidemol, Lidex, Lyderm, Topsyn); flurandrenolide (Cordran, Drenison); halcinonide (Halog); hydrocortisone (Acticort, Aeroseb-HC, Ala-Cort, Allercort, Alphaderm, Bactine, Cetacort, Cortacet, Cortaid, Cortate, Cortef, Corticaine, Cortiment, Cortoderm, Cortril, Delacort, Dermacort, DermiCort, Emo-Cort, Hi-Cor, Hyderm, Hydro-Tex, Hytone, Lanacort, Locoid, MyCort, Nutracort, Penecort, Pentacort, Prevex HC, Sential, Synacort, Texacort, Unicort, Westcort); mometasone (Elocom, Elocon); prednisone (Apo-Prednisone, Deltasone, Liquid Pred, Meticorten, Orasone, Prednicen, Sterapred, Winpred); triamcinolone (Aristocort, Flutex, Kenac, Kenalog, Kenonel, Oracort, Oralone, Triacet, Trianide, Triderm)

Natural Medicines

Aloe vera *(topical)*
Effectiveness: B   Safety: A

Berberine-containing plants
Effectiveness: C   Safety: B

Capsaicin (topical use)
Effectiveness: B+   Safety: D

***Chamomile* (Matricaria chamomilla)** *(topical use)*
Effectiveness: B+   Safety: B

Fish oils (eicosapentaenoic acid and docosahexaenoic acid)
Effectiveness: B+   Safety: A

Glycyrrhetinic acid (topical use)
Effectiveness: B   Safety: A

***Milk thistle* (Silybum marianum)**
Effectiveness: B   Safety: A

***Sarsaparilla* (Smilax sarsaparilla)**
Effectiveness: B   Safety: C

Commentary

In addition to the dietary and supplement recommendations, a number of natural herbal formulas for topical use can provide symptomatic relief. The best choices are products that contain one of the following: glycyrrhetinic acid from licorice *(Glycyrrhiza glabra),* chamomile *(Matricaria chamomilla),* and capsaicin from cayenne pepper *(Capsicum frutescens).* Of these three, preparations containing capsaicin are the easiest to find. Apply to affected areas of the skin two to three times per day.

RHEUMATOID ARTHRITIS

Definition

Rheumatoid arthritis (RA) is a chronic inflammatory condition that affects the entire body, but especially the joints. The joints typically involved are the hands, feet, wrists, ankles, and knees.

Signs and Symptoms

The onset of RA is usually gradual but occasionally is quite abrupt. Fatigue, low-grade fever, weakness, joint stiffness, and vague joint pain may precede the appearance of painful, swollen joints by several weeks. Several joints are usually involved in the onset, typically in a symmetrical fashion, that is, both hands, wrists, or ankles. In about one-third of persons with RA, initial involvement is confined to one or a few joints.

Involved joints are characteristically quite warm, tender, and swollen. The skin over the joint takes on a ruddy purplish hue. X-ray findings usually show soft tissue swelling, erosion of cartilage, and joint-space narrowing. As the disease progresses, deformities develop in the joints of the hands and feet.

Causes

There is abundant evidence that RA is an autoimmune reaction, in which antibodies formed by the immune system attack components of joint tissues. Yet what triggers this autoimmune reaction remains largely unknown. Speculation and investigation have centered around genetic factors, abnormal bowel permeability, lifestyle and nutritional factors, food allergies, and microorganisms. RA is a classic example of a multifactorial disease, wherein an assortment of genetic and environmental factors contributes to the disease process.

Dietary Factors

Diet has been strongly implicated in rheumatoid arthritis for many years. The major focus in dietary therapy is to eliminate food allergies, follow a vegetarian diet, alter the intake of dietary fats and oils, and increase the intake of antioxidant nutrients. The first step is a therapeutic fast or an elimination diet (see **food allergy**), followed by careful reintroduction of foods to detect allergens. Virtually any food can aggravate RA, but the most common offenders are wheat, corn, milk and other dairy products, beef, and foods in the nightshade family (tomato, potato, eggplant, and peppers; tobacco is also in this plant family). After isolating and eliminating all allergens, a generally healthy diet is recommended: rich in whole foods, vegetables, and fiber, and low in sugar, meat, refined carbohydrates, and animal fats. Foods particularly beneficial for the RA patient include cold-water fish (mackerel, herring, salmon, etc.) and flavonoid-rich berries (cherries, hawthorn berries, blueberries, blackberries, etc.).

The importance of a diet rich in fresh fruits and vegetables in the dietary treatment of RA cannot be overstated. These foods are the best sources of dietary antioxidants. While the benefits of vitamin C, beta-carotene, vitamin E, selenium, and zinc as antioxidant nutrients are becoming well recognized and well accepted, there are still other plant compounds that promote healthy joints. Several studies have shown that the risk of RA is highest among people with the lowest serum levels of nutrient antioxidants (vitamin E, beta-carotene, and vitamin C).

Conventional Drugs

- *Aspirin and other nonsteroidal anti-inflammatory drugs:* aspirin (Ascriptin Enteric, Bayer, Bufferin, Ecotrin); diclofenac sodium (Voltaren); diclofenac potassium (Cataflam); etodolac (Lodine); fenoprofen calcium (Nalfon); ibuprofen (Advil, IBU, Motrin, Nuprin); indomethacin (Indocin); ketoprofen (Actron, Orudis); nabumetone (Relafen); naproxen sodium (Aleve, Anaprox, Naprelan); oxaprozin (Daypro); piroxicam (Feldene); sulindac (Clinoril); tolmetin sodium (Tolectin)
- *Cox-2 inhibitors:* celecoxib (Celebrex), rofecoxib (Vioxx).
- *Antimalarial drugs:* hydroxychloroquine sulfate (Plaquenil)
- *Chelating agents:* penicillamine (Cuprimine, Depen)
- *Chemotherapy drugs:* methotrexate sodium (Rheumatrex)
- *Corticosteroids:* betamethasone sodium phosphate (Adbeon, Celestone Phosphate); cortisone acetate (Cortisone, Cortone acetate); dexamethasone (Decadron); dexamethasone acetate (Dalalone D.P.); hydrocortisone (Hydrocortone); methylprednisolone; prednisolone (Prelone); prednisolone tebutate (Hydeltra-T.B.A.); prednisone (Apo-Prednisone, Deltasone, Liquid Pred, Meticorten, Orasone, Prednicen, Sterapred, Winpred)

- *Gold salts:* auranofin (Ridaura); aurothioglucose (Solganal Suspension); gold sodium thiomalate (Aurolate, Myochrysine)
- *Immunosuppresive drugs:* azathioprine (Imuran)

Natural Medicines

Bromelain
Effectiveness: B+   Safety: A

Capsaicin (topical use)
Effectiveness: A   Safety: D

Cat's claw (Uncaria tomentosa)
Effectiveness: B   Safety: C

Cetylmyristoleate (CMO)
Effectiveness: B   Safety: B

Curcumin (from Curcuma longa*)*
Effectiveness: B+   Safety: A

Feverfew (Tanacetum parthenium)
Effectiveness: C   Safety: B

Fish oils (eicosapentaenoic acid and docosahexaenoic acid)
Effectiveness: B+   Safety: A

Gamma-linolenic acid
Effectiveness: B   Safety: A

Ginger (Zingiber officinale)
Effectiveness: B+   Safety: A

Manganese
Effectiveness: C   Safety: A

Niacinamide
Effectiveness: B   Safety: B

Pantothenic acid
Effectiveness: B   Safety: A

Phytodolar
Effectiveness: B+   Safety: A

Pregnenolone
Effectiveness: B   Safety: D

Selenium
Effectiveness: B   Safety: A

Shark cartilage
Effectiveness: C   Safety: C

White willow (Salix alba)
Effectiveness: B   Safety: C

Zinc
Effectiveness: B   Safety: A

Commentary

Defective manufacture of androgens (male hormones such as testosterone and dehydroepiandrosterone [DHEA]) has been proposed as a potential
predisposing factor for rheumatoid arthritis (as well
as for systemic lupus erythematosis). This association suggests a possible therapeutic response to
DHEA supplementation. Although there are no clinical studies in RA with DHEA supplementation, there
have been studies conducted at Stanford Medical
Center in women with systemic lupus erythematosis
(lupus or SLE) that showed DHEA supplementation
to produce some benefits. Even in the absence of
double-blind clinical studies in rheumatoid arthritis,
you may wish to discuss DHEA therapy with your
doctor.

SPORTS INJURIES, TENDINITIS, AND BURSITIS

Definition

Sports injuries refer to strains, sprains, and inflammation of supportive tissues. Tendinitis is an inflammatory condition of a tendon—the connective tissue that connects muscles to bones. Tendinitis usually results from a strain. The tendons most commonly affected are the Achilles (back of ankle), the biceps (front of shoulder), the pollicis brevis and longus (thumb), the upper patella (knee), the posterior tibial (inside of foot), and the rotator cuff (shoulder). Bursitis is inflammation of the bursa, the saclike membrane that contains fluid that lubricates the joints. Bursitis may result from trauma, strain, infection, or arthritic conditions. The most common locations are shoulder, elbow, hip, and lower knee.

Warning: For any serious injury, a physician should be consulted immediately. Conditions that indicate the need to see a physician include: severe pain, injury to a joint, loss of function, or pain that persists for more than two weeks.

Signs and Symptoms

Pain, inflammation, and limited range of motion in the affected joint are the hallmark features of tendinitis and bursitis.

Causes

The most common cause of sports injury is sudden excessive tension on a tendon or bursa, producing a strain or sprain. Repeated muscle contraction, leading to exhaustion of the muscle, can result in similar injury. Sometimes tendinitis develops when the grooves in which the tendons move develop bone spurs or other mechanical abnormalities. Proper stretching and warm-up before exercise are important preventive measures.

Dietary Factors

No specific dietary factors have been reported.

Conventional Drugs

• *Aspirin and other nonsteroidal anti-inflammatory drugs:* aspirin (Ascriptin Enteric, Bayer, Bufferin, Ecotrin); diclofenac sodium (Voltaren); diclofenac potassium (Cataflam); etodolac (Lodine); fenoprofen calcium (Nalfon); ibuprofen (Advil, IBU, Motrin, Nuprin); indomethacin (Indocin); ketoprofen (Actron, Orudis); nabumetone (Relafen); naproxen sodium (Aleve, Anaprox, Naprelan); oxaprozin (Daypro); piroxicam (Feldene); sulindac (Clinoril); tolmetin sodium (Tolectin)

Natural Medicines

Bromelain
Effectiveness: B+   Safety: A

Citrus bioflavonoids
Effectiveness: B   Safety: A

Curcumin (from Curcuma longa)
Effectiveness: B   Safety: A

Pancreatin
Effectiveness: B   Safety: A

White willow (Salix alba)
Effectiveness: C   Safety: C

Commentary

The most important treatment of a minor injury or sprain is the acronym RICE:

- Rest the injured part as soon as it is hurt, to avoid further injury
- Ice the area of pain to decrease swelling and bleeding
- Compress the area with an elastic bandage, also to limit swelling and bleeding
- Elevate the injured part above the level of the heart to increase drainage of fluids out of the injured area

Proper application of these procedures is important for optimal results. When icing, first cover the injured area with a towel, then place an ice pack on it. It is important not to wrap the injured part so tightly that circulation is impaired. The ice and compress should be applied for thirty minutes, followed by fifteen minutes without the ice to allow recirculation. After the acute inflammatory stage (twenty-four to forty-eight hours), gradually increasing range-of-motion and stretching exercises should be used to maintain and improve mobility and prevent adhesions (abnormal scar formation).

ULCER (DUODENAL OR GASTRIC)

Definition

An ulcer is a small wound that occurs in the stomach (gastric ulcer) or the first portion of the small intestine (duodenal ulcer).

Warning: Individuals experiencing any symptoms of an ulcer need competent medical care. Ulcer complications such as hemorrhage, perforation, and obstruction represent medical emergencies that require immediate hospitalization. Individuals with an ulcer must be monitored by a physician.

Signs and Symptoms

Although symptoms of a peptic ulcer may be absent or quite vague, most peptic ulcers are associated with abdominal discomfort noted forty-five to sixty minutes after meals or during the night. In the typical case, the pain is described as gnawing, burning, cramplike or aching, or as "heartburn." Eating virtually any food or using antacids usually results in great relief.

Causes

Even though duodenal and gastric ulcers occur at different locations, both appear to be the result of damage to the protective lining of the stomach or duodenum. These factors include too much gastric acid, the bacterium *Helicobacter pylori,* and various drugs, such as nonsteroidal anti-inflammatory drugs and prednisone.

Dietary Factors

Food allergy appears to be a primary factor in many cases of peptic ulcer. A diet that eliminates food allergens has been used with great success in treating and preventing recurrent ulcers.

Avoid milk and dairy products. Milk is the most common food allergen, and population studies show the higher the milk consumption, the greater the likelihood of ulcer. Milk significantly increases stomach acid production.

A high-fiber diet is associated with a reduced rate of ulcers as compared with a low-fiber diet. Fiber supplements (e.g., pectin, guar gum, psyllium) have been shown to produce beneficial effects as well.

Raw cabbage juice is well documented as having remarkable success in treating peptic ulcers. In one study, 1 liter of the fresh juice per day, taken in divided amounts, resulted in total ulcer healing in an average of only ten days.

Conventional Drugs

- *Antibiotics for elimination of H. pylori* (typically used in combination and with a proton pump inhibitor): amoxicillin (Amoxicillin, Amoxil, Trimox); clarithromycin; metronidazole; tetracycline
- *Antacids:* aluminum carbonate (Basaljel); aluminum hydroxide (ALternaGEL, Amphojel, Nephrox); aluminum hydroxide/Magnesium hydroxide (Maalox, Mylanta); calcium carbonate (Alka-Mint, Titralac, Tums); calcium carbonate/ magnesium hydroxide (Rolaids); magaldrate (Losopan, Ri Mag, Riopan); magnesium carbonate/calcium carbonate (Marblen); magnesium hydroxide (Phillips Milk of Magnesia); magnesium oxide (Mag-Ox, Uro-

Mag); magnesium trisilicate/aluminum hydroxide (Gaviscon Antacid); sodium bicarbonate (Alka-Seltzer, Arm & Hammer)
- *Histamine-2 receptor antagonists:* cimetidine (Tagamet); famotidine (Mylanta Ar, Pepcid); nizatidine (Axid); ranitidine (Zantac)
- *Proton pump inhibitors:* lansoprazole (Prevacid); omeprazole (Prilosec)

Natural Medicines

Aloe vera *gel*
Effectiveness: B   Safety: C

Bismuth subcitrate
Effectiveness: A   Safety: D

Carnosine
Effectiveness: B   Safety: B

Deglycyrrhizinated licorice (DGL)
Effectiveness: A   Safety: A

Glutamine
Effectiveness: B+   Safety: A

Zinc
Effectiveness: B   Safety: A

Commentary

The focus of treatment of peptic ulcers is moving away from inhibiting gastric acid and toward eliminating the bacterium *H. pylori*. Physicians can determine the presence of *H. pylori* by measuring the level of antibodies to *H. pylori* in the blood or saliva, or by culturing material collected during an endoscopy (the process of examination of the stomach or duodenum with a fiber-optic tube with a lens attached to it). One of the key pre-disposing factors for *H. pylori* infection is a low level of antioxidants such as vitamin C in the gastrointestinal lining. Bismuth subcitrate may be more effective than DGL in cases where *H. pylori* has been identified.

URINARY TRACT INFECTION (CYSTITIS)

Definition

Urinary tract infections occur when bacteria invade the bladder. Bladder infections are very common in women because of their anatomy; 10 to 20 percent of all women have urinary tract discomfort at least once a year. Recurrent UTIs are a significant prob-lem and can cause progressive damage, resulting in scarring and, in rare cases, kidney failure.

Warning: Although most urinary tract infections are not serious, it is important that you be properly diagnosed, treated, and monitored. If you have symptoms suggestive of a bladder infection, consult a physician immediately.

Signs and Symptoms

Burning pain on urination; increased urinary fre-quency (especially at night); cloudy, foul-smelling, or dark urine; lower abdominal pain; urine analysis that shows a significant number of bacteria and white blood cells.

Causes

Most UTIs are caused by the *E. coli* bacterium. Many factors are associated with increased risk of bladder infection: pregnancy, menopause, sexual intercourse, mechanical trauma or irritation, and structural abnormalities of the urinary tract that block the free flow of urine.

Dietary Factors

The most important dietary recommendation is to increase the quantity of liquids consumed. Ideally, the liquids should be in the form of pure water, herbal teas, and fresh fruit and vegetable juices diluted with at least an equal amount of water. If you have a bladder infection, you should drink at least 64 fluid ounces of liquids from this group, with at least half of this amount being water. You should also avoid such liquids as soft drinks, concentrated fruit drinks, coffee, and alcoholic beverages.

Conventional Drugs

- *Antibiotics:* aztreonam (Azactam); cefaclor (Ceclor); cefpodoxime proxetil (Vantin); ciprofloxacin (Ciloxan, Cipro); enoxacin (Penetrex); lomefloxacin (Maxaquin); loracarbef (Lorabid); nitrofurantoin monohydrate (Macrobid); ofloxacin (Floxin, Ocuflox); sulfamethoxazole (Gantanol); sulfisoxazole acetyl (Gantrisin)
- *Urinary pH modifiers:* methenamine mandelate/sodium acid phosphate (Uroqid-acid No. 2)

Natural Medicines

Cranberry (Vaccinium macrocarpon)
Effectiveness: A   Safety: A

Lactobacillus acidophilus
Effectiveness: B   Safety: A

Uva ursi (Arctostaphylos uva-ursi)
Effectiveness: B+   Safety: D

Commentary

There is a growing concern that antibiotic therapy actually promotes recurrent infection by disturbing the normal bacterial flora and by giving rise to antibiotic-resistant strains of *E. coli* (see *Lactobacillus acidophilus* for more information).

VARICOSE VEINS

Definition

Varicose veins are enlarged, dilated, and tortuous superficial veins in the legs. Veins are fairly fragile structures. Defects in the wall of a vein lead to dilation of the vein and damage to the valves. Normally these valves prevent blood from backing up, but when the valves become damaged, blood pools and causes the bulging veins known as varicose veins.

Signs and Symptoms

Varicose veins may be without symptoms or may be associated with fatigue, aching discomfort, feelings of heaviness, or pain in the legs. Fluid retention (edema), discoloration, and ulceration of the skin may also develop.

Causes

The following factors can cause varicose veins: pregnancy, genetic weakness of the vein walls or their valves, excessive pressure within the vein due to a low-fiber-diet-induced increase in straining during defecation, long periods of standing and/or heavy lifting, and damage to the veins or venous valves resulting from inflammation.

Dietary Factors

A high-fiber diet is the most important component in the treatment and prevention of varicose veins (and hemorrhoids). A diet rich in vegetables, fruits, legumes, and grains promotes peristalsis; many fiber components attract water and form a gelatinous mass that keeps the feces soft, bulky, and easy to pass. Individuals who consume a low-fiber diet tend to strain more during bowel movements since their smaller and harder stools are more difficult to pass. This straining increases the pressure in the abdomen, which obstructs the flow of blood up the legs. The increased pressure may, over a period of time, significantly weaken the vein wall, leading to the formation of varicose veins or hemorrhoids.

Flavonoid-rich berries, such as hawthorn berries, cherries, blueberries, and blackberries, are beneficial in the prevention and treatment of varicose veins. These berries are very rich sources of proanthocyanidins and anthocyanidins. These bioflavonoids give the berries their blue-red color and also improve the integrity of support structures of the veins and the entire vascular system. Extracts of several of these berries are used widely in Europe as medications for various circulatory conditions, including varicose veins. The procyanidolic oligomers in grape seed extract and pine bark extracts are the most popular and possibly the most effective.

Conventional Drugs

No prescription drugs are available with FDA-approved labeling for this indication.

Natural Medicines

Aortic glycosaminoglycans
Effectiveness: A   Safety: A

Bilberry (Vaccinium myrtillus)
Effectiveness: B+   Safety: A

Butcher's broom (Ruscus aculeatus)
Effectiveness: A   Safety: B

Citrus bioflavonoids
Effectiveness: A   Safety: A

Gotu kola (Centella asiatica)
Effectiveness: A   Safety: A

Horse chestnut (Aesculus hippocastanum)
Effectiveness: A   Safety: C

Procyanidolic oligomers
Effectiveness: A   Safety: A

Commentary

While small spider veins may disappear entirely, do not expect well-formed large varicose veins to magically go away. In these cases, elastic compression stockings are occasionally beneficial. Be sure to exercise and avoid standing for long periods of time. Walking, riding a bike, or jogging is particularly beneficial, as the contraction of leg muscles pushes pooled blood back into circulation. In severe cases of varicose veins the only real option is surgical excision.

References

The primary resource for evaluating the merits of the natural products featured in this book was the personal files of Michael T. Murray, N.D. To access individual articles about topics described in this book, Dr. Murray recommends accessing the Internet site for the National Library of Medicine (NLM): http://gateway.nlm.nih.gov.

The NLM gateway is a Web-based system that lets users search simultaneously in multiple retrieval systems at the NLM. From this site you can access all of the NLM databases, including PubMed. This database was developed in conjunction with publishers of biomedical literature as a search tool for accessing literature citations and linking to full-text journal articles at the Web sites of participating publishers. Publishers participating in PubMed electronically supply the NLM with their citations prior to or at the time of publication. If the publisher has a Web site that offers the full text of its journals, PubMed provides links to that site as well as links to other biological data, sequence centers, etc. User registration, a subscription fee, or some other type of fee may be required to access the full text of articles in some journals.

PubMed provides access to bibliographic information that includes MEDLINE, the NLM's premier bibliographic database covering the fields of medicine, nursing, dentistry, veterinary medicine, the health care system, and the preclinical sciences. MEDLINE contains bibliographic citations and author abstracts from more than four thousand medical journals published in the United States and seventy other countries. The file contains over eleven million citations dating back to the mid-1960s. Coverage is worldwide, but most records are from English-language sources or have English abstracts.

Conducting a search is quite easy, and the site has a link to a tutorial that fully explains the process. If for some reason you are having trouble identifying a particular reference cited in this book at the NLM Web site, you can visit www.doctormurray.com and submit a question to Dr. Murray asking for the reference to a particular study mentioned in this book.

In addition to Dr. Murray's extensive collection of original scientific articles, the following texts were also used as resources:

Blumenthal, M. (ed.). *The Complete Commission E Monographs: Therapeutic Guide to Herbal Medicines.* American Botanical Council, Austin, TX, 1998.

Gruenwald, J., Brendler, T., Jaenicke, C. (eds.). *PDR for Herbal Medicines.* 2nd edition. Medical Economics Company, Montvale, NJ, 2001.

Hendler, S. S., Rorvik, D. (eds). *PDR for Nutritional Supplements.* Medical Economics Company, Montvale, NJ, 2001.

Jellin, J. M., Batz, F., Hitchens, K. *Pharmacist's Letter/Prescriber's Letter Natural Medicines Comprehensive Database.* Stockton, CA, 1999.

Leung, A. Y., Foster, S. *Encyclopedia of Common Natural Ingredients Used in Food, Drugs and Cosmetics.* 2nd edition. John Wiley and Sons, New York, 1995

Lininger, S. (ed.). *The A–Z Guide to Drug-Herb and Vitamin Interactions.* Prima, Rocklin, CA, 1999.

Lininger, S., Gaby, A., Miller, J. (eds.). *The Natural Pharmacy.* Prima, Rocklin, CA, 1999.

McGuffin, M., Hobbs, C., Upton, R., Goldberg, A. (eds.). *American Herbal Products Association's*

Botanical Safety Handbook. CRC Press, Boca Raton, FL, 1997.

Medical Economics Company. *Physicians' Desk Reference.* 55th edition. Montvale, NJ, 2001.

Murray, M. T. *Encyclopedia of Nutritional Supplements.* Prima, Rocklin, CA, 1996.

Pierce, A. *The American Pharmaceutical Association Practical Guide to Natural Medicines.* Stonesong Press, New York, 1999.

Pizzorno, J. E., Murray, M. T. (eds.). *Textbook of Natural Medicine.* Churchill Livingstone, London, 1999.

Werbach, M. R. *Foundations of Nutritional Medicine.* Third Line Press, Tarzana, CA, 1997.

Werbach, M. R. *Nutritional Influences on Illness.* 2nd edition. Third Line Press, Tarzana, CA, 1993.

Werbach, M. R., Murray, M. T. *Botanical Influences on Illness.* 2nd edition. Third Line Press, Tarzana, CA, 2000.

About the Author

Michael T. Murray, N.D., is widely regarded as one of the world's leading authorities on natural medicine. Dr. Murray is a graduate faculty member and serves on the Board of Trustees of Bastyr University in Seattle, Washington. He is co-author of **A Textbook of Natural Medicine**, the definitive textbook on naturopathic medicine for physicians, as well as the consumer version, the **Encyclopedia of Natural Medicine**. He has also written over twenty other books, including **Dr. Murray's Total Body Tune-Up**.

Dr. Murray is Director of Product Development and Education for Natural Factors, a leading manufacturer of natural products. He has been instrumental in bringing many effective natural products to North America, including:

> Glucosamine sulfate
> Ginkgo biloba extract
> Silymarin
> Enteric-coated peppermint oil
> Saw palmetto berry extract

For the past twenty years, Dr. Murray has been compiling a massive database of original scientific studies from the medical literature. He has personally collected over 60,000 articles from the scientific literature that provide strong evidence on the effectiveness of diet, vitamins, minerals, glandular extracts, herbs, and other natural measures in the maintenance of health and the treatment of disease. It is from this constantly expanding database that Dr. Murray provides the answers on health and healing. According to Dr. Murray:

One of the great myths about natural medicines is that they are not scientific. The fact of the matter is that for most common illnesses there is tremendous support in medical literature for a more natural approach.

Unfortunately, many people are never made aware of the natural approach that can put them on the road to lifelong health. Michael T. Murray, N.D., has dedicated his life to educating physicians, patients, and the general public on the tremendous healing power of nature.

Index

Main entries appear in bold type.

thymus extracts, 498, 499
vitamin C, 91, 92–93
Allergy, food, **938–941**
aspergillus enzymes, 211, 212
pancreatin, 435, 437, 941
quercetin, 459–460, 941
Allicin. *See* Garlic
Aloe latex, whole leaf, aloin,
528–530
Aloe vera gel, **522–527,** 858, 876,
922, 983, 1038
Aloe vera (topical use), **831–832**
Alopecia (hair loss), biotin for,
37
Alpha-hydroxy acids, **832–833**
Alprazolam (Xanax): kava and,
724
Alzheimer's disease, **861–864**
carnitine, 246, 247–248, 863
DMAE, 310, 863
folic acid, 862
ginkgo biloba, 665, 667, 863
huperzine A, 710–711, 863, 864
NADH, 41, 47, 48, 863
phosphatidylcholine, 444, 445,
863
phosphatidylserine, 449, 863
silicon, 174
thiamin, 68–69, 863
vitamin B$_{12}$, 862, 863
vitamin C, 92, 862, 863
vitamin E, 103, 104–5, 862, 863
zinc, 178, 180, 863
Amiloride (Midamor): potassium
and, 164
Amino acids and their derivatives, 187
Aminoglycosides: cordyceps
and, 294, 295
Amiodarone (Cordarone): vitamin B$_6$ and, 82
Amitriptyline (Elavil, Endep)
coenzyme Q$_{10}$ and, 285
St. John's wort and, 785
Amyotrophic lateral sclerosis
(Lou Gehrig's disease): octacosanol, 432, 433
Andrographis paniculata,
530–532, 721
Androstenedione, **196–201**
Anemia, **864–866**
iron, 139, 140, 885

liver extracts, 400–401
See also Pernicious anemia
Angelica. *See* Dong quai
Angina pectoris
arginine, 206–207, 867
carnitine, 246, 248, 868
coenyme Q$_{10}$, 279, 281, 868
fish oils, 319, 321, 868
hawthorn, 702, 703, 868
magnesium, 147, 868
See also Heart disease
Antacids
bismuth subcitrate and, 233
calcium and, 125
chromium and, 131
indole-3-carbinol and, 372
iron and, 142
magnesium and, 152
manganese and, 156
vitamin C and, 98
Antibiotics
berberine-containing plants
and enhancement, 539–540
betaine and, 224
biotin and, 40
bromelain and, 558, 560, 563
caffeine and, 572
calcium and, 125
ciprofloxacin, 183
esberitox and enhancement,
644
green tea and, 693
iron and, 142
lactobacillus and, 23
magnesium and, 152
potassium and, 164
red yeast rice extract and, 465
Sinupret and, 805
tetracycline, 125, 142, 152,
180, 183, 541
vitamin B$_{12}$ and, 89
vitamin K and, 112
zinc and, 183
Anticonvulsant drugs
folic acid and, 45
vitamin B$_6$ and, 82
Antidepressant drugs
caffeine and, 572
ephedrine-caffeine combos
and, 640
folic acid and, 45
green tea and, 693